RENAL NURSING

To Shirley,
who not only stayed with me
but also corrected the English

Renal Nursing

Principally by
Robert Uldall MD, FRCP, FRCP(C)
Associate Professor of Medicine,
University of Toronto.
Director of Hemodialysis,
Toronto Western Hospital

THIRD EDITION

Blackwell
Science

© 1972, 1977, 1988 by
Blackwell Science Ltd
Editorial Offices:
Osney Mead, Oxford OX2 0EL
25 John Street, London WC1N 2BL
23 Ainslie Place, Edinburgh EH3 6AJ
238 Main Street, Cambridge
  Massachusetts 02142, USA
54 University Street, Carlton
  Victoria 3053, Australia

Other Editorial Offices:
Arnette Blackwell SA
  1, rue de Lille
  75007 Paris
  France

Blackwell Wissenschafts-Verlag GmbH
  Kurfürstendamm 57
  10707 Berlin
  Germany

  Feldgasse 13
  A-1238 Wien
  Austria

First published 1972
Second edition 1977
Reprinted 1984
Third edition 1988
Reprinted 1991, 1993, 1996

Set by Setrite Typesetters Ltd
Hong Kong
Printed and bound in Great Britain by
Hartnolls Limited, Bodmin, Cornwall

DISTRIBUTORS

Marston Book Services Ltd
PO Box 87
Oxford OX2 0DT
(*Orders:* Tel: 01865 791155
  Fax: 01865 791927
  Telex: 837515)

North America
Blackwell Science, Inc.
238 Main Street
Cambridge MA 02142
(*Orders:* Tel: 800 215-1000
  617 876-7000
  Fax: 617 492-5263)

Australia
Blackwell Science Pty Ltd
54 University Street
Carlton, Victoria 3053
(*Orders:* Tel: 03 347-0300
  Fax: 03 349-3016)

British Library
Cataloguing in Publication Data

Uldall, Robert
  Renal nursing.—3rd ed.
  1. Kidneys—Diseases
  I. Title
  616.6'1'0024613   RC902

ISBN 0–632–01728–7

Contents

List of Contributors

Carl Cardella, MD, FRCP(C), *Associate Professor of Medicine, University of Toronto, Director of Transplantation, Toronto Western Hospital*

Sharon Izatt, RN, NUA, *Renal Supervisor, Toronto Western Hospital*

Betty Kelman, RN, BA, *Clinical teacher (Renal), Toronto Western Hospital*

Ramesh Khanna, MD, *Associate Professor of Medicine, Nephrology Division, University of Missouri, Health Sciences Center, Columbia, Missouri*

Dimitrios Oreopoulos, MD, PhD, FRCP(C), FACP, *Professor of Medicine, University of Toronto. Director, Peritoneal Dialysis Unit, Toronto Western Hospital*

Jean H. Pettit, BSc, RPDt, *Renal Dietitian, Toronto Western Hospital*

Franca Tantalo, RN, *Dialysis Consultant, Cardio Med. Supplies Inc. Formerly Head Nurse, Hemodialysis Unit, Toronto Western Hospital*

Robert Uldall, MB, BS, MD, FRCP, FRCP(C), *Associate Professor of Medicine, University of Toronto. Director of Hemodialysis, Toronto Western Hospital*

Annette Vigneux, RN, *Pediatric Renal Nurse, Department of Pediatrics, McMaster University Medical Centre, Hamilton, Ontario. Formerly CAPD Coordinator, Dialysis Unit, Hospital for Sick Children, Toronto*

Alan Watson, MB, ChB, MRCP(UK), *Consultant Nephrologist, Department of Paediatrics, City Hospital, Nottingham, England. Formerly Staff Nephrologist and Director of Hemodialysis, Nephrology Division, Hospital for Sick Children and Assistant Professor, Department of Pediatrics, University of Toronto*

Catharine Isobel Whiteside, MD, PhD, FRCP(C), *Assistant Professor of Medicine, University of Toronto*

Janet Willumsen, RN, *Head Nurse, The Dialysis Unit, Hospital for Sick Children, Toronto*

Elizabeth Wright, RN, *Head Nurse, Urology and Transplant Ward, Toronto Western Hospital*

Eileen Young, RN, *Renal Nursing Coordinator for Dialysis and Transplantation, Toronto Western Hospital*

Preface to the Third Edition

Eleven years have elapsed since the publication of the second edition of *Renal Nursing*. Either the book had to be substantially rewritten or allowed to fade out completely. With each passing year the task of updating it became more formidable, and yet the need for the book seemed to have increased. As knowledge of kidney disease and renal failure has expanded the methods of managing renal failure have not only evolved and improved, but also become considerably more complex. The spate of written material on every conceivable aspect of our discipline has become a flood, yet the knowledge is widely scattered and not always very easy to read or understand. The solution seemed to be to invoke the help of other experts, and in particular to involve, to a much greater extent, the best and most experienced nurses we knew, to help us in the writing.

Dr Catherine Whiteside, the foremost physiologist in our group, has improved on Chapter 1. Eileen Young, our renal nursing coordinator, has assisted with a new chapter, Chapter 5, on an introduction to dialysis. My colleague, Dimitrios Oreopoulos, assisted by Ramesh Khanna and their two most experienced peritoneal dialysis nurses, Sharon Izatt and Betty Kelman, have between them written an entirely new chapter on peritoneal dialysis. It would be hard to envisage a more capable team than those who made such an enormous contribution to home peritoneal dialysis in North America and throughout the world. To Franca Tantalo, for so many years the head nurse in the Hemodialysis Unit at Toronto

Western Hospital, must go much of the credit for the completely revised chapter on hemodialysis. The example she set has been an inspiration to many. Carl Cardella, the director of transplantation at our hospital, has brought Chapter 9 right up to date, assisted by Elizabeth Wright, the head nurse on our urology and transplant ward.

Finally, and for the first time, we have an entirely new and separate chapter on dialysis and transplantation in infants and children. For this we are grateful to Dr Alan Watson, until recently on the staff of the Toronto Hospital for Sick Children, assisted by Annette Vigneux and Janet Willumsen. Their contribution is authoritative, fascinating and highly readable.

We hope that together we have produced the most definitive short text on practical care of the patient with kidney disease and renal failure. Though written primarily for nurses and technical staff, it will undoubtedly prove valuable to junior hospital medical staff as well as all the allied health care workers such as dietitians, social workers and hospital pharmacists.

I am indebted to Jean Pettit, our dietitian, for improving the appendix on dietary information and all the other expert colleagues and friends who have given helpful advice and information. It would be hard to imagine how the book could have been produced, had it not been for the incredible dedication and efficiency of my secretary Arlene Koteff. She led the team of medical secretaries who prepared the manuscript by making their time and skills available in spite of all their other work. I am grateful to them all.

Preface to the Second Edition

Since the publication of *Renal Nursing* in 1972 a certain amount of new information has come to light on the nature of kidney disease and a number of new methods and improvements have been developed for treating kidney disease, especially renal failure. The results in renal transplantation have generally not improved dramatically but some exciting new ideas are being tried out to assist in the diagnosis and treatment of transplant rejection. Dialysis techniques and equipment have emerged which make regular dialysis safer, more convenient and more reliable. The role of the nurse and the dialysis technician have continued to assume greater importance.

One of the most important new trends is in the management of end-stage renal failure by long-term regular peritoneal dialysis. This is not a new method but in recent years it has been more widely and successfully exploited. Renal failure is a problem of such epidemic proportions that modern kidney centres, striving as they always are to cope with more patients than they can easily manage, are employing all the different forms of treatment in order to achieve maximum flexibility. The methods should complement rather than compete with one another. The patient with renal failure may require and benefit from all these forms of treatment at different times.

It was not the intention to expand the book greatly but some increase in size was inevitable. I ask the forgiveness of my readers if the second edition proves to be more indigestible and harder on the pocket than the first.

In writing new sections for the second edition I have relied heavily on the help of colleagues who have generously shared their special expertise. Dr D. Oreopoulos, who is now an international authority on automated peritoneal dialysis and especially home peritoneal dialysis, has been my main source of information and advice on this topic. Dr A. Pierides, who is rapidly achieving eminence in the field of renal bone disease, has contributed the new section on this previously crippling but now largely treatable disability. Mr N. Hoenich gave valuable advice on technical aspects of hemodialysis. I am grateful to Miss Jean Nold, dietitian at the Western Hospital, Toronto, for the expansion recognizable in the appendix which is mainly for the benefit of North American readers. Some new illustrations (marked NT) have been added by Naomi Tummon, and also some more by Mr D.P. Hammersly of Newcastle University who did the illustrations for the first edition. Secretarial assistance was given by Mrs M. Silva and Mrs L. Cossette. Finally the enthusiasm and dedication of the renal unit nurses in both Newcastle and Toronto have been an inspiration. I trust the book will be a help to them and their colleagues everywhere.

Preface to the First Edition

This small book has been written in an attempt to help nurses who look after kidney patients. The first chapters describe the way in which normal kidneys function in relation to the rest of the body, the tests which we commonly perform and the reason for doing them, and an outline of the main kidney diseases we are likely to encounter. I have tried to keep difficult theoretical concepts to a minimum but have emphasized practical aspects of management.

The second half of the book is concerned with renal failure and methods of dealing with it. Peritoneal dialysis and hemodialysis are discussed in considerable detail since they are now established nursing procedures for which clear instructions have hitherto been sadly deficient.

The material contained in the book may be open to criticism for two reasons. Firstly some sections may be regarded as oversimplified. This is hardly avoidable when trying for example to provide a thumbnail sketch of a fascinating and intriguing disease whose various aspects could occupy a whole chapter. Those who wish to read further will have no difficulty in obtaining access to authoritative medical textbooks which discuss all the points in detail. Secondly the methods and techniques described here may vary slightly from those adopted in other centres. There are often several good ways of doing something, and for reasons of space I cannot hope to describe them all. I have described the methods which we have found reliable and safe. This is not to say that they cannot be improved upon. I hope the book is simple, clear and readable, and will take some of the fear and mystery out of what is a very demanding but at the same time rewarding form of work.

While writing the book I have received continuous advice and constructive suggestions from Miss Joan Miller SRN whose own experience of renal nursing is very extensive. I also owe a great debt of gratitude to Professor David Kerr who pioneered nephrology in the Newcastle region. Many of the methods and principles we have adopted have been the result of his influence. His criticism and advice have been invaluable. I would like to thank my other colleagues who have each given advice on the sections in which they are recognized experts—Dr J. Selkon on bacteriology, Dr W. Simpson on radiology, Dr A. Cassells-Smith on biochemistry, Professor J. Swinney and Mr R. Taylor on renal transplantation, and Dr S. Murray on tissue typing. The illustrations are the work of Mr D.P. Hammersly of the Newcastle University Medical Illustration Department.

1

Physiological Considerations

Catharine Whiteside

In order to provide expert nursing for patients with renal and urinary tract disorders it is not necessary to be familiar with minute details of renal anatomy or all the intricacies of renal physiology. Excellent and learned texts are available for those who possess the intellectual curiosity and academic ambition to study these subjects in depth. For the practical nurse it is certainly an advantage to understand roughly what normal kidneys do in relation to the rest of the body. This will help her to understand the effects of disease and the aims and principles of treatment.

Some facts about the urinary tract

The kidneys

The kidneys, which are roughly equal in size, measuring 12–13 cm in length in an average adult, lie on the posterior abdominal wall supported by some adipose tissue called the perinephric fat (see Fig. 1.1). The right lies a little lower than the left, being apparently pushed down by the liver. Occasionally one or other kidney, instead of being firmly embedded on the muscles of the posterior abdominal wall, is excessively mobile, the so-called floating kidney. Contrary to popular belief this condition is usually quite harmless. Twisting or kinking of the pedicle is very rare. Congenital absence of a kidney on one side is also rare; but the possibility must always be ruled out before a surgeon removes a kidney for any reason. The renal blood supply comes straight from the aorta usually with a single renal artery on each side but double renal arteries occur in 10–15% of normal people. This fact becomes important in renal transplantation. Accessory renal arteries also occasionally cause trouble by obstructing the ureter. The kidney may also receive a small accessory blood supply from capsular vessels as well as from the ovarian or testicular artery. This fortunate dispensation may occasionally keep the kidney alive for a period of time if the main renal artery becomes occluded. The renal veins drain into the inferior vena cava.

In comparison to their size the kidneys receive a very large amount of blood—about a quarter of the total cardiac output in the resting state. This rich blood supply is not necessary for the nutrition of the kidneys but is essential to enable them to perform all the functions which are necessary to keep the body in good health. In times of emergency such as violent exercise or acute blood loss the kidneys can manage with much less blood, which is diverted to more essential areas. The kidneys have a nerve supply which helps to govern their function and a lymphatic drainage like most other organs. These are both divided when kidneys are transplanted, yet the grafted kidney seems to function remarkably well without them. There is still some controversy as to whether the nerves and lymphatics can regenerate.

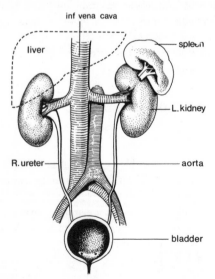

Fig. 1.1. Gross anatomy of the urinary tract.

The essential functioning units of the kidneys are the nephrons (see Fig. 1.2), of which there are altogether about one million in each kidney. The renal artery entering the kidney at the hilum divides into branches. The terminal branches, like the twigs on a tree, are called the afferent arterioles. Each afferent arteriole supplies a nephron. The arteriole actually enters the first part of the nephron called the glomerulus.

The glomerulus is a capillary bed surrounded by an open mouthed epithelial cell tube. The open end, called Bowman's capsule, leads into the tubule which, after a series of specialized tubular segments, drains into a collecting duct. The collecting ducts open out on the inner surface of the renal medulla, which is the renal pelvis, and this is drained by the ureter (see Fig. 1.3).

The formation of urine, which is the kidney's main function, starts when blood enters the capillaries of the glomeruli. About 25–30% of the plasma water and dissolved solutes smaller than protein (e.g. glucose, amino acids and electrolytes) are filtered across the glomerular capillary walls into proximal tubules. Red blood cells and protein cannot escape through the capillaries and they leave the glomeruli via an efferent arteriole to supply blood to the tubules. The volume of this glomerular filtrate is approximately 125 ml per minute in a fully grown man or 180 litres in 24 hours. It is the function of the tubules to convert this 180 litres of glomerular filtrate into 1–2 litres of urine. It comes as no surprise to learn that during its passage down the tubules most of the

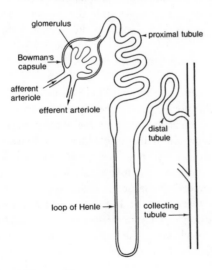

Fig. 1.2. Components of the nephron.

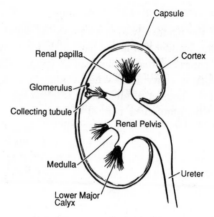

Fig. 1.3. Position of the nephron and its blood supply in relation to the whole kidney.

water and a large percentage of many of the solutes are reabsorbed back into the bloodstream. Glomerular filtration is a relatively simple physical process in which plasma water and solutes are driven across the glomerular capillary walls by the pressure with which the heart pumps blood into the kidney. The tubules, on the other hand, can be regarded as the chemical factories of the kidneys in which selective absorption and secretion are performed in a highly complicated and sophisticated way. The energy for these metabolic processes comes from the metabolism of carbohydrates and other compounds with the aid of the oxygen in the blood.

The ureters

The urine that drains into the renal pelvis is conducted by the ureters to the bladder. The ureters are not passive channels but muscular tubes with continuous peristaltic activity. The smooth muscle of the ureter massages the urine down to the bladder in a series of waves. If this peristaltic activity is defective for any reason, urine will not flow normally to the bladder but will tend to be dammed back in the renal pelvis. Where the lower end of the ureter enters the bladder, at the uretero-vesical junction, there is a valve-like mechanism which normally prevents urine from refluxing back up the ureters from the bladder. Reflux occurs when this valve mechanism is defective, and this is thought to be one of the important factors in the development of destructive pyelonephritis in childhood.

The bladder

The function of the bladder is to store the urine supplied to it by the kidneys. Once the bladder is full we have a desire to void, but this is under voluntary control so that voiding can be temporarily postponed till the time and place is convenient. When voiding occurs, it is normally complete so that no stagnant residual urine is left at the end of the act of micturition. The neuromuscular control of micturition is a complicated subject about which the experts still argue, but two simultaneous processes are required. First the muscles at the base of the bladder surrounding the urethra must relax to allow urine to enter the urethra, and second the muscles of the bladder wall must contract to expel the urine. We take all this for granted but various things may go wrong to disturb normal bladder emptying. In men the commonest problem is enlargement of the prostate causing narrowing of the prostatic urethra. In women the commonest problem is deformity of the lower part of the bladder and urethra from damage to pelvic ligaments during childbirth. Small boys are sometimes born with congenital posterior urethral valves which obstruct urine outflow. If these are not detected early, severe renal damage may occur due to back pressure. In both sexes and at all ages normal bladder function may be affected by damage to the nerve supply. This may be at the level of the spinal cord as in a traumatic paraplegia or in the sacral nerves below the cord. Any physical or neurological cause which disturbs normal bladder emptying will tend to predispose to ascending infection of the urinary tract, especially if the bladder does not empty completely. This is because any bacteria entering the bladder will multiply rapidly if their numbers are not drastically reduced by complete emptying. The mucuous membrane of a normal healthy bladder is strongly bactericidal. The male prostatic secretion is probably also highly bactericidal. Most organisms entering the bladder from below are probably killed in the normal course of events by these natural defence mechanisms. Finally, the difference in the length of the urethra in males and females, together with the fact that the opening of the female urethra is more vulnerable to contamination by coliform organisms, probably accounts to a large extent for the increased incidence of cystitis and bacterial urethritis in women.

The fluid compartments of the body

The water content of the body varies from about 75% in infants to about 45−50% in old age. The average healthy adult male consists of about 60% water. Females tend to have less water, 50−55%, and more adipose tissue, which contains very little water. The body water is contained in two main compartments, in the cells and outside the cells.

Let us take as an example an average man weighing 70 kilograms. His total body water is 60% of his body weight or 42 litres. The two major compartments are:

	Litres	*% total body water*
Intracellular water (ICW)	25	60
Extracellular water (ECW)	17	40
Total	42	100

Extracellular water is further subdivided into intravascular (plasma) and extravascular spaces. The extravascular water consists of interstitial water (about nine litres) which bathes the cells and surrounds the blood vessels, and a further five litres of extracellular water which is inaccessible because it is contained in dense connective tissue, cartilage and bone.

Extracellular water	Plasma	3
	Interstitial	9
	Inaccessible water in cartilage and bone	5
	Total	17

It can be seen that the intracellular water is about twice the volume of the plasma and interstitial water, that portion of the extracellular water which is freely available for exchange. The extracellular and intracellular water are not confined in rigid compartments but are exchanged continuously by a process of diffusion.

The composition of the body fluid compartments

The electrolytes in the different fluid compartments exist mainly in a state of ionic dissociation. For example, sodium chloride in solution does not consist of molecules of NaCl but as dissociated ions Na^+ and Cl^-. Ions with a positive electrical charge are called cations and those with a negative charge are called anions. These electrolytes are able to diffuse freely between the plasma and interstitial water. However, these ions cross cellular membranes by special transport processes. Therefore, the electrolyte composition of the two major body compartments (ICW and ECW) is very different.

The main cation in extracellular fluid is Na^+ (sodium) whereas the main cations of intracellular fluid are K^+ (potassium) and Mg^{++} (magnesium). All cell membranes contain a 'sodium pump' which continually pumps Na^+ out of cells into the ECW and at the same time pumps K^+ into cells into the ICW. This pumping is energy dependent and requires oxygen to keep it going. If cells are deprived of oxygen and cooled to low temperatures, as in the case of red blood cells stored in a blood bank, sodium will enter the cells and potassium will come out into the plasma. When the red cells are transfused into a patient's bloodstream they will regain their potassium and pump out the sodium.

The main anions in extracellular fluid are chloride and bicarbonate, whereas the main anions in intracellular fluid are phosphates and proteins. The plasma and interstitial fluid of the extracellular compartment have a very similar composition except that the plasma contains a lot of protein and the interstitial fluid very little. Because of their large molecular size proteins cannot normally escape from the plasma into the interstitial fluid. The osmotic pressure exerted by plasma proteins in the vascular compartment is important in preventing water from leaking into the interstitial compartment. If this so-called colloid osmotic pressure is severely reduced due to depletion of plasma proteins, as for example in the nephrotic syndrome, water will leak into the interstitial space and become evident as edema.

Units of electrolyte measurement

Since the first edition of this book was published the international system of units has been developed, agreed upon, and adopted generally by the international scientific bodies. The international system of units (Système International, SI) is now being used in Britain, Europe and Canada, but not yet in the United States. It seems likely that it will be adopted everywhere in due course since SI units are used for published articles in scientific journals throughout the world.

All measurements are expressed in certain basic units or in units derived from them. Some of the basic units relevant to medicine with their standard abbreviations are as follows:

Physical quantity	Name of SI unit	Symbol
length	metre	m
mass (weight)	kilogram	kg
time	second	s
temperature	Kelvin	K
amount of substance	mole	mol
pressure	pascal	Pa

Prefixes have also been agreed upon which define fractions or multiples of the basic units:

Fraction	Prefix	Symbol
10^{-1} (10th)	deci	d
10^{-2} (100th)	centi	c
10^{-3} (1 000th)	milli	m
10^{-6} (1 000 000th)	micro	µ
10^{-9} (1 000 000 000th)	nano	n

Multiple	Prefix	Symbol
10 ($\times$ 10)	deca	da
10^2 ($\times$ 100)	hecto	h
10^3 ($\times$ 1 000)	kilo	k
10^6 ($\times$ 1 000 000)	mega	M
10^9 ($\times$ 1 000 000 000)	giga	G

The main change in clinical chemistry is that with the adoption of SI units the concentrations of substances in solution are reported as mmol/l (or µmol/l, nmol/l, etc.) in place of the previous mg/100 ml (mg per cent). For the sake of American readers it is my intention to quote both systems of units when describing laboratory values. If you are used to the old system and have to adopt SI units in your hospital, conversion tables will be made available to you so that you will know what the new values mean.

In order to discuss sensibly the composition of the fluid compartments and the concentration of the electrolytes in them, we must have a unit of measurement which we understand. It is customary to express the concentration of a substance in solution as the weight of the solute in a given volume of solvent. The concentration of the plasma proteins were usually expressed under the old system as grams per 100 millilitre or grams per cent (by conversion per cent means per 100 ml). With SI units it will be quoted as grams per litre or g/l. Serum calcium may also be expressed in the traditional units as mg per 100 ml or mg per decilitre (mg/dl).

However, when we come to talk about the concentration of electrolytes in solution we face a different situation. Sodium and chloride do not combine weight for weight but according to their relative atomic weights and their ionic valence. The concentration of electrolytes in solution has traditionally been expressed as milliequivalents per litre (mEq/l).

To understand why this is so we have to learn or perhaps remind ourselves of two concepts or definitions. The first is the concept of *atomic weight*. The atomic weight of any element is the weight of one atom of that element compared with one atom of oxygen. Oxygen was chosen as the standard of reference and has an atomic weight of 16. Relative to this standard sodium has an atomic weight of 23 and chlorine an atomic weight of 35.5. When sodium and chlorine combine to form sodium chloride they do so in proportion to their atomic weights. For example, 58.5 g of NaCl contains 23 g of sodium and 35.5 g of chlorine.

The molecular weight of a compound is the sum of the atomic weights of all the elements specified in the formula, e.g. the molecular weight of NaCl is 58.5. A mole (mol) is the molecular weight expressed in grams. The mole (mol) is the new SI unit for the amount of any substance. One mole of NaCl is 58.5 g. A millimole (mmol) is the molecular weight expressed in milligrams. In biological fluids the concentrations tend to be rather small so it is convenient to talk of millimoles per litre (mmol/l). This unit of measurement is universally applicable. It can be applied to all substances in solution whether they are organic or inorganic, ionized or non-ionized.

The second concept we have to learn is the concept of electrochemical equivalence. You will remember from your chemistry that 'one equivalent of an ion is that amount which can replace or combine with one gram of hydrogen'. The standard of reference is the electrical charge (+) of one atom of hydrogen. A monovalent substance also has one electrical charge, e.g.

$$H^+ + Cl^- = HCL$$
$$Na^+ + Cl^- = NaCl$$

It is important to realize that substances react according to their electrical charges, and electrical neutrality is always preserved. An equivalent of a substance is the atomic weight expressed in grams divided by the valency. For monovalent substances like sodium and chlorine one mole (mol) is equal to one equivalent (Eq) and one millimole (mmol) will equal one milliequivalent (mEq).

Multivalent ions have greater chemical combining power than univalent ions because they have more electrical charges. One mmol of a divalent ion supplies 2 mEq, e.g. 1 mmol of magnesium (2 mEq) combines with 2 mmol of chlorine (2 mEq).

$$Mg^{++} + Cl^- + Cl^- = MgCl_2$$

In practice all the ionized electrolytes in biological fluids are expressed in milliequivalents per litre (mEq/l) or (since the advent of SI units) in millimoles per litre (mmol/l). Since electroneutrality exists the total concentration of cations is equal to the total concentration of anions.

If substances are incompletely ionized, as in the case of calcium in the plasma, their concentrations cannot accurately be expressed as milliequivalents per litre. Instead they can be expressed as milligrams per decilitre (mg/dl) or millimoles per litre (mmol/l).

Units of osmotic pressure

If two solutions of different concentrations are separated by a semipermeable membrane, the concentrations will tend to equalize because water rapidly passes through the membrane from the area of low concentration to the area of high concentration. At a slower rate, solute diffuses through the membrane from the area of high concentration to the area of low concentration. The osmotic pressure of a solution in a fluid compartment really means its power to draw water across the membrane into its own compartment. This osmotic effect of a substance in solution depends only on the number of dissolved particles and does not depend on their weight, electrical charge or chemical formula. If a molecule in solution dissociates into two or three particles, the osmotic pressure is increased two or three times respectively. Fig. 1.4 illustrates what happens when a solute is added to water on one side of a semipermeable membrane (a). Water diffuses rapidly through the membrane because of the increased osmotic pressure or drawing force caused by the higher solute concentration. The rapid diffusion of water to this side will cause a temporary rise in fluid level (b). Meanwhile solute starts to diffuse to the area of low concentration. Ultimately concentrations on both sides will be the same and the fluid levels will also equalize (c).

Units of osmotic force are called osmoles (osm) or milli-osmoles (mosm). The osmotic pressure of a solution (osmolarity) is usually expressed as milli-osmoles per litre (mosm/l).

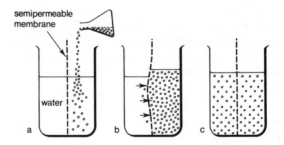

Fig. 1.4. The solute added to water on one side of a semipermeable membrane raises the osmotic pressure.

For substances which are ionized in solution such as sodium chloride, 1 mmol of NaCl will contain two osmotically active particles (Na^+ and Cl^-) or 2 mosm. But divalent cations do not exert more osmotic pressure on account of having two electrical charges. For example 1 mmol of calcium (Ca^{++}) = 1 mosm.

It is important to understand this concept of osmotic pressure in order to appreciate what determines the distribution of water in the different body compartments. Osmotic pressure must also be taken into account when providing artificial methods of dialysis using a semipermeable membrane (Chapters 5–7).

By knowing the composition of a solution the osmolarity can be calculated by adding together the milli-osmoles, the number of particles of osmotic force. Osmolarity can also be measured quickly and directly with an instrument known as an osmometer (see p.25)

The concept of tonicity

A solution is said to be isotonic if it has the same osmolarity (osmotic pressure) as plasma. Examples of isotonic solutions are 0.9% NaCl (normal saline) and 5% dextrose. Although they have an entirely different composition they contain the same number of particles in solution (mosm/l). Hypertonic solutions have a higher osmolarity than plasma. Examples are 3 or 5% NaCl or 10% mannitol. Because of their high osmotic pressure they tend to draw the water out of red cells which become crenated in their presence. They should never be mixed with blood in an intravenous infusion for this reason. When infused intravenously they are rapidly diluted in the bloodstream so that hemolysis does not occur.

Hypotonic solutions have a lower osmolarity than plasma (e.g. 0.45% NaCl). Such solutions cause red cells to swell, so the same precautions apply to mixing with blood in intravenous infusions. Hypotonic saline is in fact used as a test for red cell fragility. Intravenous infusion with hypotonic solutions may be indicated in certain cases of hypertonic dehydration, especially in infants.

Pure water is never infused intravenously but occasionally accidents have occurred when a patient's blood has mistakenly been dialysed against pure water in an artificial kidney machine. This causes almost immediate and massive hemolysis and will quickly prove fatal if it is not detected at once.

Fig. 1.5 illustrates the appearance of red cells in normal (isotonic) plasma (a); in hypertonic solution (b), e.g. mannitol, in which they

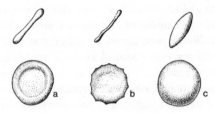

Fig. 1.5. Red cells in (a) isotonic plasma, (b) hypertonic solution, and (c) hypotonic solution.

become shrunken and crenated; and in hypotonic solution (c) in which they become swollen and in danger of hemolysis because of entry of water.

The functions of the kidney

The main functions of normal kidneys are listed below. The order in which they appear in the list is quite arbitrary and for purposes of descriptive convenience only. They cannot really be separated artificially in this way since they are all occurring simultaneously and are intimately connected with one another.
1 Excretion of nitrogenous waste products.
2 Regulation of body water.
3 Regulation of major body electrolytes.
4 Regulation of acid−base balance.
5 Excretion of drugs and poisons.
6 Regulation of blood pressure.
7 Erythropoiesis.
8 Vitamin D metabolism.

1 Excretion of nitrogenous waste products

Perhaps the best-known function of the kidneys is 'excretion of the poisons which would otherwise accumulate in the bloodstream'. This popular phrase usually refers to the end products of protein breakdown of which the best known is urea.

The rate of production of urea by the body depends on several factors, the most obvious of which is the amount of protein consumed in the diet. The greater the protein intake, the greater the protein breakdown and the more urea and other substances which will have to be excreted. In situations in which protein is being synthesized rapidly to build new tissues, as for example during pregnancy, there will be less urea production since amino acids, which would otherwise be broken down into urea, are being incorporated into the new proteins. This is called an *anabolic* state (anabolism means protein synthesis) and the blood urea and urea excretion will tend to be low. If, on the other hand, proteins in the diet as well as the body's own proteins are being broken down rapidly, for example, during high fevers or as a result of extensive muscle injury or high doses of steroid therapy, urea production will be high—perhaps many times higher than usual. This is called a *catabolic* state. The state of anabolism or catabolism should always be taken into consideration when assessing the cause for a particularly high or low level of blood urea.

Under normal circumstances the kidneys excrete urea entirely by means of glomerular filtration. Some solutes which enter the glomerular filtrate from the bloodstream, such as glucose and amino acids, are completely reabsorbed by the tubules and do not appear in the urine at all. In contrast to this approximately half the filtered urea is reabsorbed by the tubules while the other half appears in the urine. Healthy individuals have a large reserve of normal functioning nephrons. If dietary protein intake is increased and urea production is high the blood urea level will rise slightly and there will be a corresponding increase in the amount of urea in the glomerular filtrate.

With quite wide fluctuations in urea production there may be very little alteration in blood urea concentration because of the big reserve of healthy renal tissue. Only when the glomerular filtration rate is substantially reduced as a result of renal damage will there be a significant rise in blood urea.

Rarely one may encounter quite startling elevations of blood urea due to excessive protein intake in individuals with normal renal function. A notable example was the case of an eccentric lady who was found to have a blood urea of 150 mg% (25.0 mmol/l) (normal 3.5–6.0 mmol/l). It transpired that she was in the habit of eating 400 g protein daily, mainly in the form of boiled cod! Her renal function was normal and she had no symptoms of uremia. Dietary indiscretions have more serious effects in patients with impaired renal function.

Creatinine, another well-known breakdown product of muscle metabolism, depends for its excretion on glomerular filtration but it is not significantly reabsorbed or secreted by the renal tubules. Furthermore, creatinine excretion tends to be remarkably constant in any particular individual from day to day. It is hardly affected by dietary protein intake but seems to be related mainly to an individual's muscle mass. Women with a small muscle mass have a lower blood creatinine level than men with a large muscle mass. Because of its special property of passing down the renal tubules without being significantly absorbed or secreted, creatinine is especially useful for making an estimation of glomerular filtration rate (see p.30). For the other reasons just mentioned, blood creatinine is a more reliable indicator of renal function than blood urea.

There are many other less well-known end-products of nitrogen metabolism which are much more toxic than urea, and whose accumulation in 'uremia' is serious, but in practice urea and creatinine are simple and convenient to measure and together they serve as an excellent guide to progress in any individual patient.

2 Regulation of body water

During health the composition of the body fluids remains remarkably constant from hour to hour and day to day, though mild fluctuations occur in relation to meals and the rhythm of sleep. The fluid requirements of infants are somewhat precarious since their immature kidneys have only moderate concentrating ability. Adult kidneys on the other hand are remarkably efficient at conserving water when there is a shortage and excreting large volumes when there is an excess. About 80% of the water presented to the tubules in the glomerular filtrate is reabsorbed in the proximal convoluted tubules. The urine concentration is performed by variable reabsorption of water by the collecting tubules under the influence of antidiuretic hormone (ADH). ADH is liberated from the posterior pituitary gland after stimulation of so-called osmoreceptors which are special nerve endings in the hypothalamus. Hypertonic plasma is the stimulus for more ADH secretion leading to more water reabsorption and therefore a more concentrated urine. When the plasma is diluted by a generous water intake, ADH secretion is suppressed and a brisk water diuresis occurs.

If the posterior pituitary is damaged by trauma or disease, so that ADH secretion is defective, the patient continuously passes a large volume of dilute urine and is correspondingly thirsty. In this condition, known as diabetes insipidus, the thirst and polyuria can be corrected by use of one of the synthetic preparations of ADH. There is no defect in the kidneys themselves in diabetes insipidus and the only danger is dehydration if water is withheld. The synthetic vasopressin analogue dDAVP taken intranasally once or twice a day is very effective in controlling the polyuria.

Inappropriate ADH secretion

In recent years a syndrome of dilutional hyponatremia (hyponatremia means low serum sodium) has been increasingly recognized particularly in association with bronchogenic carcinoma and certain endocrine abnormalities such as myxedema. This is due to continuous and inappropriate secretion of an ADH-like substance which causes abnormal water retention and consequently a low serum sodium concentration due to dilution. The characteristic finding is a low serum osmolarity in association with a continuously high urine osmolarity. It is best managed by simply limiting the patient's water intake.

Recently good results have been reported from a drug called demeclocycline which appears to act as an effective antagonist of ADH.

3 Regulation of the major body electrolytes

Sodium

Sixty to eighty per cent of the major electrolytes are reabsorbed in the proximal tubules along with water. Selective reabsorption and secretion of the remainder takes place in the distal tubules according to the needs of the body. Sodium and water largely regulate blood volume and the osmolarity of the extracellular fluids. It is therefore fortunate that healthy kidneys conserve sodium very efficiently if there is a shortage and can excrete large amounts if there is an excess. Urinary sodium excretion may vary from 10 mEq (10 mmol) per day, if salt is withheld from the diet, to 150 mEq (150 mmol) per day on a high salt intake. If a severe deficit of body sodium occurs the circulating blood volume will be decreased, the blood flow to the kidneys will be reduced and renal function will become impaired. Renal diseases which damage the tubules may be associated with inability to conserve sodium normally.

Potassium

The renal handling of potassium is not as efficient as that of sodium nor is potassium conserved so well when there is a shortage. Furthermore, urinary potassium excretion is somewhat at the mercy of both sodium and hydrogen ions (H+). (You may remember from your chemistry that hydrogen ions in practice means acid.) Both a high sodium diet and the administration of alkali will increase urinary potassium loss. A low sodium diet and administration of acid will both tend to cause potassium retention. Potassium loss is also increased by adrenal cortical steroids. It is not uncommon to find a low serum potassium in a patient taking high doses of prednisone. Nearly all diuretics cause increased urinary potassium excretion which in time leads to potassium deficiency. This is why diuretics should always be accompanied by potassium supplements, except in chronic renal failure when the serum potassium may already be high.

The bulk of body potassium is contained in the cells and the level of serum potassium often does not truly reflect deficiency or excess. There is a reciprocal relationship between potassium and hydrogen ions which in simple terms can be explained as follows. They are both cations carrying a positive electrical charge. If one of them enters the cells the other has to come out because electrical neutrality must be preserved. If serum potassium becomes elevated due to excessive potassium administration, potassium enters the cells and hydrogen ions come out into the plasma. This makes the plasma more acid. If serum potassium is low, potassium comes out of the cells into the extracellular fluid and hydrogen ions go into the cells. The loss of ionic hydrogen will make the plasma more alkaline. Changes in potassium are no longer thought to be the major causes of these acid–base disturbances: extracellular fluid volume and chloride are the major factors. This explains why administration of alkali is an excellent way of acutely lowering serum potassium. Sodium bicarbonate will neutralize the hydrogen ions in plasma and cause hydrogen ions to come out of the cells. Potassium will then enter the cells to preserve electrical neutrality.

4 Regulation of acid–base balance

The metabolic processes of the body can only function within narrow limits of alkalinity and acidity. Blood pH, which reflects the H^+ concentration in plasma water, never varies much from 7.4 in normal circumstances. A pH below 7.0 or above 7.7 is not compatible with life for very long. There is a generally accepted normal range from 7.35–7.45. If the pH falls below 7.35 an acidosis is said to exist. A pH above 7.45 indicates an alkalosis. Maintenance of a steady pH depends on three interconnecting systems:
- buffers,
- the lungs (compensation),
- the kidneys (correction).

A buffer is a substance which takes up an acid or alkali without a significant change in pH. If an acid (H^+ load) is added to the body, e.g. during diabetic ketoacidosis, the pH of the body is held relatively constant by buffers. The buffers in the intracellular water are predominantly proteins. The major buffer system in the extracellular water is bicarbonate (HCO_3^-). Bicarbonate combines with H^+ to form carbonic acid (H_2CO_3)

which dissociates to CO_2 and H_2O:

$$HCO_3^- + H^2 \rightleftharpoons H_2CO_3 \rightleftharpoons CO_2 + H_2O$$

The intracellular and extracellular buffers act simultaneously to 'defend' the pH against sudden changes in H^+ concentration.

A fall in pH (acidosis) stimulates the respiratory center in the brain to increase the ventilation rate. Increased ventilation results in more CO_2 being blown off or excreted from the lungs. This causes the above equation to shift to the right. This respiratory compensation for acidosis is limited by the mechanics of ventilation. It should be noted that alkalosis results in a decreased ventilatory rate, a subsequent retention of CO_2 and net H^+ production (the above equation shifts to the left). The respiratory compensation in this direction is limited because of ensuing anoxia (an overriding stimulus for ventilation).

An excess acid or alkali load is excreted by the kidneys—referred to as the *renal correction* of an acid–base disturbance.

In the normal course of events our diet, when broken down in the body, contains more acid than alkali, and the main route of excretion of acid is through the kidneys. Renal acid excretion is a slow process, going on all the time, the rate of acid elimination being increased or decreased according to the needs of the body. Hydrogen ions are excreted into the distal tubules and disposed of in three main ways.

• By combination with bicarbonate to produce CO_2 and water. Carbon dioxide diffuses back into the bloodstream.

• By excretion with buffers, especially phosphates, which take up hydrogen ion.

• By combination with ammonia (manufactured in the renal tubules) and excreted as an ammonium salt: $NH_3 + H^+ = NH_4^+$.

In patients with chronic renal failure there are not enough surviving nephrons to excrete all the acid adequately and a mild metabolic acidosis may develop. It is not really surprising that renal diseases associated primarily with tubular damage, such as pyelonephritis, tend to be accompanied by more severe acidosis than diseases such as glomerulonephritis which affect primarily the glomeruli.

There is an interesting and rare group of diseases characterized by specific inability of the distal tubules to excrete hydrogen, even though all other aspects of renal function are quite adequate. These conditions may be congenital or acquired and are characterized by chronic metabolic acidosis which leads to osteomalacia and nephrocalcinosis. This is because calcium, which is more soluble in an acid medium, tends to dissolve out of the skeleton (because of the acidosis) but crystallizes in the urine, which is always alkaline. The condition is called *renal tubular acidosis* and it is important to recognize it because it can be treated very effectively by oral administration of alkalis.

Respiratory causes of acid–base disturbance

Not all acidosis or alkalosis is determined by metabolic factors. Chronic lung disease with CO_2 retention can lower the blood pH by increasing carbonic acid. The other features will be a raised PCO_2 on blood gas analysis, and a raised plasma bicarbonate. The patient will also have clinically obvious lung disease. The condition is called *respiratory acidosis*. A respiratory alkalosis is sometimes seen in hysterical hyperventilation and in the early stages of aspirin poisoning, when overbreathing causes CO_2 to be blown off by the lungs. The patient may develop tetany from the alkalosis and his plasma bicarbonate will be low.

It may be apparent from reading this that respiratory alkalosis in many respects resembles metabolic acidosis. Both are accompanied by hyperventilation and a low plasma bicarbonate. If it is not possible to distinguish them by their clinical features, measurement of the pH of an arterial blood sample will certainly clear up any doubt.

Finally, it is worth remembering that although respiratory mechanisms are normally very efficient in helping to compensate the acid–base disturbance of a metabolic defect (e.g. hyperventilation helps to correct the acidosis of renal failure) the same will not be true for a patient with chronic chest disease such as chronic bronchitis and emphysema or for a patient with an acute pneumonia. Such a patient may already have a respiratory acidosis from this cause, so that the two defects will compound each other.

Hence renal failure is always much more dangerous if it is accompanied by chest disease.

5 Excretion of drugs and poisons

The kidneys share with the liver the important job of disposing of drugs and poisons that enter the body. Water-soluble drugs tend to be excreted mainly in the urine while fat-soluble drugs are usually dealt with predominantly by the liver. Having entered the liver they may be excreted in the bile or changed into water-soluble inactive components which are then excreted in the urine.

In general, the morphine group of powerful analgesics, as well as most antidepressives and tranquillizers, are dealt with mainly by the liver. The long-acting barbiturates, aspirin, digitalis and nearly all antibiotics are excreted mainly by the kidneys. Some drugs, such as the penicillins, can be given in very large doses to produce high blood levels with little fear of toxicity. Others such as digitalis have a comparatively narrow margin between their therapeutic level and their toxic level.

Nearly all drugs are dangerous if taken in overdoses either accidentally or for attempted suicide. Hospital admissions for self-administered drug overdoses have reached epidemic proportions in recent years, so much so that a working knowledge of the mode of excretion of drugs is very valuable to all medical and nursing staff, especially on medical wards. The management of drug overdosage is a large subject in itself, but it should be mentioned here that certain groups of drugs can be eliminated more quickly by the technique of diuresis. This involves the use of generous intravenous fluid infusion and diuretics such as mannitol or furosemide (frusemide). Alkalinization of the urine with intravenous sodium bicarbonate greatly increases the excretion of some drugs such as phenobarbitone and aspirin. Forced diuresis must be used with great discretion, however. It offers no advantage in cases of poisoning with the tricyclic antidepressives and may actually be dangerous by precipitating pulmonary edema.

Hemodialysis may be indicated in selected cases of very severe poisoning when there is a danger of death in spite of good conservative treatment including assisted ventilation. In general, drugs that are excreted by the kidneys can be removed faster with an artificial kidney machine. Hemodialysis is particularly effective in severe aspirin poisoning and should be considered whenever the serum salicylate level approaches 12.5 mmol/l.

Recently, a technique known as hemoperfusion has tended to replace hemodialysis as a means of eliminating drugs and poisons. In essence this consists of passing the patient's heparinized blood through activated charcoal to adsorb the toxic substance. It is much faster and more efficient than hemodialysis and will be described in more detail in Chapter 9.

These remarks about drugs also apply to domestic and industrial poisons which may be taken deliberately or accidentally. The kidneys provide a way of removing noxious substances from the body but they themselves are peculiarly vulnerable to toxic damage for two main reasons. First they have a very rich blood supply in proportion to their weight, and second the process of excretion involves concentration of the poison in the renal tubules to many times the concentration that exists in the blood.

This is why the renal tubules, which are composed of sensitive and highly differentiated cells, tend to take the brunt of the damage in many cases of poisoning. This will be referred to in the causes of acute renal failure in Chapter 4.

If patients are already suffering from some degree of impaired renal function due to another cause, drugs excreted by the kidneys must be given with extreme caution for two reasons.

• The drug, because of inadequate excretion, may build up to toxic blood levels and damage other organs, e.g. deafness from the aminoglycoside group of drugs, cardiotoxicity from digitalis.

• The high blood levels may be toxic to the kidneys and further aggravate existing damage.

This subject will be discussed further under the management of chronic renal failure in Chapter 4.

6 Regulation of blood pressure

The mechanism of control of normal blood pressure as well as the explanation for the development of essential hypertension are still the subject of controversy among experts, and will no doubt be debated for many years. From a practical point of view it is important to know that nearly all kidney diseases, whether bilateral or unilateral, may at some point be associated with hypertension, though certain kidney lesions seem more likely to produce hypertension than others. Hypertension is more common in diseases that produce glomerular damage in the cortex than in those that produce tubular damage in the medulla. The classical form of experimental renal hypertension was produced by Goldblatt in dogs by partially occluding the renal artery. It now seems likely that anything which prevents the normal pulsatile flow of blood to the kidneys can produce hypertension in man. Well-known examples are renal artery stenosis and coarctation of the aorta. However, this sort of ischemia is only one mechanism because many diseases of the renal substance itself cause hypertension even before there is any significant renal artery narrowing. It is also known now that a hormone called renin is manufactured in the kidneys at some site close to the afferent arterioles and probably in a group of cells next to the glomerulus called the juxtaglomerular cells. Renin apparently acts on a plasma globulin called angiotensinogen to produce a substance called angiotensin II. Angiotensin II has a vasoconstrictor effect on blood vessels, thereby increasing the resistance to flow and causing a rise in blood pressure. High concentrations of renin have been found in the renal vein blood as well as in the systemic circulation in many forms of renal hypertension. Removal of diseased kidneys or by-passing a renal artery stenosis has frequently cured or improved renal hypertension, and in these cases the blood renin levels have usually returned to normal.

Unfortunately it is not always as simple as this. The results of arterial reconstructive surgery for renal artery stenosis are frequently disappointing, and removal of unilateral diseased kidneys is not always followed by a return to normal blood pressure. In some cases this may be due to the fact that the blood pressure has been elevated long enough to produce permanent damage in the small blood vessels. Furthermore, the renin—angiotensin system is interrelated with other important factors such as the sodium content of the body and the secretion of aldosterone, the salt retaining hormone of the adrenal cortex. Information in this field is rapidly increasing and it may not be too long before all the pieces of the puzzle fit together.

7 Erythropoiesis

The manufacture of red blood cells takes place in the bone marrow—especially the vertebrae and flat bones in adult humans. A substance called erythropoietin, which is produced by normal kidneys, stimulates the bone marrow to make erythrocytes. In some renal disorders such as renal carcinoma and some cases of polycystic kidney disease and hydronephrosis there appears to be an over-production of red blood cells.

Of greater numerical importance is the anemia which invariably occurs in patients with chronic renal failure (see Chapter 4). Part of this anemia is probably due to lack of erythropoietin production by diseased kidneys. There is certainly a reduced production of red cells in uremia but it has also been shown that red cells do not survive so long in uremic serum and clearly this is an important additional factor. The anemia is not cured by administration of iron or other hematinic factors.

8 Vitamin D metabolism

The kidneys play an important role in maintaining the mineralization of normal bone by calcium and phosphate. This is at least partly due to the fact that the conversion of vitamin D (so vital in bone metabolism) to its most active metabolic end-product takes place in the kidneys. This also partly explains why patients with chronically damaged kidneys tend to develop defects of bone mineralization. This is discussed more fully in later chapters.

2

Tests and Investigations

Robert Uldall

In assessing disorders of the urinary tract the history and physical examination are no less important than in any other branch of medicine. A well-taken history will often immediately indicate the right diagnosis, especially if one knows which questions to ask. For example, the cause of a patient's chronic renal failure may remain a mystery until one takes the trouble to enquire carefully into the patient's consumption of mixed analgesics. A housewife may have taken eight codeine tablets a day for four years—at first for some trivial reason and later because it became a habit. It might not occur to her to mention it, perhaps because she did not think it was important. We now know that regular and prolonged consumption of mixed, phenacetin-containing analgesics can cause interstitial renal damage of severe degree. Fortunately most advanced countries have banned the use of phenacetin in mixed proprietary analgesic preparations. Hence the only cases we see now are in patients coming from less advanced countries.

Physical examination in the case of renal and urological disorders is often disappointingly unrewarding, but nevertheless should not be neglected. For example, polycystic kidney disease can often be diagnosed confidently by simple palpation of the abdomen.

After the history and physical examination have been completed, several more tests will be required to make a complete assessment of the problem. The responsibility for ordering the tests and investigations will usually be that of the doctor in charge of the case. It often falls to the nurse to see that the tests are properly carried out. Her responsibilities in this respect can be listed as follows:

• She must be able to explain to the patient what is involved. Anxious or apprehensive patients may need reassurance. Regrettably it is not uncommon for busy medical staff to omit this important duty.

• In investigations which demand the cooperation of the patient she must be able to instruct the less intelligent patient exactly what to do.

• She must make sure that the patient is adequately prepared, e.g. bowel preparation and fluid deprivation before an intravenous urogram and shaving the pubic hair before cystoscopy.

• She must be able to supervise the accurate collection of samples and make sure they are delivered to the right place.

• In investigations such as renal biopsy which carry a risk, she should be aware of the risks and know what routine observations are required to spot the danger signs.

• As nurses become more experienced they will learn to anticipate which tests will be required. Such things as fluid balance charts and regular urine testing in certain patients and initiation of 24 hour urine collections in other patients will become second nature.

• Correct and legible labelling of specimens and accurate completion of request cards is very important. For example, a request for blood grouping for transfusion should always be accompanied by the patient's hospital record number. The name alone may not be enough to prevent mistakes such as giving the patient the wrong blood.

• All blood samples from regular dialysis patients should be regarded as potentially capable of transmitting hepatitis. Blood should not be allowed to get on to the outside of the tube. The tube should be sealed in a plastic bag and clearly labelled as coming from a dialysis patient. The laboratory can then take appropriate special precautions in dealing with it.

The supervision and conduct of investigations may be tedious and time consuming, especially when they have to be fitted into the routine of a busy out-patient clinic or ward. The tests will seem less of a nuisance if their purpose is understood and the information gained from them has some meaning. The main points about each of the common tests and investigations will be described. The chapter can either be read straight through, or the index can be used to refer to any particular test at the time it is being done.

Recording fluid balance

Perhaps the most simple and fundamental of all ward investigations is the measurement of fluid intake and urine output. We completely depend on knowledge of these volumes to tell us what is going on. It is probably true to say that any patient with any disease of the urinary tract should be on an intake and output chart, at least until it is deemed unnecessary by the doctor. The same applies to every patient in hospital who is seriously ill. Elderly people may become apathetic and stop drinking. Febrile patients may become dehydrated. Shocked patients may become oliguric and then accidentally over-transfused.

It is important if possible to obtain the patient's cooperation to maintain an accurate fluid balance chart. All fluid volumes should be listed accurately in columns and totalled at the end of each 8 hour shift or at the end of the 24 hour period. In acute situations hourly urine volumes may have to be measured. Hourly urine volume measurement is only feasible if the patient has an indwelling urinary catheter, as for example in the immediate post-operative period after renal transplantation or perhaps when one suspects the onset of acute renal failure.

The logical accompaniment of a fluid balance chart is daily weighing, preferably at the same time each day. Large changes of weight from one day to the next are nearly always due to positive or negative fluid balance, so that weight measurement is the ideal way of checking the accuracy of gain or loss of water.

A serious obstacle to sensible recording of fluid balance is the old-fashioned habit of clinging to ounces and pints instead of talking about millilitres and litres. The volumes of the different body compartments are all measured in litres, so it no longer makes sense to record fluid volumes in ounces and pints or weights in stones and pounds. All wards and clinics should now have scales which weigh in kilograms, and measuring cylinders which are calibrated in millilitres.

Examination of the urine

Routine urinalysis to check for abnormal urinary constituents is usually a nurse's responsibility. This is made easy now by the availability of a whole series of paper dip tests. The routine tests on urine which she may be expected to perform are as follows.

Specific gravity

This is a measurement of the weight of solute in the urine. The measurement is performed with a urinometer which is floated in the urine in a cylindrical flask. The level to which the urinometer sinks is read on the scale. A low figure such as 1003 means a dilute urine. A high figure such as 1028 means a concentrated urine. If the specific gravity never varies very much from 1010 one should suspect the possibility of chronic renal failure. This is because patients with chronic renal failure are unable to concentrate or dilute their urine. The small amount of healthy renal tissue is working at maximum capacity to get rid of solutes such as urea which are continuously present in the blood in abnormally high concentrations. The urine specific gravity will be raised by the presence of abnormal constituents such as protein and sugar. The importance of this is that specific gravity may be hard to interpret in the presence of proteinuria. The specific gravity may be quite high even though the urine is not concentrated.

A refractometer is a useful small portable instrument which can measure the refractive index of a solution by using only one drop. This is useful if there is not enough urine to fill the urinometer. However, refraction is also a measure of density and therefore suffers from the same limitations described above for specific gravity.

Osmolarity

A more reliable measurement of urine concentration than specific gravity is the osmolarity. This is a measurement of the number of particles in solution. It is measured by means of an osmometer, an instrument which makes use of the fact that the freezing point of a solution is strictly in proportion to the number of particles in it. The osmometer actually measures the freezing point but the osmolarity can be read directly on the instrument dial. Osmometers are normally kept in the hospital laboratory. Only 2 ml of urine are required to get a reading. Although anybody can be taught to use an osmometer reliably with a few minutes tuition, nurses are not usually expected to operate the instrument.

pH

Urine pH can be measured roughly with indicator papers which show a range of different colors with varying pH. On a normal diet urine is usually acid, pH 4−6. In some forms of treatment we may deliberately aim to make the urine alkaline, pH 7 or more, and indicator papers can be used to check this.

Protein

It is more accurate to talk about protein in the urine than albumin. What we measure with the Albustix test is hardly ever pure albumin but a mixture of different proteins. A trace of proteinuria should always be rechecked on another sample. Remember that a small amount of proteinuria may be undetectable when the urine is very dilute but is readily detected if the urine is concentrated. The early morning urine sample is nearly always fairly concentrated and this is why it has traditionally been used for routine ward testing. If there is still doubt after testing this sample with Albustix it is worth checking with salicylsulphonic acid or by boiling. 3+ or 4+ means heavy proteinuria which will need to be measured accurately. If one really needs to know how much urinary protein a patient is passing, a 24 hour urine sample should be collected and sent to the laboratory where it will be tested by one of the accurate quantitative methods.

Glucose

Clinistix is the specific ward test for glucose in the urine and when this is positive we naturally think of the possibility of diabetes. Several other conditions are also associated with glycosuria, especially any disease which damages the renal tubules. A common and harmless condition which causes glycosuria is the renal glycosuria of pregnancy. This condition which is also called a *low renal threshold* is caused by leakage of glucose into the urine at a lower level of blood sugar than normal. The glucose leak disappears after delivery. Clinitest tablets are used for measuring the amount of glucose in the urine. They are not specific for glucose but will measure any reducing substance.

Acetone

If glucose is found in the urine, a test should always be made for acetone. This is also routinely available as a dip test on the strips which we use to carry out several tests simultaneously. Acetone is present in the urine in any diabetic who is becoming ketotic, so it may be a sign of diabetic precoma. Ketones in the urine are also very common in children who have been starved due to some intercurrent illness. When ketones are due to starvation there will usually be no glycusuria. Many entirely healthy patients may have a positive test for ketones simply as a result of missing a meal.

Blood

Chemical tests for blood in the urine actually detect hemoglobin. Hemoglobinuria can sometimes occur without hematuria, so it will be necessary for the medical staff to view the urine with a microscope to be sure that it actually contains red blood cells rather than just hemoglobin. Blood which is evenly mixed with the urine is usually coming from one or both kidneys. Bleeding from the bladder or urethra is usually more pronounced at the beginning or end of the act of micturition. It may help the diagnosis considerably if these observations are made and recorded.

Small numbers of red blood cells in the urine may be missed by the routine paper test (a) because they are diluted in a large volume and (b) because they are not hemolysed to hemoglobin. In order to avoid missing small numbers of red cells if slight hematuria is strongly suspected, one can do two things. First the urine can be centrifuged in a tube and the supernatant can be poured away. Then add two drops of acetic acid to the deposit in the bottom of the tube. This will hemolyse any red cells that are present. The acidified deposit should be shaken up and tested.

Bile

Bile in the urine is usually evident as a yellowish color of the froth as well as a yellowish-brown of the urine itself. If this is confirmed by a paper test or chemical test it usually means obstructive jaundice. Myoglobin in the urine is also a golden brown color. It can be distinguished from bile and hemoglobin by spectroscopic examination in the laboratory. The importance of myoglobinuria is that it is sometimes a sign of extensive muscle damage which may lead to acute renal failure.

Urine microscopy

Any patient being examined for any kidney disease should have his urine examined microscopically by the doctor who conducts the physical examination. Failure to do so will repeatedly result in unnecessary mistakes. Sending the specimen to the laboratory for microscopic examination by a technician is no substitute. An interested physician will wish to look for the diagnostic clues in a fresh urine specimen himself. Very often it will be necessary to centrifuge the urine in a tube to find the important evidence which may be impossible to find in an uncentrifuged specimen. A nurse assisting in a renal out-patient clinic may be asked to spin down the fresh urine sample for the doctor to examine after he has examined the patient. After labelling the tube, centrifugation at 2 000 revolutions per minute for five minutes is usually satisfactory for concentrating the particulate matter in a small 'button' at the bottom of the tube. An excellent example of the value of microscopy is in distinguishing the origin of the red blood cells in a patient with hematuria. If there are red blood cell casts in the urine we know that they assumed that shape by being passed through the glomeruli and down the tubules. We then know that the patient's bleeding is glomerular in origin and the patient will not need a cystoscopy to look for a bleeding source in the bladder.

Biochemical tests

It is impossible to discuss fully the reasons for and significance of all the different biochemical tests we do, but some practical points about each of the main ones deserve mention.

Urea and electrolytes (blood urea (20−40 mg per cent) (about 3.0−6.0 mmol/l) (mmol/1 × 6 = mg/100 ml))

This is the most commonly used overall screening test for impaired renal function. It does not always accurately reflect renal function because the level of blood urea is determined by the rate of production as well as by the rate of excretion. Impaired excretion due to diseased kidneys will cause the blood urea to rise, but so also will increased production due to excessive protein intake, tissue breakdown from muscle injury, any infection, and absorption of blood from the gastro-intestinal tract. The blood urea also tends to be high in patients who are dehydrated. Under these conditions more urea is reabsorbed into the bloodstream from the tubules. Decreased urea production during pregnancy and in patients with liver disease may cause the blood urea to be abnormally low.

Sodium (normal value 130−145 mEq/l) (mmol/l)

Sodium is the main positively charged ion (cation) in extracellular fluid and it is the main electrolyte which determines blood volume. A high serum sodium level may be due to too much sodium or too little water, while a low serum sodium may be due to sodium deficiency or too much water. Combinations of these factors may also exist. It is often necessary to know the clinical circumstances before making a correct assessment.

Chloride (95−105 mEq/l) (mmol/l)

Chloride is the main negatively charged ion (anion) in extracellular fluid. Sodium and chloride usually move together—either they are both high or they are both low. Occasionally, however, chloride alone may be low if a lot of chloride has been lost as hydrochloric acid from the stomach during vomiting. Chloride alone may also be high in conditions of metabolic acidosis and in this case the plasma bicarbonate (quoted on the report as CO_2) will be low. Well-known causes of metabolic acidosis are chronic uremia, congenital renal tubular acidosis and ureterosigmoidostomy.

Potassium (3.5–5.0 mEq/l) (mmol/l)

Potassium is the main intracellular cation and only small concentrations are present in extracellular fluid. If this small extracellular concentration varies above or below a rather narrow range there may be devastating physiological consequences. The commonest cause of a high concentration is renal failure, either acute or chronic, with consequent failure to excrete potassium in the urine. Additional causes may be tissue destruction, infection, and gastro-intestinal blood absorption. The commonest causes of a low potassium level are the use of diuretics which increase urinary potassium loss, and prolonged diarrhea which causes loss of potassium in feces. Habitual use of laxatives may bring this about. The main effects of a high serum potassium are muscle weakness and cardiac arrest. Low serum potassium tends to cause even more profound muscle weakness and cardiac arrhythmia. Prolonged potassium depletion can also cause renal tubular damage. This is largely reversible if treated in time. Clearly the most dangerous complication of all these is cardiac arrest from hyperkalemia. Fortunately even this disaster can usually be reversed if cardiac resuscitation is started at once and measures are adopted immediately to lower the serum potassium.

All nurses should always pay immediate attention to a high serum potassium level. Any level above 6 mmol/l should be reported at once to the medical staff who can then take steps to remedy the situation.

If blood for serum potassium estimation is sent to the laboratory for an urgent result it should be the responsibility of the chief nurse to make sure the result is phoned back urgently to the ward. Unfortunately one cannot always rely on busy laboratory technicians to report to the ward at once if they find a dangerously high figure.

Failure to draw attention to a high serum potassium level may be the cause of entirely preventable death.

Plasma bicarbonate (20–30 mEq/l) (mmol/l)

The plasma bicarbonate is affected by metabolic factors (the relative amounts of acid and alkali in the body) and also by respiratory factors such as the degree of CO_2 retention in people with chest disease. See Chapter 1 on the control of acid−base balance.

Serum creatinine $\left(\dfrac{\mu mol/l}{88.4} = mg/100\,ml \right)$

In healthy individuals who have no kidney disease the level of the serum creatinine depends largely on body size, especially the amount of muscle. The range is approximately from 35 μmol/l in small children to about 115 μmol/l for a large man. Average for a woman would be about 75 μmol/l and for a man about 97 μmol/l. Apart from the size of one's muscle mass, the only thing which affects serum creatinine is renal function. It is only slightly affected by protein intake and tissue damage, and not at all by infection or blood absorption. It is therefore generally a much more reliable index of renal function than the blood urea. Creatinine is now being estimated in all hospital laboratories as a routine test. It is particularly helpful for following the progress of patients with kidney disease to see whether renal function is improving, stable or deteriorating.

Creatinine clearance

When blood enters the glomeruli of the kidneys a filtrate is formed by passage through the capillary walls of water and solutes, but not protein. (The protein molecules are too large to pass through unless the patient has some glomerular disease.)

The filtrate of water and solutes passes down the tubules eventually to be formed into urine. The rate of formation of this filtrate for an average healthy man is in the region of 180 l/day or about 125 ml/minute. This glomerular filtration rate (GFR for short) is a convenient measurement to make in any particular kidneys. Any disease which destroys glomeruli or their tubules will decrease the glomerular filtration rate. What has all this got to do with creatinine clearance? It has been shown that the creatinine in the blood is filtered off at the glomeruli and when it enters the tubules it is not significantly reabsorbed. Neither is creatinine appreciably secreted by the tubules into the urine. So, by measuring the amount of creatinine in the urine over a timed period, we can estimate how much has been filtered by the glomeruli.

The creatinine clearance, which is calculated by knowing the blood creatinine concentration, the urine creatinine concentration, and the urine volume over a timed period, is actually a very close approximation to the glomerular filtration rate. It is not the only way of measuring the

GFR, but it is the most convenient routine method which has been found so far.

For the laboratory to calculate the creatinine clearance it must have a carefully timed urine specimen (a 24 hour urine sample has various advantages) and a small sample of clotted blood in a plain tube collected sometime during or near to the 24 hour period. It is most convenient for the laboratory if these arrive taped together with the request card. The total period of the urine collection should also be clearly marked. More or less than 24 hours volume may serve equally well as long as the period of the collection is accurately known. An inaccurately timed urine collection is the commonest cause of an inaccurate creatinine clearance. Some of the practical points about 24 hour urine collections are discussed on p.35.

Magnesium (1.5–2.0 mEq/l) (mmol/l × 2 = mEq/l)

Next to potassium, magnesium is the most important cation in the cells. Like potassium, it is present in extracellular fluid in low concentrations. Conditions of magnesium deficiency and excess are much less common than in the case of potassium, and the effects are also usually less serious. Magnesium deficiency can occur occasionally when there is prolonged starvation accompanied by loss of gastro-intestinal contents through diarrhea or vomiting. The symptoms of magnesium deficiency are not clearly defined but weakness, nervousness and tremor have all been described.

Hypermagnesemia (high blood magnesium) is uncommon except in renal failure, especially when magnesium-containing medicines are administered. Very high levels of serum magnesium cause first weakness and then total paralysis. This has occurred when a patient with chronic renal failure was given Epsom salts (which contain magnesium sulphate). Magnesium trisilicate should be avoided in these patients for the same reason though, being less soluble, it is less readily absorbed and not so dangerous as magnesium sulphate.

Calcium (9.0–10.5 mg/dl) (2.3–2.7 mmol/l) (mmol/l × 4 = mg/dl)

Calcium is the main mineral in bone. High blood levels of calcium are found in hyperparathyroidism, a condition in which excessive secretion of parathyroid hormone, usually from an adenoma, causes excessive loss of calcium and phosphate in the urine. Calcium is lost from bones (osteitis fibrosa cystica) and deposited in the kidneys where it tends to form calculi. Hyperparathyroidism is treated by surgical removal of the adenoma. The other main cause of high serum calcium is cancer which has spread to cause metastases in bone.

The commonest cause of a low serum calcium is chronic renal failure in which there is defective calcium absorption from the gastro-intestinal tract. The renal osteodystrophy (bone disease) which tends to accompany chronic renal failure is probably partly due to the acidosis which tends to be present. Fortunately this condition usually responds well to administration of vitamin D.

Serum phosphorus (2−4 mg/dl) (mol/l × 3.1 = mg/dl)

Serum phosphorus or phosphate is closely and inversely related to calcium. It tends to be low in hyperparathyroidism when the calcium is high and it is usually high in chronic renal failure when the calcium is low. The product of calcium and phosphorus tends to be roughly constant; but if for some reason the product is high, calcium tends to precipitate in various soft tissues; and this is dangerous if it is allowed to continue. A warning sign of soft tissue calcification may appear as small deposits in the cornea of the eyes. The patient has red, itchy eyes and looks as though he has conjunctivitis. Soft tissue calcification in the heart can cause cardiac arrhythmias and eventually complete heart block.

Uric acid (3.0−6.5 mg/dl) (μmol/l = mg/dl × 59.5)

The level of serum uric acid is usually high in renal failure due to inadequate renal excretion. In the absence of renal failure a high serum uric acid usually means gout. Gout is a familial disease which may affect both the joints and the kidneys, though in any one individual one or other of these areas may be quite free of trouble for a long time. The arthritis of gout is thought to be due to chemical inflammation of the synovial membranes by uric acid crystals. Renal damage from gout may take various forms including the formation of urate calculi as well as diffuse renal parenchymal damage involving glomeruli and tubules. In addition to familial or primary gout there are some disorders, especially certain blood diseases such as certain leukemias, in which there is a high rate of uric acid production due to rapid formation and destruction of cells. Serum uric acid may rise even higher when these conditions are treated and a lot of abnormal cells are rapidly destroyed. Under these circumstances we talk of secondary gout. The most extreme form of this is acute uric acid nephropathy. The patient develops renal failure due to widespread crystallization of uric acid in the renal tubules.

Fortunately the drug allopurinol can block the formation of uric acid in the body, so lowering the blood level. This has been shown to exert protective effects on both joints and kidneys.

Alkaline phosphatase (20–90 iu/l)

A raised level of alkaline phosphatase in the blood may be a sign of bone disease, such as renal osteodystrophy, or the bone disease which sometimes develops in patients on regular long-term hemodialysis. The level will gradually return to normal if and when the bones heal.

Alkaline phosphatase is also raised in obstructive jaundice. There is nearly always a slight element of obstructive jaundice in an attack of hepatitis so that a moderate elevation may occur in this condition.

Acid phosphatase (1–3 iu/100 ml)

When a carcinoma of the prostate starts to extend beyond the prostatic capsule there may be elevated levels in the blood of an enzyme called acid phosphatase. This test is therefore worth doing in any suspected case of prostatic carcinoma when the diagnosis is in doubt. A raised level probably confirms cancer with extraprostatic spread. It is, however, worth remembering that prostatic massage will raise the level in normal men and the same applies to recent rectal examinations or enemata. Conversely, a normal acid phosphatase does not exclude a small carcinoma which is still confined to the gland. If prostatic cancer is suspected, blood for acid phosphatase estimation should be drawn before the rectal examination is performed.

Plasma renin assay (and plasma renin activity)

Renin is a hormone produced by the cells of the juxtaglomerular apparatus (specialized cells next to the glomeruli). Its physiological role is in the control of normal blood pressure. Under conditions of hypotension, blood volume depletion or sodium depletion, it is secreted in greater amounts. It is converted by an enzyme to angiotensin I, then to angiotensin II which causes arteriolar vasoconstriction and a rise in blood pressure. Any process which restricts the flow of blood to renal tissue stimulates renin secretion and causes a rise in blood pressure. The classical cause is constriction or stenosis of a main renal artery. Parenchymal renal damage, particularly in the region of the glomeruli, also causes excessive renin production and it is now believed that increased plasma renin activity is the common factor in all cases of hypertension due to renal disease. This may partly explain why renal diseases with primary glomerular damage (and hence involvement of the juxtaglomerular cells) are more commonly associated with hypertension than renal diseases with primarily tubular damage.

Measurement of plasma renin is assuming increasing importance in the investigation of hypertension due to renal disease. Before blood is drawn for this purpose the patient normally rests horizontal for 24 hours and is kept on an adequate dietary sodium intake. Both sodium depletion and the upright position can increase renin secretion.

In order to determine whether one kidney rather than the other is responsible for causing hypertension in an individual patient it is possible to obtain blood from each renal vein for plasma renin assay. This is done by selective renal vein catheterization under X-ray control.

Serum aminotransferase (transaminases)

The serum aminotransferases, SGOT and SGPT, are raised when tissue destruction occurs in almost any organ but they are especially useful in detecting cardiac muscle necrosis in myocardial infarction and hepatic cell necrosis due to an attack of hepatitis. If any patient on regular dialysis develops an unexplained rise in serum transaminase the suspicion of hepatitis should immediately be raised. Most dialysis units perform serum transaminase estimations on all their patients at regular intervals.

Hepatitis B antigen (Australia antigen)

This is a difficult and specialized test, only performed in certain laboratories, the value of which lies in the detection of patients carrying the virus of serum hepatitis. A positive test probably means that the patient is either incubating the disease, is actually suffering from it, or has got over it but is still a carrier and is therefore potentially infective. A patient with a positive test is a very serious danger to other patients and staff who have to handle his blood. It is now generally agreed that such patients must be isolated and cannot be allowed to share facilities with uninfected patients. Improved techniques have made the test very sensitive and very reliable, and it is now possible to obtain a quick result within a few hours in any major medical center.

Occasionally an individual may have a positive hepatitis B antibody.

This implies a previous infection and residual immunity. If the antibody is present in high titer it confers protection from further attacks. This may be useful in medical or nursing staff who are called upon to treat patients who are hepatitis B positive.

Active vaccination against hepatitis B is now available. It is hoped that the majority of patients and staff will in future be antibody positive and therefore immune to hepatitis B because of vaccination.

The 24 hour urine collection

This means all the urine that an individual's kidneys produce in a 24 hour period. Collection is usually started first thing in the morning. The patient rises, empties his bladder and discards the urine. He must start with an empty bladder and note the time of emptying. From this time for the next 24 hours *all* urine must be saved and collected in the container, *including* the last specimen at the same time the next day.

The commonest causes of error are:
- The patient retains instead of discarding the first specimen at the beginning of the test, so keeping the urine that his kidneys have made during the previous night. This will give an erroneously large volume.
- The patient voids urine at the same time as he empties his bowels, and so loses some of the urine into the lavatory bowl. He should be advised to empty his bladder into a container before going to move his bowels.
- The patient forgets to save one of the specimens or a nurse pours it out instead of adding it to the 24 hour collection.

It is a sad fact that 24 hour urines collected from in-patients are more prone to inaccuracy than those collected at home by out-patients. Most experienced head nurses find that it usually pays to make an intelligent and cooperative in-patient responsible for his own collection. He is less likely to make a mistake than several different nurses in the 24 hour shift.

The uses of the 24 hour urine collection

Quantitative protein estimation (normal less than 100 mg/24 hours)

Patients tend to have a heavier loss of urine protein when they are up and about than when they are in bed. Thus a 24 hour collection will be representative of both phases. It may be of interest in an individual patient to estimate proteinuria quantitatively over timed periods at night and during the day. This has particular relevance to the syndrome of orthostatic proteinuria in which proteinuria is only detectable in the upright position and disappears during the recumbent position. It is a generally benign and in most cases quite harmless condition which is not uncommon in otherwise healthy young adults.

The correct method of testing for postural or orthostatic proteinuria is to use the sample voided when the individual first steps out of bed in the morning. If this is negative for protein on three different days, while the sample obtained after the patient is up and about is positive, then the patient can be assumed to have orthostatic proteinuria.

Small amounts of urinary protein, less than 1 g/day, are very common in nearly all forms of kidney disease. Heavy proteinuria, more than 3 g/day, nearly always signifies disease affecting the glomeruli of the kidneys and is the main feature of the nephrotic syndrome. See p.66.

The actual measurement of total urine protein can be performed accurately in the laboratory in various ways. In practice it is convenient and in many centers customary to use the same 24 hour urine collection for measuring total protein, creatinine clearance and any other urinary constituents.

Bence-Jones protein

This is a very special type of protein usually only found in the urine of patients suffering from multiple myeloma. Characteristically it forms a precipitate when urine is heated to about 60°C and the precipitate disappears again as the temperature rises further. However the isolation and identification of this protein is quite delicate and specialized and can only be done reliably in a good hospital laboratory.

Urinary calcium

Normal women—not more than 250 mg/24 hours
men—not more than 300 mg/24 hours
(mmol/period × 40 = mg/period)

This is usually measured at some stage in any patient who is suspected of having a calcium-containing renal calculus. Conditions which particularly predispose patients to this are hyperparathyroidism, in which there is a parathyroid adenoma causing calcium to come out of the bones and be passed in large quantities in the urine; and idiopathic hypercalciuria in which the excessive urinary calcium excretion is due to a primary defect of excessive calcium absorption from the gastro-intestinal tract.

In both these diseases there is a tendency for abnormally high rates of urinary calcium excretion. Hypercalciuria can also be caused by excessive ingestion of calcium and vitamin D.

Urinary uric acid

It is sometimes of interest to measure urinary uric acid excretion in patients with gout and it may help to distinguish between primary gout and secondary gout.

Urinary amino acids

In patients who suffer from cystinuria, who have renal stones composed of cystine, the urine contains an excess of the amino acids cystine, lysine, arginine and ornithine. A rare disease of the renal tubules in children, called the Fanconi syndrome, is characterized by the excretion of glucose, phosphate and amino acids in the urine in abnormal amounts. There may be an associated renal tubular acidosis.

Urinary electrolytes

Measurement of urinary sodium and potassium may be of great value in determining the cause of abnormalities of serum sodium and potassium. For example, some renal diseases, especially those that affect mainly the tubules, such as pyelonephritis, are associated with an abnormal urinary loss of sodium. The resulting depletion of sodium may further impair renal function.

Measurement of urinary sodium is also of value in determining the cause of low urine output. See p.99.

Investigation of various renal tubular disorders

There are a number of rather uncommon or rare abnormalities of renal tubular function, which may be congenital or acquired, which can be investigated by estimating the amounts of substances excreted in the urine. These values, considered together with the serum values, will usually reveal the nature of the abnormality. For example, there is a well-known congenital abnormality of the renal tubules resulting in failure of normal reabsorption of phosphate. There is an excessive urinary phosphate loss, a low serum phosphate, and a tendency to demineralization of the skeleton presenting as rickets in childhood or adolescence. Treatment is usually quite satisfactory once an accurate diagnosis is made.

The urinary concentration test

Healthy kidneys respond to fluid deprivation by conserving water. This function of producing a small volume of concentrated urine is performed by the tubules (see p.14). Impaired concentrating ability is a sensitive sign of renal tubular damage. The test consists of depriving the patient of water in any form for a given period and measuring the degree to which the urine is concentrated.

A commonly used standard test employs an 18 hour period of fluid deprivation following the evening meal at 6 p.m. The early morning urine as well as the 9 a.m. and 12 noon specimens are kept and tested. In at least one of these specimens the specific gravity should exceed 1028 and the osmolarity should exceed 800 mosm/l.

Fluid deprivation followed by tests of serum and urine osmolarity can also be used to confirm a suspected diagnosis of diabetes insipidus. Failure to concentrate the urine in this condition is due to lack of antidiuretic hormone. Water should not normally be withheld for more than a few hours because of danger of severe dehydration. Weight loss and increasing tonicitiy of the serum occur during the test in a true case of diabetes insipidus. Concentrating ability returns as soon as the patient is given an injection of vasopressin.

Serum cholesterol (100−280 mg per cent) (mmol/l × 38.7 = mg/dl)

Cholesterol in the blood tends to be raised in conditions such as diabetes and myxedema which are associated with a high incidence of atheroma in the arteries. For reasons which are not fully understood the cholesterol is also high in renal disease which leads to low plasma protein levels caused by prolonged and heavy urinary protein loss. See nephrotic syndrome, p.70.

Plasma triglycerides (normal 30−180 mg/dl)
(mmol/l × 88.6 = mg/dl)

When red cells are separated from blood the plasma is normally a clear yellowish color. If the plasma is turbid or milky it indicates the presence of increased concentrations of fatty substances called triglycerides. These will be raised in patients with nephrotic syndrome (p.70) and also in patients with familial hyperlipidemia. Hyperlipidemias, whatever their cause, tend to predispose to premature atheroma in blood vessels and hence the early onset of coronary and cerebral as well as peripheral arterial disease.

Lipids also tend to be raised to some extent in some patients with chronic renal failure. This may partly explain the tendency of patients with long-standing renal failure to have an increased incidence of heart attacks and strokes. Blood for trigyceride estimation should be taken in a fasting state.

Plasma proteins

The normal plasma protein pattern is disturbed in conditions such as the nephrotic syndrome in which there is prolonged and heavy urinary protein loss. Albumin tends to be lowered more than globulin because more albumin is usually lost in the urine. Electrophoresis is a technique which separates and identifies the plasma proteins, and demonstrates which fractions are reduced or increased. This may have diagnostic value in distinguishing different diseases. Immunoelectrophoresis of plasma proteins will give a determination of the concentrations of the various immunoglobulins, IgG, IgA, IgM, etc. This may have great diagnostic importance in distinguishing different types of glomerulonephritis. For example, the level of IgA is high in patients with IgA nephritis. This is the commonest type of glomerulonephritis in most parts of North America.

Urine protein selectivity

It has been shown that, in patients with heavy proteinuria due to glomerulonephritis, the relative amounts of different proteins in the urine give an indication of the severity of the underlying disease. In so-called minimal change nephritis in which the glomeruli look normal on ordinary light microscopy, the urinary protein consists mainly of the low molecular weight fractions such as albumin. This is called selective proteinuria and usually indicates a good prognosis for response to steroids or immunosuppressive drugs. In nephritis where there are obvious changes visible on light microscopy the urinary protein consists of both low and high molecular weight fractions and this type of proteinuria is called unselective. It usually indicates a poor response to specific therapy.

The samples needed by the laboratory are a few millilitres of clotted blood and a urine sample the volume of which depends on the amount of protein in it. If not much protein is present a large volume of urine will be needed so that it can be concentrated. Urine protein selectivity is also recognized as being important in diabetic glomerulosclerosis. When the condition first starts there is very selective proteinuria. As the condition progresses the proteinuria becomes progressively non-selective.

Serum complement

The immunological mechanisms involved in the primary glomerular disease known as glomerulonephritis are extremely complicated and still not fully understood (see pp.66−80). However, the experts are gradually identifying the part played by a very complex group of protein substances called complement.

Serum complement is now commonly measured in most renal centers from a blood sample; and when the result is reported we know we are actually talking about a specific type of serum complement for which an agreed standard exists. The importance of the test in practical terms is that when it is found to be abnormally low it is usually due to one of three well-known forms of glomerulonephritis (GN). These are post-streptococcal GN, mesangiocapillary GN and lupus nephritis (see pp.66−80 in Chapter 3).

Bacteriology

Although symptoms and signs may lead us to suspect urinary tract infection, and the presence of polymorphonuclear leukocytes in the urine is evidence of inflammation, we depend on culture to prove the existence of bacterial infection. We also know that significant infection can be present in the absence of symptoms or signs and even when no leukocytes are present in the urine.

Mid-stream urine culture

A mid-stream urine sample in a male can be used for culture on the assumption that the urine has come straight from the bladder without contamination by the skin. In an uncircumcised male the foreskin should be drawn back and the penis washed before voiding. It is important to emphasize to the patient that the urinary stream should not be interrupted to catch the specimen. If the act of micturition is stopped and restarted to obtain the specimen contamination may occur. It is more difficult for obvious reasons to obtain an uncontaminated specimen in a female. In practice this can be done by cleaning the perineal area and then sitting with the legs wide apart while the labia are held apart with one hand.

Again the specimen should be caught in mid-stream. If the specimen cannot be sent for culture at once it should be refrigerated at 4°C until it can be sent. If it is left standing at room temperature for more than an hour there is a danger of growth of contaminants. In a refrigerator it can be left safely overnight. Because cultures obtained from voided urine samples are prone to be contaminated the British Medical Research Council defines bacteriuria as more than 100 000 organisms per ml. The organisms are counted by seeing how many colonies they form when the urine is spread on a culture surface by a standard method. So the bacterial count is expressed as the number of colony forming units (CFU). It is assumed that each organism forms one colony. A significant infection would be 100 000 CFU/ml. Although this number of organisms would always be expected to be present in a case of acute pyelonephritis, and although healthy patients with asymptomatic bacteriuria will have 100 000 CFU/ml, this definition is too restrictive for certain other types of urinary tract infection. For example, woman with acute symptomatic cystitis requiring, and responding to, appropriate antibiotics may only have 100 CFU/ml at the time that she presents asking for help. The same thing may apply to infection limited to the urethra.

So the colony count must be interpreted in the light of the clinical situation.

The biggest causes of inaccuracy in mid-stream urine culture are:
1 poor technique in collection of the specimen,
2 delay in sending the specimen to the laboratory.

If the laboratory receives a fresh or refrigerated uncontaminated specimen it should be able to provide a bacterial count, identification of the organism involved, and details of antibiotics to which the organism is sensitive. The laboratory request form should always carry details of any antibiotic therapy which the patient is already receiving.

Other methods of obtaining urine for culture

Under certain circumstances it is difficult to obtain uncontaminated specimens for culture by the mid-stream technique, as for example in menstruating or post-partum women, in small babies and in patients with neurogenic loss of bladder control.

Infants and neonates can sometimes be persuaded to micturate 'to order' by holding them up with a hand under the abdomen while gently stroking the back with the other hand. An assistant must try deftly to catch the urine when the infant voids. Some infant nurses become very good at obtaining specimens by this method but not infrequently the infant fails to oblige. Suprapubic pressure may be helpful. Many pediatricians are now using sterile disposable bags. The adhesive neck of the back holds it in place over the perineum.

Suprapubic bladder aspiration

In recent years the technique of aspiration of urine by a suprapubic needle puncture has been shown to be both successful and safe. The method can be used for any age group including neonates. In this technique the patient must have a full bladder and lie on his back. The doctor percusses the pubic area to confirm that the bladder is full. The skin above the pubic symphysis must be cleaned with antiseptic. A venepuncture needle on the end of a sterile syringe is then passed vertically through the abdominal wall, in the midline, into the bladder. As soon as the cavity of the bladder is reached, urine can be aspirated into the syringe. No local anesthetic is needed nor any dressing on the abdomen afterwards. The puncture causes only minor discomfort. The presence of any organisms in the urine is certain evidence of infection since contamination cannot occur. Therefore, the specimen should be clearly labelled as having been obtained by suprapubic needle aspiration. This will avoid mistakes in interpretation.

Catheterization

Catheterizing the bladder to obtain urine specimens for culture can hardly ever be justified nowadays because of the risk of introducing infection and because good alternatives exist. If, for some reason, it should prove to be necessary it should be done with the most meticulous aseptic technique and it is probably wise to instill some aqueous chlorhexidine into the bladder after the culture has been obtained before removing the catheter. This should dispose of any bacteria which may have been introduced inadvertently.

The dip-slide method

When considerable delay is anticipated in the urine specimen reaching the laboratory as, for example, when it has to be sent from some distance outside the hospital, by post or some form of transport, an ingenious device can be used consisting of a glass microscope slide which carries a culture medium on both sides. The slide is provided with a small sealed container. The patient voids the mid-stream urine specimen into a sterile bowl of some kind, such as a china bowl sterilized by boiling. The glass slide is carefully taken out of its container, without touching the culture surface, and dipped once into the urine. It is immediately replaced in the container, sealed up and despatched to the laboratory with a clear record of the patient's name and the date and time of obtaining the specimen. Any organisms in the freshly voided urine, having become impregnated on the culture surfaces will start to form colonies which can be identified in due course by the laboratory.

The boric acid method

This is an alternative to the dip-slide method and is used for the same reason, to overcome the problem of delay in reaching the laboratory. With this method the mid-stream specimen is voided into a sterile universal culture bottle containing about half a gram of boric acid, usually in the form of a tablet. The boric acid does not destroy organisms which are present in the urine, nor will it allow multiplication of the organisms or any contaminants. The bacteria are kept as it were in suspended animation until the urine is plated out in the laboratory on culture media.

These methods have revolutionized the culture of urine in a domiciliary setting and each has its enthusiastic advocates. The boric acid method has the advantage of cheapness. It also allows microscopy of the sample. The dip-slide equipment, though slightly more expensive to buy, does most of the work for the laboratory; and negative cultures need no further attention since they are immediately apparent as clean culture surfaces.

Culture for tubercle bacilli

When urinary tuberculosis is suspected, the whole of the early morning urine specimen should be collected and sent to the laboratory on three different mornings for culture and guinea pig inoculation. The culture, which is carried out on special media, takes 6−8 weeks. Occasionally the organism will be seen under the microscope in a specially stained centrifuged specimen, but other non-pathogenic acid-fast bacilli such as the smegma bacillus are occasionally found in urine so that the findings of a direct smear must be interpreted with caution.

Serum antibodies

Considerable interest has been focused on the finding of antibacterial antibodies in the serum of patients with active pyelonephritis. The method can be used to identify different strains of *E. coli*, so it should be possible to tell whether one is dealing with a new infection or a relapse of a previous infection inadequately treated.

Visualizing the urinary tract and diagnostic imaging

Plain X-rays of the abdomen

A good quality plain abdominal X-ray which includes the kidneys, ureters and bladder may be surprisingly informative. Careful examination will often reveal the renal outlines. A large kidney shadow may be due to hydronephrosis or perhaps compensatory hypertrophy. A very small kidney usually means disease in an advanced stage. If both kidneys are small the patient almost certainly has chronic renal failure with little prospect of recovery. A plain X-ray will also show up radio-opaque material. Nearly all renal calculi are radio-opaque and these may appear within the kidneys, in the line of the ureters or in the bladder. The exception is uric acid stones which are radiolucent. These will only show up as a filling defect in a study using opaque contrast medium. Diffuse calcification of kidney tissue may be due to such causes as hypercalcemia from a parathyroid adenoma or renal tubular acidosis. Localized calcification can be caused by renal tuberculosis.

Intravenous urogram (IVU)

If a contrast medium such as Hypaque or Conray is injected intravenously it is excreted by the kidneys and appears in high concentration in the urine. The atoms of iodine in the contrast medium make it radio-opaque. It thus outlines the pelvicalyceal system of the kidneys, the ureters and the bladder. Contrast medium in the tubules increases the overall radiographic density of the kidney producing an appearance called a nephrogram. The best pictures are usually obtained 5–15 minutes after the injection. The IVU is the best overall test for demonstrating the structure of the urinary tract. It will reveal any significant abnormality in shape or size as well as deformity, dilatation or obstruction. Many kidney disorders such as pyelonephritis, polycystic kidneys and renal tuberculosis can often be diagnosed at a glance by means of an IVU. Renal artery stenosis may be suspected from the finding of a smaller kidney on one side with delayed excretion and increased concentration of the contrast medium on the same side. It would take too long to list all the conditions in which an IVU is useful. It is enough to say that if a disease alters the gross appearance of the urinary tract, when seen in silhouette, an IVU will help demonstrate it.

In this investigation, perhaps more than most, a great deal depends on careful preparation. A constipated, gas-filled bowel will tend to obscure the urinary tract shadows. This is why laxatives and enemata may be needed. Secondly, better pictures will be obtained if the urine is concentrated, and this is usually achieved by a period of fluid deprivation before the test. A cup of tea just before the examination will probably ruin the result and waste everyone's time. The exception to this is in the case of a patient with chronic renal failure and a high blood urea. These patients have a fixed low urinary concentration which is not improved by dehydration. Dehydration may even be dangerous. The only way to obtain good pictures in these patients is to use a large dose of contrast medium— sometimes as much as 150 ml intravenously. This is remarkably free of side-effects; and it has recently been shown that the same technique can be successful even in acute renal failure with very low urine output. Ureteric compression to dam back the contrast medium is sometimes useful. Filling the stomach with gas, by giving an effervescent drink, may be helpful in showing up the contrasting renal shadows— especially in small children. There is an increasing tendency to use the IVU in emergency investigation of renal and ureteric colic. Slight abnormalities such as a degree of ureteric dilatation may be present during an attack of pain, indicating the presence of a small stone for instance, which may not be visible when the pain has subsided days later.

Just about the only contra-indications to the use of an IVU are:
- sensitivity to iodides,
- multiple myelomatosis,
- diabetes.

In a patient with multiple myelomatosis an IVU will very frequently precipitate acute renal failure. It is probably a combination of the contrast material and the dehydration reducing the rate of tubular flow and causing precipitation of myeloma proteins in the renal tubules. The kidneys may never recover from this insult.

Intravenous urograms or indeed any contrast study are a risk in diabetics. The risk is particularly high in diabetics who already have chronic renal impairment from diabetic glomerulosclerosis. If an IVU is essential in a diabetic the risk can be greatly reduced by performing the study under conditions of liberal fluid administration and high urine flow.

When intravenous urograms or indeed any abdominal X-rays are ordered for women in the reproductive age group they should only be done in the first half of the menstrual cycle when we know that a pregnancy could not have started. Any time after the middle of the cycle we may inadvertently irradiate a very early embryo. We are less concerned if we know that the patient is on an oral contraceptive or has an intrauterine device.

Cystogram

This is an X-ray of the bladder performed by introducing contrast medium via a urethral catheter. It will reveal any defect in the outline of the bladder such as a diverticulum or a large tumor. If the patient is asked to micturate it is possible to demonstrate the urethra. This is called a urethrogram. A urethral diverticulum may be demonstrated in this way. Ureteric reflux may occur during filling of the bladder but sometimes is seen only during micturition. This condition is important to detect since it is known to predispose to pyelonephritis.

Retrograde pyelogram

If, for some reason, the urinary tract cannot be demonstrated by an IVU, as, for example, when one or both kidneys are totally non-functioning, fine catheters can be passed up the ureters from below by visualizing the ureteric orifices of the bladder through a cystoscope. Contrast medium injected up the catheters outlines the ureters and pelvicalyceal systems. The procedure is painful enough to require a general anesthetic, so the patient must be starved. Both hematuria and infection are occasional complications. It is a good practice to take the opportunity, while ureteric catheters are *in situ*, to collect urine samples for culture from each ureter. The specimens should be labelled as left or right before they are sent to the laboratory. Ureteric catheters are expensive and should not be disposed of when removed. They should be retrieved to be sterilized again.

Cystoscopy

A slim tubular metal instrument called a cystoscope is used by the urological surgeon to examine the interior of the bladder. See Fig. 2.1.

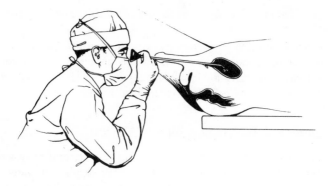

Fig. 2.1. Examination of the bladder with a cystoscope (cystoscopy).

There are two main types of cystoscopes, those in which there is direct vision through a simple window, and those providing indirect vision through a system of prisms in a telescope. With the latter type of instrument a magnified view of the interior of the bladder is obtained. Cystoscopes are adapted for passing fine catheters up through the ureters to the renal pelvis on each side. Urine samples can be obtained from each kidney and contrast media injected for retrograde pyelography. Other instruments are modified to enable endoscopic operations to be performed on the bladder or prostate gland. The urethra can be similarly examined by an instrument called a urethroscope. For these procedures a general anesthetic is usually given but local anesthesia of the urethra can be obtained by instilling an anesthetic jelly. The preparation of the patient's skin and genitalia for these examinations is the same as for abdominal surgery.

Renal arteriogram

The blood supply of the kidneys can be outlined by introducing contrast media into the aorta close to the mouths of the renal arteries. This procedure, performed under local anesthesia by a radiologist, is usually done by passing a catheter up the aorta through a femoral artery in the groin. The main indications are for the diagnosis of renal artery stenosis and in the elucidation of possible tumors of the kidney. An arteriogram will, for example, differentiate a simple cyst from a tumor. The diagnosis and definition of renal tumors has now been largely taken over by CAT scans, so arteriography is being used less and less for tumor investigation. After the investigation, a firm dressing is applied to the groin and the patient is kept in bed for 24 hours to reduce the risk of bleeding from the arterial puncture.

Digital subtraction angiography is a refinement in which the arterial supply of an organ can be demonstrated after an intravenous injection of contrast material. It is a big advantage to be able to avoid arterial puncture, which requires a 24 hour hospital admission.

Computerized axial tomography (CAT scan)

The advent of CAT scans has been a giant leap forward in diagnostic radiology in the last few years. The CAT scan supplies the radiologist with an extraordinarily detailed cross-section of the body in one plane. For any intra-abdominal organ the transverse plane is used and the radiologist is free to choose the level of the cross-section and at what intervals he would like to see the cuts. Fig. 2.2 shows a typical cross-section which represents one film on a CAT scan at the level of the kidneys. The right kidney is invaded by a renal cell carcinoma (hyper-nephroma). The supreme advantage of the CAT scan is that in any particular cross-sectional plane it can, with a sensitivity undreamed of a few years ago, distinguish where one tissue ends and another begins. For example, it will demonstrate accurately the outline of a uric acid calculus which would not show up at all on a plain abdominal X-ray. The CAT scanner has revolutionized the radiology of the urinary tract as well as the radiology of practically every area of the body. The radiation received by the patient is clearly more than that of a plain X-ray but is in most cases no greater than that of a barium contrast study. CAT scans are expensive because of both the capital equipment costs and the running costs. CAT studies are not ordered indiscriminately (and usually a radiologist is consulted about whether the study should be done or not). For the differentiation of mass lesions they are nothing short of miraculous.

Magnetic resonance imaging (MRI)

This is still largely an experimental technology which uses a very powerful magnetic field to obtain a result rather similar to that of a CAT scan. It depends on the fact that a magnetic field reacts in different ways to tissues of different chemical composition. The equipment has not yet found its way into routine clinical practice in most of the major North American centers, at least at the time of writing. At present it is fiendishly expensive both to buy and install. Somehow one has to prevent the

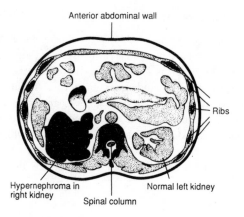

Fig. 2.2. CAT scan showing a hypernephroma in the right kidney.

powerful magnetic field from influencing all electrical equipment within its vicinity. The technology is still in its infancy, and the long-term effects of working with it are not yet known. It does have the inherent advantage of producing no ionizing radiation.

The radiation hazard

When ordering any urinary tract X-rays in women in the reproductive period of life one should always bear in mind the timing of the X-rays in relation to the menstrual cycle. If X-rays are done in the second half of the cycle (after ovulation but before the next period) there is a possibility of irradiating a recently fertilized ovum of an unplanned pregnancy. This could lead to deformities in the child. Because of this potential danger, well-organized X-ray departments insist on knowing the date of the last menstrual period before planning the X-rays. If necessary and unless it is an emergency the X-rays can be postponed till after the onset of the next period.

The use of radio-active isotopes

Radio-active isotopes are used in two main ways for diagnostic purposes. The renogram studies function in the kidneys and the renal scan gives an indication of structure. The tests are performed by the medical physics department (sometimes called the department of nuclear medicine).

Radio-isotope renogram

In this test an injection of ^{131}I hippuran is given intravenously. Special scintillation counters are placed carefully over the patient's back, one for each kidney. The progress of the radio-active material is followed as it enters the renal arteries, undergoes glomerular filtration, and is then excreted by the tubules. When both kidneys are normal the renograms are symmetrical and normal. The test has considerable value in detecting a poorly functioning kidney, and especially a kidney which is affected by renal artery stenosis. It will also distinguish a kidney which has an intact blood supply but no function from one in which the blood supply is completely occluded.

The renal scan

A radio-active mercury compound is usually used for this investigation and a picture is obtained showing both kidneys rather like a pointillist painting. Structural lesions such as infarcts or tumors show up as areas differing in density from the rest of the normal kidney tissue.

In recent years the renal scan has assumed considerable diagnostic importance in the assessment of kidneys after renal transplantation. It is very useful in the differential diagnosis of causes of poor function in the early post-operative period. Frequently help is obtained in distinguishing rejection from other causes of renal damage or failure.

Diagnostic ultrasound

Ultrasonic diagnosis, which works on the same principle as the ultrasonic ASDIC recorder used by submarines, is well developed in relation to some systems of the body—for example, detecting the presence of the fetal head in obstetrics. Centers are now employing ultrasonic diagnosis in relation to the urinary tract. In the hands of skilled operators it is possible to distinguish several different structural renal lesions such as polycystic kidneys and hydronephrosis. Its advantage lies in its complete harmlessness. No X-ray or injections are needed and the patient experiences no discomfort. It suffers from the same shortcomings as the renal scan, i.e. other diagnostic methods are often more reliable and accurate. Ultrasound is also invaluable in localizing the position of a kidney for renal biopsy. We use it in any situation in which there is not enough function for the kidneys to be visualized on an IVU. The value of ultrasound still depends a lot on the skill of the radiologist.

Renal biopsy

Next to the intravenous urogram, renal biopsy is probably the most informative special investigation performed by the renal physician. It is potentially a dangerous investigation for which signed consent is always obtained.

The technique involves obtaining a minute cylinder of kidney tissue for histological examination. Nowadays this is usually done percutaneously by means of a needle. Previously, open operation with a small loin incision was required. Biopsy is helpful in any renal disease in which the disease process is evenly distributed through all the kidney tissue. In practice, this usually means diseases affecting primarily the glomeruli which cause proteinuria and hematuria—especially any form of glomerulonephritis or nephrotic syndrome. It is also appropriate when one suspects a diffuse tubulointerstitial condition such as allergic interstitial nephritis. In a patchy or focal disease such as pyelonephritis the renal biopsy may not hit a representative area of the kidney. Other diagnostic methods are more appropriate in such conditions.

Preparation for renal biopsy includes careful control of blood pressure, and tests of blood coagulation. It is common practice to have a unit of blood crossmatched and ready in case of bleeding. If blood coagulation is abnormal because of uremia it may be necessary to dialyse the patient before a biopsy is performed. If the blood pressure is unacceptably high the biopsy should be postponed until the blood pressure has been controlled. All patients for renal biopsy should be put on a blood pressure chart on admission. A complete contra-indication to percutaneous renal biopsy is a recent history of malignant hypertension. This is because the vessels in the kidney can be assumed to be so abnormal that they will not stop bleeding when they are cut. This is despite the fact that the blood pressure may be perfectly controlled at the time of the biopsy. In the past when we ignored this rule we had cause to regret it.

Most operators perform renal biopsy with some form of X-ray guidance to localize the kidneys accurately so that the biopsy can be obtained from a safe area of the cortex, away from the hilum where the main blood vessels are located. It is normally performed under local anesthesia. The need for premedication depends entirely on what kind of patient one is dealing with. We use it more often than not, but the patient must remain sufficiently alert to hold the breath in inspiration both during the X-ray and during the procedure. See Fig. 2.3. The patient lies in the prone position with a pad or pillow under the abdomen. The two main types of needle used are the Menghini, originally developed as a liver biopsy needle, and the Vim-Silverman or some modification of it. The Menghini is a simple cylindrical needle which cuts a biopsy with the aid of suction by a syringe. The needle must be kept very sharp. If the cutting end is damaged it will be useless.

The Vim-Silverman needle has a pair of cutting blades which grasp the biopsy. An outer tube is advanced over the blades to enclose the specimen before withdrawal. Each type of needle has its enthusiastic advocates, and operators tend to stick to the method which they find successful. The equipment required for a renal biopsy procedure is as follows:

biopsy needle,

exploring needle (used for gauging depth of the kidney below the surface),

syringe, needles, local anesthetic,

scalpel blade,

gauze swabs, skin antiseptic, sterile towels,

sterile saline for use with Menghini needle.

It is best if the histology technician is in attendance during the biopsy to receive the sample. He or she can scan the tissue immediately under a low power microscope to see if it is adequate for all the examinations which will be required.

The main risk of biopsy is bleeding. Once the biopsy is obtained a dry dressing is placed over the back and the patient is returned to the ward where he must stay resting in bed for 24 hours. Pulse and BP are recorded every 15 minutes for two hours and then every hour until

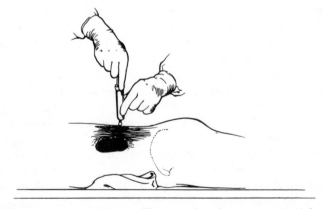

Fig. 2.3. Percutaneous renal biopsy. The core of renal tissue is aspirated from the lower of the kidney.

further notice is given by the medical staff. Urine samples should be examined for hematuria. Any undue pain, hematuria or change in vital signs should be reported at once to the medical staff. The patient should not be allowed up until examined by the doctor the next day and he is normally advised to take things easily for a couple of days afterwards.

If bleeding does occur it usually takes the form of a perirenal hematoma or rather profuse continuing hematuria. Both these complications usually settle with conservative management. Surgical exploration may occasionally be necessary to stop the bleeding and on rare occasions it has been necessary to remove a kidney which has been badly damaged. For this reason it is generally considered unwise to perform a renal biopsy on a solitary kidney. The calculated risk of this procedure must be weighed against the possible benefit to the patient of the information gained by it.

Hematuria from renal biopsy may occasionally cause clot obstruction of the ureter which fortunately is usually only temporary. Very occasionally after renal biopsy hematuria is prolonged and heavy, leading to the need for blood transfusion; and there is a danger of exsanguination if it were to continue. This unusual complication has, in our experience, always settled down after administration of an antifibrinolytic drug called epsilonamino-caproic acid. The rationale for this is based on the belief that a puncture wound connecting with the renal pelvis cannot form a firm plug of thrombus because the urine contains a natural fibrinolytic substance called urokinase which lyses the fibrin clot. The drug probably works by neutralizing the urokinase. Whether this is the mechanism or not, the drug is magically effective in stopping the hematuria. It may have to be given for a prolonged period. A much less common complication is the production of a traumatic intrarenal arteriovenous fistula. This may be suspected from the development of an audible bruit over the kidney and it may lead to the development of hypertension.

In most renal centers, percutaneous needle biopsy is performed in selected cases in renal transplants, mainly in order to diagnose rejection or distinguish this from other conditions. In transplants, X-ray guidance is unnecessary since the kidney is easily palpable under the anterior abdominal wall. The biopsy can be done while the patient stays in his own bed in the ward. Only if the kidney is hard to feel may we have to resort to ultrasound to guide us accurately. We have no hesitation in using this guidance if necessary. It is not unusual for a patient after a kidney transplant to have two or more renal biopsies. The complication rate is extremely low provided that the same careful precautions are taken as with a biopsy in the normal anatomical site.

Processing and examination of renal biopsy material

Until a few years ago the tissue obtained by renal biopsy was placed immediately in a simple fixative such as 10% formaldehyde and prepared for study by light microscopy only. Although very valuable, this technique is not always adequate on its own to distinguish fine differences in kidney disease, especially glomerular diseases. Modern renal centers therefore make use also of electron microscopy to study glomerular morphology (structure) at very high magnification, and fluorescence microscopy to study the immunological processes which may be occurring in kidneys. Briefly what this means is that antigen−antibody reactions in relation to glomeruli can be studied by showing up the presence of these antibodies in the immunoglobulins which may be deposited there. By special vital staining techniques the immunoglobulins can be shown to shine brightly in vivid colors under the ultraviolet light. This is called fluorescence and the demonstration of immunoglobulins by this method is called immuno-fluorescence.

Biopsy material for immunofluorescent staining techniques has to be fresh rather than fixed, and the tissue for electron microscopy needs a different fixative (usually glutaraldehyde) from the tissue for light microscopy.

Thus, the tissue obtained by renal biopsy has to be adequate for enough to be available for examination by all three methods, namely light microscopy, electron microscopy and immunofluorescence microscopy.

In practice this means that either a laboratory technician must come to the bedside or X-ray table where the biopsy is being taken so that he or she can receive the material and divide it up; or the whole biopsy must be taken fresh to the laboratory without any delay to be examined and divided there.

3

The Main
Kidney Diseases

Robert Uldall

The normal person has a large reserve of functioning kidney tissue. A volunteer kidney donor suffers no loss of health or vigour if he loses one kidney, provided that the remaining one is normal. The kidney that is left behind almost immediately increases in size and provides about 70% of the function which was previously available when both kidneys were working normally. This phenomenon is called compensatory hypertrophy and also occurs whenever kidney tissue is destroyed by disease. The healthy tissue which is left behind works harder so that the ill-effects of disease are reduced. In advanced diseases a relatively small number of intact healthy nephrons are able to adapt to the situation of a higher blood urea and other waste products. By these adaptive mechanisms a small fraction of the original population of healthy nephrons is able to sustain life. Despite these fortunate dispensations of nature, kidney diseases are one of the largest natural causes of death in men and women between the ages of 20 and 40 in the affluent countries of the world. The disease processes that affect the kidneys are many and varied, but only a handful of diseases are numerically important in terms of kidney destruction. One of the main reasons why these diseases are so dangerous is that they can reach an advanced stage without ever causing symptoms. Insidious destruction of nephrons can be an entirely silent process until the patient begins to suffer from the effects of renal failure—by this time the damage is done. Nevertheless it is always worth making a correct diagnosis even at a late stage, in the hope that enough renal tissue can be preserved to maintain health. The kidneys have considerable powers of regeneration. Naturally we always try to detect diseases early and, by appropriate treatment, hope to avert serious damage.

There are five major disease categories which account for the majority of cases of what are called end-stage renal failure. These are glomerulonephritis, diabetes, pyelonephritis, hypertension, and polycystic kidney disease.

Table 3.1. shows the approximate incidence of these diseases amongst young adult patients as well as all age groups with total kidney destruction. In all age groups combined, glomerulonephritis is the leading cause of renal failure and diabetes comes next. Non-fatal infections of the urinary tract (including pyelonephritis) are extremely common in all forms of medical practice. Because of their great numerical importance these major diseases will be discussed first and at greater length than the others. For information about rare renal disorders it will be necessary to refer to a comprehensive medical text.

Table 3.1. Causes of end-stage renal failure in Canada. Young adults (age 15–44) and all ages combined

Disease type	Percentage	
	Young adults (15–44)	All ages combined
Glomerulonephritis	34	26
Diabetes	22	17
Pyelonephritis	15	12
Hypertension	4	12
Polycystic kidneys	5	7
Drug-induced nephropathy	1	2
Miscellaneous	16	14
ESRF (etiology unknown)	3	10
	100	100

Urinary tract infection

Urinary tract infection endangers life by causing pyelonephritis, which is bacterial invasion of the kidneys. To put this in perspective it should be said at once that the vast majority of urinary infections are of nuisance value only and not in any sense life-threatening. About 50% of all women have a urinary infection at some time in their lives and only a very small proportion develop significant renal damage. Infections of the urinary tract are mainly caused by coliform organisms or other organisms which normally colonize the gastro-intestinal tract. These organisms which also tend to colonize the skin of the perineum are sometimes called Enterobacteriaceae.

Cystitis and urethritis

Cystitis strictly means inflammation of the bladder from any cause but is most commonly due to bacterial infection. The symptoms which suggest cystitis are frequency, an uncomfortable feeling of incomplete emptying, and dysuria. Frequency, which means frequent passage of small amounts of urine (larger volumes cannot be retained comfortably in the inflamed bladder) should be distinguished from polyuria which means a large urine output causing frequent passage of normal or increased volumes of urine. Dysuria means discomfort on voiding and this usually has a burning quality. Urgency or inability to delay the act of micturition, and strangury, which means pain after micturition, occur in some cases. The urine may have a strong smell and look cloudy; and hematuria may occur especially at the end of micturition when the bladder is nearly empty. Cystitis is very many times more common in women than in men for several reasons. First, the short urethra has an opening which is vulnerable to contamination by coliform organisms in the perineal region. Second, the conspicuous tendency in some women for cystitis to start shortly after intercourse suggests that intercourse may actually massage organisms through the urethra into the bladder. Third, pregnancy and childbirth distort the anatomy of the urethra and bladder neck. Fourth, the prostatic secretion in men is thought to be strongly bactericidal. No equivalent protection has been discovered in women. Finally, damage to the pelvic ligaments and pelvic floor muscles by childbirth may lead to a degree of prolapse with further deformity in this area. The characteristic symptom of this type of prolapse is stress incontinence—urine leaks out of the bladder momentarily when intra-abdominal pressure is suddenly raised as in coughing or laughing or sudden exertion of any kind. When prolapse is diagnosed, the urinary symptoms can often be improved by surgical operation.

Cystitis in males is very uncommon unless there is some defect in normal bladder emptying such as may be caused by congenital urethral valves in small boys or enlargement of the prostate in middle-aged and elderly men. Spinal cord injury or disease may cause bladder dysfunction in both sexes.

The diagnosis of cystitis can be confirmed by finding an excess of leukocytes (more than 20 cells per mm^3) on microscopy of the urine. In some cases red cells will also be present. The organism should be isolated whenever possible by culture of a mid-stream specimen of urine though this may not always be feasible in a domiciliary setting. In any event treatment need not be delayed until the culture report is available. If cystitis recurs on more than two occasions, the patient should be examined for some underlying cause such as pyelonephritis, calculi or bladder abnormality. This will require cystoscopy and is best postponed until after the acute attack has settled. Instrumentation of the urethra in the presence of active infection occasionally leads to development of Gram-negative septicemia—so called because the responsible organisms, usually *E. coli*, stain pink with a Gram stain. Organisms such as streptococci and staphylococci which stain blue with a gram stain are Gram-positive. These are seldom responsible for urinary infections.

That certain Gram-negative rod-like organisms such as *E. coli* manage to infect the urinary tract so successfully is probably related to the fact that they have little sharp projections protruding from their surfaces which allow them to adhere to the lining cells of the renal pelvis, ureter and bladder. These appendages are called fimbriae and their importance may lie in the ability they confer on bacteria to attach to surfaces where they will not be washed away by the urinary stream. This then allows multiplication and invasion.

Some women frequently develop symptoms resembling cystitis which repeatedly respond to antibiotic therapy yet urine culture is repeatedly negative. It is becoming realized that in the majority of these cases the infection and inflammation is limited to the urethra. The condition can conveniently be called the urethral syndrome. Benefit has been obtained in some of these patients by urethral dilatation.

A different form of urethritis is the type associated with a purulent urethral discharge in association with a prickling or burning sensation in the urethra. This is nearly always venereal in origin, due to gonorrhea or one of the other sexually transmitted diseases. In these cases examination and culture of the urethral discharge is extremely important before any treatment is started and it is naturally wise to obtain expert advice. It is worth noting here that in women gonorrhea may often be present without causing symptoms.

Pyelonephritis

Pyelonephritis means bacterial infection of the kidney substance and renal pelvis. It is nearly always an ascending infection due to organisms reaching the kidney in the urine from the bladder. Just occasionally the infection may be carried to the kidneys in the blood, so-called hematogenous infection. Characteristically the infection affects the tubules in the medulla and the interstitial tissues surrounding the tubules. In severe cases micro-abscesses can be seen histologically.

Clinically, pyelonephritis may be acute or chronic, symptomatic or completely asymptomatic. It is a good generalization that the severity of the symptoms is inversely related to the danger of the disease. Acute pyelonephritis in a young adult woman may cause very distressing symptoms without significant damage or loss of function whereas pyelonephritis in a young child may be completely silent or unaccompanied by any symptoms which localize the infection to the urinary tract, yet renal damage may be extensive and severe. Symptoms are not a reliable guide to diagnosis. Some of the ways in which pyelonephritis may present will now be considered.

Acute symptomatic pyelonephritis

Pyelonephritis is often, but not always, preceded by symptoms of lower urinary infection such as frequency and dysuria. When it is, the diagnosis is easy because attention has already been focused on the urinary tract. The main symptoms of pyelonephritis are an aching pain in the renal angle, fever, rigors, malaise and anorexia. Physical examination may reveal a high temperature, 39–40°C, and tenderness over the affected kidney in the loin. If both kidneys are affected, pain and tenderness will be correspondingly bilateral though usually one side is worse than the other.

Acute pyelonephritis in small children is frequently misleading in the sense that symptoms and signs seldom point to the urinary tract. The child may simply be ill and feverish or just listless. In infants, urinary tract infection may present as jaundice, or even as septicemia with renal failure. The true explanation is not found until the urine is subjected to microscopy and culture.

Pyelonephritis in the elderly may present as an acute confusional state with incontinence or simply as general deterioration of physical condition and behaviour. Diagnosis at the two extremes of life will not therefore be made unless one is always suspicious that pyelonephritis may be the cause. Suspicions can be confirmed by microscopy of the urine to find numerous leukocytes. Infection is proved by culturing the urine to find the organism, which can then be tested for its sensitivity to the different antibiotics. Usually we do not wait for the culture before starting antibiotic therapy but the results of the culture may show that a different antibiotic should be used.

Chronic pyelonephritis

This term implies continuing pyogenic infection of the kidneys which is usually rather patchy or focal in different areas of the kidneys. When nephrons or groups of nephrons are destroyed they are replaced by scar tissue. Intervening tissue may be quite healthy.

If an individual reaches adult life with two healthy kidneys and an anatomically normal urinary tract, the chance of developing chronic destructive pyelonephritis is remote, unless he or she acquires some structural abnormality which causes obstruction or stagnation. Normal pregnancy causes a minor acquired abnormality by producing dilatation and tortuosity of the ureters. This is probably why pyelonephritis tends to be so common and severe during pregnancy, and damage occurring at this time may lead to chronic infection or scarring.

Other common abnormalities, as age advances, are renal stones, and various forms of obstruction and deformity of the ureters and bladder, and in older men enlargement of the prostate. Once a kidney becomes scarred as the result of a bad attack of infection, the scarring and consequent deformity predispose to further attacks of infection, and a vicious circle is set up in this way.

We know that the truly dangerous age for the development of destructive pyelonephritis is during infancy and childhood. It seems that the child's immature kidneys are extremely vulnerable to the damaging effects of pyogenic infection. The danger is greatly increased by the difficulty of diagnosis at this age. There may be no localizing symptoms or signs. Diagnosis depends on alertness and suspicion. Unfortunately there may not be much sign of any illness to arouse suspicion. Many cases of advanced pyelonephritic damage presenting for the first time in early adult life, perhaps as toxemia of pregnancy, probably originated in infancy and childhood. If chronic pyelonephritis is untreated it tends to advance progressively to chronic renal failure. It is frequently complicated by hypertension which in turn increases the renal damage.

The best way of showing that urinary infection has reached the point of chronic pyelonephritis is by means of an intravenous urogram. The signs that one may see are a decrease in thickness of the kidney cortex, blunting of the calyces, irregularity of the renal outline and asymmetry in the size of the kidneys (see Fig. 3.1). In general, pyelonephritis causes visible shrinking of kidney tissue in the area where it strikes. The other advantage of an IVU is that it will show up abnormalities such as renal stones or ureteric dilatation which may be predisposing to infection in the first place.

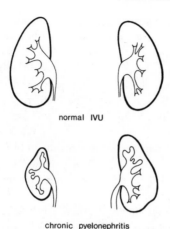

normal IVU

chronic pyelonephritis

Fig. 3.1. The appearances of a chronic pyelonephritis as shown on an IVU contrasted with a normal kidney.

The presence of free reflux of urine from the bladder up one or both ureters is a factor which increases the severity of pyelonephritis at all ages, but especially during childhood. This can best be demonstrated by a micturating cystogram (see p.46). Renal biopsy is a rather unreliable way of diagnosing the disease because one may hit a normal area. In order to determine the extent of the renal damage one should perform tests of renal function such as blood urea and creatinine. A very sensitive test in this condition is the urinary concentration test. This may detect minor degrees of renal tubular damage which are not shown by other investigations.

Asymptomatic bacteriuria

This means a positive urine culture in the absence of symptoms. It seems that females in nearly all age groups have a higher incidence of bacteriuria than males. Healthy non-pregnant women with normal urinary tracts seem to be no exception and in the majority of these the bacteria do not appear to do any harm. In certain special groups the bacteriuria is likely to become associated at some time with damaging urinary tract infection. Of these the best known is pregnant women. If they are left untreated a proportion will develop overt pyelonephritis before the end of the pregnancy. Administration of a short course of an appropriate antibiotic with a repeat urine culture after treatment will greatly reduce this problem.

Because of this there is now an increasing tendency to screen all pregnant women by mid-stream urine cultures at their first ante-natal attendance. The problem is a serious one because urinary infections during pregnancy are associated with an increased incidence of spontaneous abortion, prematurity and impaired fetal growth, quite apart from any permanent damage which may be sustained by the mother.

The second obvious group is patients who are already known to be suffering from chronic pyelonephritis or any other urinary tract abnormality such as renal stones or an abnormality in bladder emptying. Once these patients have been identified they should have urine cultures at regular intervals and appropriate antibiotic treatment for any positive culture which is found.

The third and most doubtful group which is receiving attention at present is infants and young children, especially young girls. About two per cent of all girls of school age have asymptomatic bacteriuria and a proportion of these are found to be suffering from hitherto unrecognized pyelonephritis. It is hoped that by discovering these cases early, severe damage from chronic pyelonephritis will be prevented by regular follow-up and antibiotic treatment. It may be that the best age at which to carry out large-scale screening is during infancy but here we have the difficulty of obtaining uncontaminated urine specimens suitable for culture. Suprapubic bladder puncture to aspirate urine in all healthy infants is a somewhat radical procedure and has yet to be justified.

Reflux nephropathy

In recent years it has come to light that renal damage almost indistinguishable from pyelonephritic scarring can be caused by ureteric reflux even in the absence of infection. It is thought that gross reflux, either unilateral or bilateral, present from the time of birth, causes a forceful retrograde flow of urine into the renal pelvis every time the bladder contracts. Damage is caused to the papillae of the renal medulla by means of a back pressure effect. Cystoscopy will show that the ureteric orifice in the bladder on the affected side is not a normal valve-like slit but a wide open hole, the so-called 'golf-hole' ureteric orifice. It is not generally diagnosed at an early stage because it causes no symptoms. Fortunately there is a tendency for ureteric reflux to decrease as a child matures, provided that infection does not occur, and some of these cases probably resolve spontaneously. The severely affected case may progress until the condition reveals itself with the onset of chronic renal failure. What we need is a harmless and cheap screening test to show up all cases of ureteric reflux at birth but as yet no such test is available.

Management of urinary infections

The mainstay of treatment of urinary infections is antibacterial therapy. The choice of which antibacterial agent to use should be governed as far as possible by testing the sensitivity of the organism. A sensible approach is to obtain the mid-stream urine for culture and then start treatment immediately with the drug which is likely to be effective. Occasionally there is a good response to treatment even when *in vitro* sensitivity tests indicate bacterial resistance. In this case it may not be necessary to change the antibiotic.

A few years ago there was a vogue for using very long courses of antibiotics to treat urinary infections. More recently it has been shown that the cure rate and relapse rate are not significantly different if one uses antibiotics for ten days, six weeks or six months. Success has even been reported with a single dose. It is common to give a two week course followed by a repeat urine culture when treatment is completed. A high urine output is probably an advantage because frequent emptying of a full bladder gets rid of a lot of organisms, and so discourages their multiplication. The fact that bacterial growth is discouraged by a very concentrated urine might argue in favor of restriction of fluids but this advantage is probably outweighed by the disadvantage of stagnation. Most authorities in fact advocate a high fluid intake; some even suggest the additional use of diuretics.

Changing the pH of the urine to the alkaline side used to be important in the old days of the insoluble sulphonamides but this is hardly ever indicated with current antibiotics. There is a theoretical reason for making the urine acid when treating *Proteus* infections but in practice this is quite difficult to do and the benefit is probably slight.

The choice of which antibiotic to use should be based on knowledge of which one is likely to be effective and on the *in vitro* sensitivity tests. Tetracyclines should not be used in patients with renal failure because they increase uremia by increasing urea production. It must be remembered that antibiotics accumulate to high blood levels in patients with impaired renal function. Nitrofurantoin (Furadantin) should be avoided in renal failure because the high blood levels may cause permanent polyneuritis with foot-drop.

Great care must be exercised when using aminoglycoside antibiotics such as tobramycin and gentamicin in patients with impaired renal function because the high blood levels may cause permanent nerve deafness and vestibular damage as well as renal damage. Others, such as the polymyxins, thiosporins or colomycin, will also aggravate renal damage under these circumstances. Doses of all these drugs must be given at less frequent intervals when kidney function is impaired and if necessary we may have to enlist the help of the laboratory in estimating blood levels and excretion rates. The widely used sulphamethoxazole–timethroprim combination may occasionally aggravate renal damage in patients who already have chronic renal impairment. It should be given in half doses in these patients.

Apart from antibiotic therapy, attention should also be given to simple hygienic considerations such as frequent washing of the perineal area with soap and water, and making sure that there is no associated vaginal infection such as candidiasis or 'thrush', which predisposes to ascending infection. Women who tend to get urinary infections after intercourse should be encouraged to empty their bladders as soon as possible after intercourse in order to wash out any organisms which may have been introduced. Some of these patients successfully stay free of trouble by taking one tablet of an antibiotic every time they have intercourse.

Finally, for recurrent urinary infections two further measures are sometimes helpful. Hexamine hippurate (Hiprex) 1 g twice a day before meals can be used as prophylactic suppression therapy. It is not an antibiotic but an antiseptic. It is thought that under the influence of a normally acid urine a dilute solution of formaldehyde is formed. This is bactericidal and kills organisms that gain entrance to the bladder. Hiprex is of no value in treating an established infection but may effectively prevent recurrent infections.

Secondly, for women with recurrent urinary infections the drug cycloserine given in a dose of 250 mg on alternate evenings (this is a very small non-toxic dose) can be taken continuously. The main value lies in the fact that *Escherichia coli*, the most common urinary pathogen, never becomes resistant to cycloserine. Cycloserine also effectively kills most of the other urinary tract organisms. Unlike many other antibiotics, such as ampicillin, cycloserine does not tend to cause allergic reactions if taken for a long time.

Correction of mechanical and structural defects

Eradication of urinary infection may be difficult or impossible in the presence of certain structural abnormalities such as renal calculus, partial ureteric obstruction or free ureteric reflux. The decision whether or not to interfere surgically to correct these abnormalities must be made in each case on its own merits. Many of the problems just mentioned can be cured or improved by operation.

The urinary catheter and catheter technique

For various reasons and at different times catheters must be used to drain the urine from the bladder. Catheters should never be used unless there is a compelling reason. If a catheter is used it should be treated with great respect because it is a potentially dangerous instrument. Catheters, even if used in a most meticulous way, are liable to cause urinary infections. One of the reasons for this is that organisms may lurk just inside the urethral orifice where they cannot be wiped off by antiseptic. The catheter may inoculate these organisms into the bladder as it advances up the urethra. If catheters are used in a slipshod way infection will certainly occur. Here are some suggestions on points of catheter technique.

• Do not use catheters in males just to prevent wet beds. A Paul's tube will do this just as well.

• When inserting a catheter the aseptic technique should be of the standard required for any major surgical operation.

• Once a catheter is connected to a urine drainage bag it should not normally be disconnected until the catheter is removed. Urine is removed by an outlet tube at the bottom of the bag so that the sealed drainage circuit is not broken. Drainage bags without outlet tubes should never be used for bladder drainage because in order to empty the urine the bag has to be disconnected from the catheter. This may allow entry of pathogenic organisms up the catheter.

• The drainage bag should have a non-return valve so that urine from the bag cannot run back into the bladder when the bag is lifted for emptying.

• It is quite a good idea to have the catheter running through a piece of sponge foam soaked in antiseptic. This can be advanced up to the urethral orifice to keep it clean and moist and free of infection.

• The greater the volume of urine output the less will be the chance of infection ascending through the catheter.

• Catheters should not be used only in order to measure urine volume accurately in oliguric patients, for example patients with acute renal failure. This is a dangerous practice and the information gained can be obtained in other ways.

• When indwelling catheters have to remain in position for a long time the urine should be cultured at regular intervals and always before the catheter is removed. Urine for culture should be aspirated with a sterile needle and syringe through the wall of the catheter rather than from the bag where it may be contaminated.

• During prolonged catheter drainage it may be worth injecting a small volume of 1/5 000 aqueous chlorhexidine solution into the bladder through the wall of the catheter with a fine needle about twice a day. This is done with a clamp on the catheter below the site of injection. The clamp is removed after the antiseptic has been in the bladder for a few minutes. A positive culture in the presence of a catheter should, in the absence of symptoms, be left untreated until the catheter is removed. Earlier therapy leads to the development of resistant organisms. Antibiotics are given on removal of the catheter, and follow-up cultures should be taken to make sure the infection has been eradicated.

• An alternative way of carrying out bladder irrigation, one which is frequently employed by urological surgeons after prostate operations, is irrigation through an extra lumen in the catheter by gravity from an iv stand, with a Y-connection leading down to the drainage bag. This is particularly useful in preventing clot obstruction of the catheter from bleeding.

Glomerulonephritis and nephrotic syndrome

Unlike pyelonephritis, which is a bacterial infection mainly of kidney tubules, glomerulonephritis is a non-bacterial inflammation of glomeruli. Glomerulonephritis takes various forms but all the types have two things in common. First, the glomeruli are in some way abnormal so that protein leaks through to appear in the urine. Proteinuria is therefore a more or less constant sign. Second, the basic trouble in all cases is an antigen—antibody reaction in relation to glomeruli. In other words there is an immunological or allergic reaction affecting the glomeruli. The allergic factor or antigen cannot often be identified but occasionally it can. One well-known antigen which is capable of causing glomerulonephritis is the hemolytic streptococcus, though only certain strains have been implicated. The streptococci do not infect the kidneys but form antigen—antibody complexes which become trapped in the glomerular capillaries of the kidneys. Once there, they set up an allergic inflammation which may heal or continue to smoulder causing progressive glomerular damage and perhaps eventually renal failure. A number of other micro-organisms as well as certain drugs and poisons have been implicated in this way, but in many, if not the majority of, cases of human glomerulonephritis the initial allergic insult cannot be identified. Instead we must be content with defining glomerulonephritis according to the histological appearance on renal biopsy and by the way it behaves clinically. Some types of histological appearance will accurately predict a certain type of

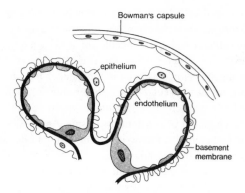

Fig. 3.2. Ultrastructure of glomerular capillary loops.

clinical illness. In others the clinical progress is very variable. There are, however, some useful generalizations, though naturally there are exceptions in all groups and at all ages.

First, glomerulonephritis tends to be a mild disease in young children, more severe in young adults, and rapidly fatal in the elderly. This contrasts with pyelonephritis, which is most dangerous in infants and young children and comparatively harmless in healthy adults.

Second, when glomerulonephritis causes proteinuria but no hematuria, or hematuria without significant proteinuria, it is usually a mild disease with a good prognosis. When heavy proteinuria co-exists with hematuria it is usually a more serious disease with a bad prognosis.

Glomerulonephritis can be divided by renal biopsy into three main histological types. These are:

- minimal change,
- proliferative,
- membranous.

The pictures in Fig. 3.3 are intended to illustrate the reasons for these names. *Minimal change* means what it says, that the abnormalities of the glomeruli on light microscopy are so slight as to appear normal. Electron microscopy in these cases actually shows minor abnormalities which we need not concern ourselves about. *Proliferative* means that there is proliferation of various kinds of cells in the region of the glomeruli. The glomeruli look abnormally cellular, and this proliferation may be focal or diffuse. Proliferative glomerulonephritis exists in all grades of severity and there are probably about six different subgroups under the heading of proliferative. *Membranous* means thickening of the

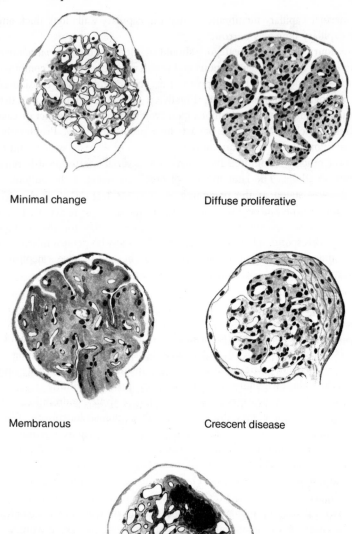

Minimal change

Diffuse proliferative

Membranous

Crescent disease

Focal sclerosis

Fig. 3.3. Typical appearance of glomeruli as seen on biopsy in various forms of glomerulonephritis.

glomerular capillary membrane so that the capillary walls look thick and the capillary lumen is narrow.

A fourth histological category should be mentioned called *membrano-proliferative* in which membranous and proliferative changes are combined in the same glomeruli. For purposes of description this is best considered as a subgroup of proliferative. Finally, it should be pointed out that minimal change and membranous glomerulonephritis are distinct disease entities which by and large behave in a predictable way. Proliferative glomerulonephritis is not an entity but a group of diseases which tend to recover quickly in children but progress at a variable rate towards renal failure in adults. The later the age of onset the worse is the outlook.

As was stated at the beginning, a constant feature of glomerulo-nephritis is proteinuria. This may be slight, moderate or heavy. By heavy proteinuria we usually mean more than 3 g per day for the average adult—correspondingly less for children. Anyone who persistently passes more than 3 g per day of urinary protein can be said to have a nephrotic syndrome. This bald statement deserves some explanation.

Nephrotic syndrome

Since you will hear this term used repeatedly in relation to kidney diseases it is important to understand its meaning. The first thing to realize is that nephrotic syndrome is not a distinct disease. It really only means the clinical picture brought about by heavy proteinuria.

Secondly, this heavy proteinuria of the nephrotic syndrome can be caused by several kidney diseases other than glomerulonephritis. Glo-merulonephritis is by far the commonest cause of the nephrotic syndrome but other well-known causes are amyloidosis, diabetic nephropathy, renal vein thrombosis, certain forms of heavy metal poisoning and allergic reactions to drugs and poisons. There are also several rather rare causes.

The feature which these diseases have in common is that they increase the permeability of the glomerular capillaries to protein. The histological appearances of the glomeruli under light microscopy vary greatly and may be normal or grossly abnormal. The most useful single investigation in the diagnosis of these conditions is renal biopsy. A good renal biopsy may contain twenty glomeruli and this number will be sufficient to demonstrate the abnormalities which are representative of the process which is present in both kidneys. The primary defect is heavy urinary protein loss—in some cases up to 20 g of protein in 24 hours. This has the effect of depleting the proteins in the plasma, especially the albumin fraction of the plasma proteins. This is a relatively small molecule and therefore leaks out more readily. The liver manufactures plasma proteins faster to make up the deficit but there is a limit to what the liver is able to do. The result is a fall in plasma proteins or hypoproteinemia. This in turn results in a fall in the colloid osmotic pressure of the plasma (see p.10) so that water tends to leak into the interstitial space to become apparent as edema. The edema of nephrotic syndrome is distributed according to gravity. The patient's eyes tend to be puffy in the mornings after lying down but during the day this puffiness disappears and is replaced by swelling of the feet and ankles, most troublesome towards the evening. If the patient is in bed the edema goes to the sacral area. The fourth classical feature of the nephrotic syndrome is the high blood cholesterol and high level of other plasma lipids which makes the plasma milky in appearance. No one knows exactly why this occurs but a simple way to explain it is that the liver is working so hard manufacturing plasma proteins that it inadvertently synthesizes cholesterol and lipids, the manufacture of which depends on related metabolic mechanisms. The diagram in Fig. 3.4 illustrates some of the consequences and mechanisms of the nephrotic syndrome.

To summarize, the classical features of the nephrotic syndrome are heavy proteinuria, hypoproteinemia, edema and hypercholesterolemia. Of these the only essential feature required to make a diagnosis is heavy proteinuria. Any of the other features may be absent in a particular patient at certain times. For example, treatment with diuretics may get rid of the edema but the patient still has a nephrotic syndrome. Well-known complications of the nephrotic syndrome are increased susceptibility to various kinds of infection (perhaps caused by loss of plasma globulins which contain antibodies) and premature atheroma formation thought to be due to long-standing increase in plasma lipids and cholesterol. When a nephrotic syndrome is cured or remits spontaneously so that proteinuria ceases, the plasma proteins return to normal, edema disappears, and the plasma lipids and cholesterol also revert to normal levels.

Having side-tracked to discuss nephrotic syndrome we must get back to glomerulonephritis. The main histological categories will be considered in turn.

Minimal change

This is by far the commonest form of glomerulonephritis in children. It usually presents with a rapid onset of classical nephrotic syndrome with proteinuria and edema in the toddler age group. Puffy eyes and frothy urine (a high protein content makes urine frothy) may be the first signs,

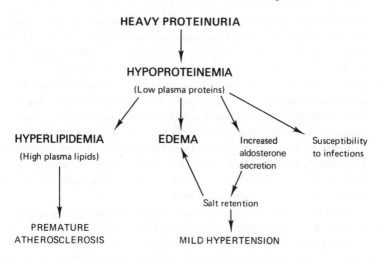

Fig. 3.4. Interacting factors in the nephrotic syndrome.

soon to be followed by generalized edema of the whole body. Ascites and pleural effusions may cause respiratory difficulty. The child becomes very prone to infections of various kinds. Before the advent of effective therapy these infections were not infrequently fatal. Urine microscopy will show no red cells. Laboratory examination usually shows that the proteinuria is highly selective (see p.39). After obtaining an initial baseline of investigations it is justified to start treatment as soon as possible with prednisone. This usually brings about a remission within a few days. After this, the dose of prednisone can be lowered to a main-tenance level which is relatively non-toxic. Diuretics are frequently employed while waiting for the prednisone to take effect. The majority of children respond satisfactorily to prednisone and undergo complete re-mission without relapse. A proportion, however, relapse every time the dose is lowered so that it is not possible to maintain a remission without toxicity from prolonged high dosage. Fortunately there is now an effective alternative treatment in the form of cyclophosphamide. Nearly all those who relapse frequently on prednisone can be rendered protein-free with cyclophosphamide. This allows prednisone to be withdrawn and only a very few relapse when the cyclophosphamide is stopped. The total course of cyclophosphamide is usually limited to six or eight weeks.

Cyclophosphamide is an immunosuppressive and cytotoxic drug and its mode of action in glomerulonephritis is not really understood. It causes suppression of the bone marrow, particularly the white blood cells, and this effect depends on the dose. Fortunately it is usually possible to give a dose which is effective in treating the glomerulonephritis without causing too much white cell suppression. With prolonged treatment alopecia often occurs but this recovers when the treatment is discontinued or the dose lowered. Sometimes the head hair regrows a slightly different color or may become curly when formerly it was straight. A rare and very dangerous side-effect of cyclophosphamide is hemorrhagic cystitis—a profuse and sometimes life-threatening bleeding from the bladder mucosa which has occasionally necessitated surgical removal of the bladder. We have not experienced this complication when treating renal disorders and it seems more likely to occur whem massive doses of cyclophosphamide are used for cancer.

Women on cyclophosphamide develop amenorrhea on average after about six months and men taking the drug develop loss of sperm formation after about the same period. Both sexes become permanently sterile if the drug is continued for too long after this. This has to be taken into account if cyclophosphamide is prescribed for prolonged periods for other diseases.

Renal biopsy is not usually necessary for the diagnosis of minimal change glomerulonephritis in children unless the lack of response to prednisone makes one doubt the diagnosis. It may, however, be very helpful in certain parts of the world where quartan malaria is endemic. In these areas there is a high incidence of nephrotic syndrome which is an allergic reaction to the malarial parasite. Renal biopsy shows proliferative changes in these cases and there is no benefit from steroid therapy.

Minimal change glomerulonephritis in adults is less common than in children (about 20% of all adult glomerulonephritis). It has the same symptoms and signs of nephrotic syndrome without hematuria but the response to prednisone is generally less satisfactory. The necessity for prolonged steroid therapy to keep patients free of proteinuria is attended by the risk of serious steroid side effects. Of those who fail to respond, most will obtain a complete remission with cyclophosphamide. If it is not possible to obtain a complete remission, most patients can be kept free of edema by judicious use of diuretics. Susceptibility to infection will remain but patients do not develop renal failure because the histological lesion does not progress.

Focal glomerulosclerosis

This condition, because it may cause nephrotic syndrome in childhood, tends to be mistaken for minimal change disease. It is more serious and fortunately less common. There are other important differences. A clue to diagnosis may be given by the presence of microscopic hematuria, which is nearly always present, and this never occurs in minimal change. The deep glomeruli next to the medulla, the juxtamedullary glomeruli, are the first to become affected; and in the early stages of the disease a wedge renal biopsy obtained by open surgical technique containing only superficial cortex may fail to diagnose the condition. The condition may respond well to steroids but usually not at all to cyclophosphamide. All the glomeruli become affected as the disease progresses, and there is a strong tendency to hypertension, as well as progressive renal failure after a variable period—usually years. Focal glomerulosclerosis may sometimes cause congenital nephrotic syndrome, though actually the commonest age of onset of focal sclerosis is during the teens. It has a tendency to recur in grafted kidneys after renal transplantation.

Proliferative glomerulonephritis

Although this condition is usually benign and recoverable in children, with occasional exceptions, it is generally a progressive destructive disease in adults and the biggest cause of renal failure in the young adult age group. It has been said that whoever discovers a vaccine to prevent glomerulonephritis will achieve far more good during his life-time than a hundred transplant surgeons. The types and natural history of proliferative glomerulonephritis are very varied and there are already known to be several antigen–antibody combinations which can cause it. Many more will doubtless be discovered. In all forms of proliferative glomerulonephritis the proteinuria tends to be of the unselective variety. Some of the commoner clinical presentations of proliferative glomerulonephritis will now be mentioned.

Acute post-streptococcal glomerulonephritis

This is known to be an immunological response to a hemolytic streptococcal infection, usually of the throat, but sometimes of the skin, 10–14 days before. It is commonest in children of school age and presents as an acute illness with puffy eyes and red or smoky urine. Often there is oliguria and hypertension in the first few days. The blood urea may be raised and it may be necessary to restrict salt, water and protein intake in the acute phase. The streptococcal infection should also be eradicated with penicillin. The condition usually settles rapidly but proteinuria and microscopic hematuria may persist for up to a year. When it occurs in the older age groups, complete healing is the exception. The disease tends to progress and become chronic, leading ultimately to renal failure. The incidence of post-streptococcal glomerulonephritis seems to be declining in countries with advanced systems of health care, perhaps because of earlier treatment of streptococcal infections.

IgA nephritis (Berger's disease)

This form of glomerulonephritis is associated with the name of Dr Berger who is credited with first describing it. Now that it is being diagnosed accurately by renal biopsy it is turning out to be numerically the commonest form of glomerulonephritis in many parts of the world.

The disease is called IgA nephritis or IgA nephropathy because IgA is identified in the glomeruli on immunofluorescence microscopy and the level of IgA is found to be elevated if one performs immunoelectrophoresis of the patient's plasma proteins. It is common in both children and adults and its most consistent feature is continuous microscopic hematuria accompanied by red cell casts. This gives the clue that the red cells are glomerular in origin. The other main feature is that it has a very long course over many years. For many years it was believed to be a benign condition but as more long-term follow-up studies have been published the more it seems that the majority progress ultimately to end-stage renal failure. Children with IgA nephritis rarely progress to renal insufficiency during childhood; it will be carried on into adult life and cause renal failure later.

IgA nephritis is commoner and also seems to have a worse prognosis in males. Heavy proteinuria, greater than 2 g per day, seems to be associated with a downhill course but there are exceptions to this. In some published series the feature of recurrent macrosopic hematuria seems to be a favorable prognostic indicator.

Because it is such a common entity it is an important contributory cause of end-stage renal failure. So far there is no specific therapy which has been shown to produce any benefit.

Mesangiocapillary glomerulonephritis (membranoproliferative)

Although the commonest age of onset of this disease is in the late teens, it causes the most trouble in young adults. It is associated with hematuria and proteinuria, which may be slight or heavy, and a slowly progressive course to terminal renal failure after about 5–12 years. Hypertension is often an early feature and difficult to control. Renal function may be well maintained despite bad histological appearances until late in the course of the disease, but once renal impairment appears renal failure usually occurs rapidly.

The diagnosis can be confirmed by the characteristic appearance on renal biopsy (see p.68). As its name implies, this form of glomerulonephritis has abnormalities of mesangial cellular proliferation, as well as glomerular basement membrane thickening. The other well-known and helpful diagnostic feature is the peculiar tendency for the serum complement (see p.40) to be low throughout the course of the disease.

The most important aspect of management is meticulous control of blood pressure to prevent further renal damage. There is as yet no general agreement about the benefit of specific therapy such as immunosuppressive and anticoagulant therapy, which are potentially harmful.

Most patients with this disease will ultimately be suitable for dialysis and/or renal transplantation. Unfortunately the disease has an unpleasant propensity to recur in the transplanted kidneys. This may happen even if the original diseased kidneys are removed first.

Rapidly progressive glomerulonephritis (crescent disease)

This, the most devastating form of glomerulonephritis, is a subgroup of proliferative GN. It is usually confined to adults and it is noted for its rapidly downhill course with renal failure occurring in days or weeks rather than in months or years. It may occur in the guise of acute renal failure, especially in men over the age of 60. It is sometimes called crescentic nephritis because of the characteristic appearance of the glomeruli obtained by renal biopsy. The majority of the glomeruli are seemingly surrounded, as if being strangled, by large crescentic growths of epithelial cells arising from the epithelial lining of Bowman's capsule, see Fig. 3.3, p.68. These epithelial crescents are in some way associated with intraglomerular deposition of fibrin and they are the histological hallmark of the disease.

Small, insignificant crescents occur in other forms of glomerulonephritis. It is the large occlusive nature of the crescents in this disease, more like collars than crescents, which sets it apart from other conditions. Crescentic nephritis is usually an isolated entity of quite unknown etiology, but a similar appearance may be seen in severe forms of other conditions as, for example, in the glomerulonephritis of Henoch–Schonlein syndrome (both in children and adults) and in polyarteritis nodosa (usually in elderly men).

This disease still has a bad prognosis but most authorities now report gratifying responses to treatment in the form of high doses of soluble methyl prednisolone injected intravenously, e.g. 10 mg/kg/day for about three days followed by oral prednisone. This treatment is sometimes accompanied by immunosuppressive drugs such as cyclophosphamide and azathioprine and sometimes by courses of intensive plasma exchange. There is still a lot of debate about which components of this treatment are really necessary but there is general agreement that the outlook in the absence of treatment is almost uniformly grim.

Goodpasture's syndrome

This rare and terrifying disease is of great interest because of the distinctive mechanism of its causation and the fact that there is now a brilliantly effective treatment for it where previously it was almost uniformly fatal. The disease presents as a form of rapidly progressive glomerulonephritis accompanied by hematuria, proteinuria, hypertension and progressive renal impairment. At about the same time as the onset of glomerulonephritis, patients have episodes of alarming bright red hemoptysis. These episodes are accompanied by dyspnea and evidence of impaired blood gas exchange.

The cause is now known to be the development of an antibody against glomerular basement membrane as well as against the alveolar capillary membrane. The natural history in the absence of treatment is progressive renal failure with hypertension and progressive damage to the lungs leading to respiratory failure after many distressing episodes of hemoptysis. If dialysis alone is employed for the renal failure, most patients still die from the pulmonary complications. The treatment, which is dramatically life-saving, was worked out at the Royal Postgraduate Medical School in London. Intensive plasma exchange is started as early as possible to remove the offending antibody, and at the same time immunosuppressive treatment is administered to suppress the cells which are forming the antibody. With this treatment the lung condition quickly improves. The prognosis for the kidney condition largely depends on whether the treatment is started before the patient develops oliguric renal failure. If treatment is not started before this, the kidneys usually do not recover.

Opportunistic infections in immunosuppressed patients

In any patient treated with combined immunosuppressive therapy there is loss of resistance to infection and an increased incidence of what we call opportunistic (also called nosocomial) infections.

These are infections which are not normally sufficiently virulent or pathogenic to attack healthy people but which become pathogenic and sometimes dangerous in people with reduced immunity.

The commonest opportunistic infections you will see are candidiasis and herpes simplex.

Herpes simplex is easy to diagnose at a glance because we are all familiar with it. Candidiasis must be looked for systematically, the commonest place being in the patient's mouth, especially under a denture. It looks like curdled milk but cannot be scraped off the mucous membrane without causing bleeding, and the mucous membrane round about is always red and inflamed. It may also occur in moist areas of the skin such as under the breasts and in the perineum. Nurses can play an important role in detecting candidiasis so that treatment can be started before it spreads to cause esophageal candidiasis and even *Candida* septicemia.

A more serious opportunistic infection, commonly seen in North America, is *Pneumocystis carinii*. This is a protozoan parasite which causes a diffuse bilateral infection of the lungs leading rapidly to death from respiratory failure if it is not diagnosed and treated early enough. Diagnosis may depend on an open lung biopsy. In this part of the world *Pneumocystis* is so common that susceptible (immunosuppressed) patients are treated prophylactically with sulphatrimethoprim (Septra) to prevent the condition from establishing itself. Since adopting this policy we have hardly seen a single case.

Malarial nephropathy

Numerically the most important form of glomerulonephritis in those parts of the world where quartan malaria is endemic, this disease is caused by an immunological reaction to *Plasmodium malariae*, the same mechanism whereby post-streptococcal glomerulonephritis is caused by streptococcal infection.

The condition usually presents as a nephrotic syndrome and histologically there is a diffuse proliferation of cells in the glomeruli. There is a high incidence of progression to renal failure usually with hypertension. There is some evidence of benefit from the use of azathioprine.

Other forms of proliferative glomerulonephritis

Although the above forms of proliferative glomerulonephritis are mainly distinct disease entities we still come across patients with proliferative glomerulonephritis who in the light of present knowledge we are not able to categorize. Unhappily, because of lack of effective treatment, an exact histological diagnosis may be largely academic anyway. Only occasionally in such patients do we find a possible etiological factor. For example, cancers of various kinds have been shown to cause membranous glomerulonephritis. The probable mechanism is that the tumor protein becomes antigenic. The nephritis may actually go into remission if the tumor is removed by surgery. There is also some circumstantial evidence of glomerulonephritis being caused by exposure to hydrocarbons such as petroleum products. These cases are the exceptions and in the majority we never discover the precipitating cause.

Membranous glomerulonephritis

The disease is comparatively rare in childhood and fairly common in adults. It usually presents as a nephrotic syndrome with very few or no red cells in the urine. A minority of patients simply have modest proteinuria and are completely asymptomatic. Renal biopsy shows thickened glomerular capillary loops and a narrowed capillary lumen. In contrast to proliferative glomerulonephritis there is no increase in glomerular cellularity. The capillary loop thickening is a characteristic and individual process which requires a special silver stain to demonstrate it convincingly. The natural history of the disease is variable. About 25% of sufferers undergo complete clinical remission, and a similar proportion progress within a few years to terminal renal failure resulting in death or regular dialysis. Of the remainder, about half continue with asymptomatic proteinuria and the other half remain nephrotic with heavy proteinuria. Heavy proteinuria in this disease (as in most forms of glomerulonephritis) seems to indicate a worse prognosis than mild proteinuria. Hypertension tends to be a late phenomenon. Children have a more benign course than adults so that renal failure from this cause in children is rare.

Although steroid therapy has been suggested by various authorities to be valuable in membranous glomerulonephritis, it now seems more likely that apparent good results were in patients who were due to undergo spontaneous remission had they not received treatment at all. No other form of treatment is of any proven benefit. Non-specific measures such as control of hypertension and edema should always receive attention.

Hereditary nephritis

It has been known for a long time that nephritis may occur in more than one child in a family, being present at or shortly after birth or occurring later but at the same age in each child. There is an association with deafness in some families and in most cases the disease has led inexorably to renal failure. The course is uninfluenced by any treatment.

Renal vein thrombosis

Spontaneous thrombosis of the renal veins is an occasional cause of nephrotic syndrome. It may also complicate the condition in any patient who already has nephrotic syndrome, probably because the blood of such patients is more than normally inclined to clot. The symptoms are loin pain followed by hematuria and oliguria. In the event of recovery massive proteinuria follows. Renal vein thrombosis can also be an entirely silent complication of nephrotic syndrome, and since both conditions cause heavy proteinuria the diagnosis may be missed completely. There is still considerable debate about how commonly nephrotic syndrome is complicated by renal vein thrombosis. The general consensus is that it is relatively uncommon.

The condition can be confirmed radiologically by the use of contrast medium introduced into the inferior vena cava. Renal biopsy in such patients shows appearances similar to those of membranous glomerulonephritis. Anticoagulant therapy is beneficial.

Renal vein thrombosis may also occur acutely in small infants who become dehydrated and hence hypercoagulable from such conditions as gastroenteritis. There is usually a life-threatening acute renal failure and the kidneys are palpably enlarged and tender. Dialysis may be needed until the renal failure recovers under the influence of anticoagulant therapy.

Glomerulonephritis in association with collagen diseases

Renal involvement in the form of glomerulonephritis is a frequent accompaniment of the collagen diseases, such conditions as systemic lupus erythematosus (SLE), polyarteritis nodosa, Wegener's granulomatosis and scleroderma. Of these lupus nephritis in SLE is the most common and the one of which we have the most experience. SLE is a multisystem disease affecting skin, blood, joints, serous membranes, the nervous system and the kidneys. Once renal involvement occurs the outlook is bad because the nephritis nearly always progresses to renal failure in the absence of treatment. Most authorities are agreed that steroids benefit both the general disease and the renal lesion; and recently several

workers have found further benefit from combined steroid and cyclophosphamide therapy. Cyclophosphamide may have to be given for a long
time to prevent relapse.

Other aspects of management in glomerulonephritis

Even if there is no effective specific treatment for the renal lesion in a
patient with glomerulonephritis or nephrotic syndrome, a lot can be done
to make the patient's life more comfortable. Edema can nearly always be
controlled by a judicious combination of diuretics with salt and water
restriction if necessary. The diuretics most commonly used for this
purpose are furosemide (frusemide) (Lasix) and spironolactone (Aldactone
A). Furosemide, except in rare cases, is apparently completely non-toxic
and can be given safely in large doses. Spironolactone works by counter-
i.ng the action of aldosterone, the salt-retaining hormone of the adrenal
medulla, which is produced in large amounts in patients with hypoproteinemia. In a patient with very resistant edema due to extremely decreased
plasma proteins it is sometimes possible to provoke an excellent diuresis
with intravenous infusions of albumin or plasma. Unfortunately the effect
tends to be only temporary since the plasma proteins fall again as a result
of urinary protein loss.

The hypertension which often occurs in association with glomerulonephritis should always be meticulously controlled with hypotensive drugs
to prevent further aggravation of the renal damage.

Finally patients with diffuse diseases of kidney tissue have an increased
susceptibility to urinary tract infections. Urine cultures should be performed regularly and infections promptly treated when they are detected.

Hypertension

The extent to which hypertension damages kidneys is not accurately
known because it is so often present in combination with, or as a
consequence of, other diseases such as glomerulonephritis or gout, which
may be the initial provoking cause. Moreover, it is often impossible to say
how much damage has been caused by the underlying disease and how
much by the hypertension. Essential hypertension means high blood
pressure with no recognizable underlying cause other than perhaps a
constitutional or hereditary predisposition. This, as well as secondary
hypertension, may become severe and enter a malignant phase with
accelerated renal destruction. In a late stage it may be impossible to rule
out the presence of an underlying renal lesion. The effects of severe
hypertension are widespread, with damage to blood vessels in almost

every organ, but the most conspicuous injury is to cerebral blood vessels, the heart and the kidneys. Stroke, heart failure and renal failure are the three common causes of death in hypertension. In the kidneys the damage is evident as progressive thickening of arterial walls, narrowing of the lumen, and progressive ischemia of the renal tissue. This ischemia tends to lead to release of renin and further aggravation of the hypertension so that a vicious circle is started. Hypertension may be slight and comparatively harmless for many years but it tends to gather momentum with an accelerating rate of deterioration.

Essential hypertension is mainly a disease of the middle-aged and elderly but hypertension secondary to other causes can occur at any age and even in young children. The actual levels of blood pressure seem to be less important than the effect the hypertension has on the organs of the individual. Statistics show that women tolerate high levels better than men.

The severity of the hypertension in a particular patient can be judged in three main ways:
- by the degree of cardiac enlargement,
- by its effects on the blood vessels of the optic fundi as seen through an ophthalmoscope,
- by the presence of proteinuria and impairment of renal function.

Efforts should be made to assess the severity of the hypertension as well as to look for and, if possible, treat the underlying cause. Well known but uncommon causes of hypertension are coarctation of the aorta, Cushing's syndrome (over-secretion of adrenal cortical hormones), pheochromocytoma (a benign tumor of the adrenal medulla which secretes noradrenaline and adrenaline) and Conn's syndrome (an adrenal tumor which secretes an excess of the salt-retaining hormone aldosterone). More common than these is renal artery stenosis, usually due to atheromatous narrowing of the origin of the renal artery and occasionally caused by a congenital abnormality of the renal artery wall called fibromuscular hyperplasia. Most common as causes of hypertension are various forms of renal disease either unilateral or bilateral. It is occasionally possible to cure hypertension by excising a tumor, surgically correcting a renal artery stenosis, or removing a small diseased kidney, and this may be very rewarding but is very much the exception in the mass of clinical practice. In the last few years considerable experience and some success has been gained in dilating renal artery stenoses by means of intra-arterial balloon catheters. This method, which is called transluminal angioplasty, is less risky than vascular by-pass surgery, and also considerably less of an ordeal for the patient.

The majority of hypertensive individuals must be managed by means of hypotensive drugs. We now have an excellent range of drugs at our disposal so that inability to control blood pressure is distinctly uncommon. The incidence of side-effects from the agents currently available is slight and it is nearly always possible to find a drug or combination of drugs which suits the patient. One of the commonest side-effects is postural hypotension, a fall in blood pressure to abnormally low levels in the standing position. This is why it is important, when starting a patient on hypotensive therapy, always to check blood pressure in lying and standing positions. It is pointless to obtain perfect control with the patient lying in bed if he faints every time he stands up. One may have to settle for less than perfect control in the recumbent position in order to obtain a tolerable pressure on standing. Nearly all drugs cause some postural hypotension but some are more guilty in this respect than others. It may be worthwhile raising the head of the bed on blocks to make use of this postural response to tilt. This simple measure may assist in lowering the recumbent level. Weakness, lethargy and, in men, impotence are common symptoms at the start of treatment, which is partly why patients so often stop taking their tablets.

Hypotensive therapy has been greatly improved by the advent of a group of drugs called the beta-adrenergic blocking agents (the beta-blockers for short), examples of which are propranolol (Inderal) and oxprenolol (Trasicor). These agents have the great advantage of not causing postural hypotension, neither do they often cause impotence. They may be effective either on their own or in combination with other anti-hypertensives, and they can be used safely in large doses with two exceptions. They may not be given to patients with heart failure or incipient heart failure because this will be made worse. Secondly they aggravate any tendency to asthma or bronchospasm. Beta-blockers are therefore contra-indicated in these conditions. In addition to lowering the blood pressure they also slow the heart rate. This may be very useful when they are given in conjunction with vasolidator hypotensive drugs such as Apresoline, Prazosin, Diazoxide and Minoxidil, all of which are inclined to cause tachycardia. On the other hand the bradycardia caused by beta-blockers may limit the dose one is able to give.

Many hypertensive patients have a casual disregard for their own welfare. It may be difficult to convince them of the need for treatment if they feel better without it. Because of this hypertensives should be followed up with the same zeal as patients with active pulmonary tuberculosis. Renal function should be checked from time to time and also the serum potassium in those who are taking diuretics. Persistence of proteinuria even after good control of hypertension implies continuing renal parenchymal damage and suggests the presence of some underlying disease which also needs attention.

The most severe form of hypertension is malignant hypertension, in which hemorrhages, exudates and papilledema can be seen in the optic fundi. Treatment is urgent in order to prevent complications, but the blood pressure should never be lowered too rapidly. Rapid reduction of blood pressure to normal or hypotensive levels in a patient with malignant hypertension may result in cerebral infarction, permanent blindness, or acute renal failure. If oliguric renal failure occurs in such circumstances there is only a small chance of recovery. Thereafter, the patient may be dependent on dialysis. Gradual reduction of blood pressure in easy stages is always wiser since it allows adequate renal perfusion to continue.

Refractory hypertension

Occasionally, even with the present excellent range of hypotensive drugs, a patient will be found whose blood pressure seems uncontrollable without severe or disabling side-effects such as profound postural hypotension. Oral treatment with Diazoxide may control blood pressure in these cases, but hyperglycemia is a constant complication requiring treatment with oral hypoglycemic agents. It also causes troublesome hypertrichosis (excessive growth of hair). A similar drug, Minoxidil, appears to be even more powerful than Diazoxide. It does not cause postural hypotension, impotence or hyperglycemia though it does produce hypertrichosis. It seems to bring about blood pressure control in the majority of even the most severely hypertensive patients. It is a useful agent in selected cases. Minoxidil occasionally causes pericardial effusions, especially in the presence of fluid retention elsewhere. All the drugs which act as vasodilators also cause fluid retention, and Minoxidil seems to cause more fluid retention than most. It is therefore wise to warn patients about the development of edema and be prepared to use a diuretic to prevent it.

Captopril

Captopril is the best known of a group of drugs which act to inhibit the conversion of renin to angiotensin. Hence, in theory, any hypertension which depends on the presence of high renin production should be helped by the administration of captopril. In practice this means any case of renal hypertension and any case of renal artery stenosis. Captopril has been a very useful addition to our antihypertensive drugs in the last five years but there are two notes of caution which should be sounded.

Firstly, captopril should always be started in small doses. We use half of a tablet, 12.5 mg, as the initial dose until we see what the response to treatment is going to be. Secondly, in renal artery stenosis captopril decreases glomerular perfusion pressure rather dramatically by dilating the efferent arterioles. This can cause a sudden reduction in renal function. In cases of bilateral renal artery stenosis or in a solitary kidney with renal artery stenosis captopril may precipitate acute renal failure. Fortunately it seems to be recoverable when the captopril is stopped.

Diabetic nephropathy

Patients who have had diabetes mellitus for many years are liable to develop a whole series of complications including generalized arteriopathy, cataracts, peripheral neuropathy, retinopathy and nephropathy. Diabetic retinopathy, a major cause of blindness, and nephropathy, the specific renal lesion of diabetes, are frequently found together in the same patient, though one may precede the other. The renal lesion is diabetic glomerulosclerosis. The first suspicion that the patient may be affected by this condition is usually aroused by the finding of proteinuria for the first time on routine urine testing in the out-patient clinic. The proteinuria may be intermittent at first and later persistent and heavy. Renal biopsy, even in the early cases, usually reveals extensive glomerular and arteriolar involvement. The glomeruli gradually lose their delicate structure and become replaced by shapeless masses of tissue which can no longer act as filters. The time scale of the disease is measured in years, and there is often heavy proteinuria amounting to a nephrotic syndrome at the height of the disease. Diuretics may be required to control the edema and hypotensive drugs for the hypertension. In fact meticulous control of blood pressure is the only therapeutic intervention which is widely accepted as being of benefit in slowing down the progress of the renal damage.

However, some of us also believe that meticulous control of blood glucose, such as can be obtained by continuous subcutaneous insulin infusion with an insulin pump, guided by frequent estimations of the capillary blood glucose, also has an effect in stabilizing the renal function. Some patients have also lost their proteinuria in response to this therapy.

Special care must be used when any X-ray contrast studies are ordered in diabetics because there is a danger that they may induce acute renal failure. This danger can be reduced by making sure that the patient is well hydrated.

Diabetics are also more prone than the normal population to development of urinary infection and pyelonephritis. They may also occasionally develop renal papillary necrosis as a further complication of urinary infection. In this condition a renal papilla breaks off in the renal pelvis, often with pain and hematuria, and it may temporarily block the ureter. Urinary infections in diabetics are a common and troublesome cause of loss of control of the diabetes.

The management of renal failure in these patients has undergone a revolution in the last few years. Very good results have been obtained with both hemodialysis and long-term peritoneal dialysis in the form of CAPD (see Chapter 6). Excellent results have also been obtained with renal transplantation. Unfortunately long-term survival rates are still disappointing because of the high incidence of ischemic heart disease. Myocardial infarction is the commonest cause of death in both the dialysis population and transplant recipients. The transplant recipients are also disconcertingly prone to development of peripheral vascular disease requiring amputations of the lower limb.

In spite of these difficulties the management of diabetics with end-stage renal failure has become a cheerful and optimistic exercise such that the patients can retain a remarkable degree of independence and rehabilitation. For example many totally blind diabetics have learned very successfully to do their own CAPD.

Analgesic nephropathy

For a long time now it has been known that regular consumption of large numbers of mixed phenacetin-containing analgesics over a prolonged period can cause severe renal tubular damage and eventually renal failure. This probably occurs because of repeated episodes of renal papillary necrosis leading to scarring and fibrosis in the medulla, called interstitial nephritis. Aspirin−phenacetin−codeine mixtures have been sold all over the world in drug stores under proprietary names without a doctor's prescription. Patients presenting with renal failure due to analgesic nephropathy may admit to taking 6−8 such pills daily for several years. Analgesic nephropathy reached epidemic proportions in Australia where consumption of analgesics became an accepted part of daily living. The role of phenacetin in this condition is not entirely clear because phenacetin is hardly ever taken alone. Aspirin and other simple analgesics when taken alone are probably not entirely harmless to the renal tubules but the weight of present evidence points clearly to mixed phenacetin-containing analgesics as the main cause of damage. Diagnosis is made on the history and the finding of renal tubular damage. Patients hardly ever admit spontaneously to taking these drugs and the information has to be obtained by firm and persistent questioning. In a mild case there may be no loss of glomerular filtration rate but only an impairment of urine concentrating ability. With continued consumption there will be progressive damage and finally chronic renal failure. Not infrequently episodes of renal colic may be caused by fragments of necrotic renal papilla becoming detached and passing down one or other ureter. If the condition can be detected before the damage is too far advanced the patient can usually be persuaded to give up taking analgesics and the disease process will be arrested. There may even be some initial improvement in renal function perhaps due to recovery of nephrons only partially destroyed. The renal tubular damage often causes substantial urinary salt loss so that a high sodium diet may be an important aspect of management. The real answer to this problem lies in proper education of the public to an awareness of the danger of regular analgesic consumption. In countries such as Britain and Canada where phenacetin has been excluded by law from all mixed analgesic preparations, analgesic nephropathy has virtually disappeared, except among immigrants from countries where the drugs are still available.

Polycystic kidney disease

A comparatively common disorder, polycystic kidney disease is inherited as an autosomal Mendelian dominant characteristic. That is to say that it occurs in equal numbers in, and can be transmitted by, both sexes. If either parent has the disease, there is a 50% chance of any of the offspring being born with it. Although congenital, it does not give trouble until adult life when the myriads of tiny cysts in the kidneys start to get big enough to compress the normal kidney tissue. It commonly presents as pain, macroscopic hematuria, or a palpable renal mass. As the cysts get bigger the kidneys may become very large and a proportion of patients develop chronic renal failure progressing to end-stage renal failure by middle age. The occurrence of renal failure is not closely related to kidney size. The disease tends to run a similar course in different members of the same family. For example if the father developed renal failure in his forties the son will probably do the same—though there are exceptions to this. In the early stages patients may need admission to hospital for the hematuria, which may be heavy enough to require blood transfusion, and may occasionally cause clot obstruction of a ureter. Other complications are secondary hypertension and a tendency to superimposed urinary tract infection. There may also be normal or low blood pressure with a sodium-losing stage secondary to failure of sodium reabsorption by the abnormal tubules. Some patients may need a high sodium intake. Young women with polycystic kidneys tend to go through pregnancy quite uneventfully. There is unfortunately no test for diagnosing the condition in the baby either before or after birth. The cysts may be big enough to show up on ultrasound or on a CAT scan by the late teens or early twenties. The disease is not usually considered by the patients or their doctors as a reason for not having children.

The chronic renal failure of polycystic kidney disease is treated like any other cause of chronic renal failure, special attention being paid to treating urinary infection promptly, controlling the blood pressure, and dealing conservatively with any episodes of hematuria.

Management of end-stage renal failure in this condition is more problematical. Long-term peritoneal dialysis may be difficult or impossible because of the presence of the large kidneys. Hemodialysis is usually very satisfactory except during episodes of hematuria when the heparin required for dialysis may aggravate the bleeding. See the section on reduced heparin for hemodialysis, p.249. The kidneys should never be removed except for life-threatening reasons such as recurrent septicemia or massive local infection unresponsive to antibiotics. These patients usually have the advantage of high hemoglobins despite their renal failure, probably because of high erythropoietin production from their kidneys.

The problem of whether or not nephrectomy will be required will have to be debated again if and when the patient is keen to have a kidney transplant. Kidneys should only be removed for specific and compelling reasons and then, if possible, only one. If the transplant fails and the patient has to go back on dialysis with no kidneys at all, the anemia will be severe and disabling. At least one kidney should always be preserved if possible.

Patients with polycystic kidney disease usually have a few cysts in the liver. Generally these cause no trouble but occasionally they also may become infected. More serious is the increased incidence of aneurysms in the cerebral arteries because these may cause death from subarachnoid hemorrhage, though in our experience this has been rare.

Renal amyloidosis

Amyloid is a peculiar infiltrating protein-like material, in the form of a meshwork of fibrils, which has a waxy texture. It tends to localize around blood vessels. It infiltrates various organs of the body including the kidneys, liver, spleen, heart and gastro-intestinal tract. Involvement of the kidneys can be confirmed by renal biopsy. It causes proteinuria, usually of nephrotic degree, and eventually renal failure. The condition is either primary, in which no cause can be found, or secondary to various other conditions, the commonest of which are long-standing sepsis, chronic tuberculosis, and rheumatoid arthritis. If the underlying condition can be eradicated it is sometimes possible to arrest the progress of the amyloid infiltration. Unfortunately it is often not possible to cure the underlying disease.

It is not sufficiently recognized that renal failure from amyloid used to be one of the main causes of death in paraplegics who developed chronic suppurating bed-sores.

Gout

Gout is a familial, in-born error of metabolism in which there is an abnormally high level of uric acid in the blood. This is caused partly by over-production of uric acid and partly by inadequate renal excretion. The part which each of these factors plays varies from one individual to another. Gout damages the body in two main areas, the joints and the kidneys. In the joints it causes a very painful inflammatory arthritis due to the presence of urate crystals. In the kidneys urate crystals may aggregate to form urate calculi. These may grow to fill the renal pelvis or pass down the ureter where they may cause obstruction with ureteric colic. In addition gout may have a progressive destructive effect on renal tissue—mainly the tubular and interstitial tissue which is damaged and replaced by scar tissue, but glomeruli are also involved to some extent in some patients.

Secondary gout is a condition in which a raised uric acid level is due to other diseases which cause excessive uric acid production. Leukemias and the various reticuloses are the commonest causes of secondary gout and the highest uric acid levels are often produced during treatment. Very high levels may result in extensive intrarenal urate crystallization with anuria. This is called acute uric acid nephropathy and requires treatment by dialysis. Less dramatic gouty renal damage, of the chronic or calculous variety, can now be treated very satisfactorily by the drug allopurinol. This blocks the conversion of xanthine in the body to uric acid and so diminishes uric acid production. The drug has very few and infrequent side-effects and always succeeds in lowering blood uric acid levels.

A simpler method of avoiding formation of uric acid calculi is to take sufficient sodium bicarbonate to keep the urine alkaline at all times. This is because sodium urate is much more soluble than uric acid. This method may be adequate by itself in somè cases.

Renal tuberculosis

This disease is fortunately disappearing but we must still be on the alert for it because occasionally it turns up unexpectedly. It used to be associated with long-standing pulmonary tuberculosis which may not have been treated. Nowadays patients discovered to have renal tuberculosis often have no pulmonary involvement. The disease usually starts with caseating tubercles in the papillae of the renal medulla of one or both kidneys. Later the infection may spread down to involve the ureter and bladder. From here the infection may spread up the opposite ureter to involve the other kidney. Tuberculosis of the ureter and bladder causes scarring and deformity and loss of bladder capacity. Troublesome frequency is therefore common. Another characteristic finding is leukocytes in the urine but no bacteria on culture—so called sterile pyuria. This should always raise the suspicion of urinary tuberculosis. Later hematuria may also occur. An IVU may suggest the diagnosis which can be confirmed by culture and guinea pig inoculation. It should always be remembered that urinary tuberculosis may be masked by the presence of superimposed pyogenic infection. Suspicion may be aroused if heavy pyuria persists after eradication of bacterial infection. Prolonged antituberculosis therapy for at least two years will be required. Occasionally a severely damaged kidney must be removed surgically.

Urinary schistosomiasis (bilharzia)

This is a protozoan infestation caused by the parasite *Schistosoma haematobium*. The parasite, which is found mainly in parts of Africa and Asia, is carried in small fresh-water snails in stagnant ponds and rivers. It penetrates the skin of children paddling or bathing in the water so that in some regions as many as 70% of the children are affected. Damage occurs to the bladder and ureters with a low-grade inflammatory process causing extensive scarring. The main symptom is hematuria. Treatment is by compounds of antimony, the most successful of which has been sodium antimonyl dimercaptosuccinate given as an intramuscular injection in a dose of 10 mg per kg body weight. In endemic areas patients are given one injection every six months. Schistosomiasis is not normally seen in temperate climates unless the patient has spent time living in an endemic area abroad. There is now a reliable serological test for the diagnosis of schistosomiasis, so that a negative test can safely be used to exclude the disease.

Renal calculi

If kidney stones are properly dealt with they should never lead to renal failure; but stones in the urinary tract are the commonest cause of renal colic (also called ureteric colic). Ureteric colic, one of the most agonizing pains people may be called upon to suffer, is caused by painful muscular contractions of the ureter which is trying to propel the stone down towards the bladder. The majority of stones which form on or close to the renal papillae as a result of solutes in the urine coming out of solution are aggregates of crystals which slowly get larger until they break off and pass down the ureter. The majority are expelled spontaneously with attacks of ureteric colic, sometimes accompanied by visible hematuria and very often by microscopic hematuria.

Nearly all renal calculi have a metabolic cause in the form of too much of some substance in the urine, so that the urine cannot keep it in solution and it precipitates or crystallizes out. The main causes are too much calcium, too much oxalate, too much uric acid and, more rarely, too much cystine. The pH of the urine is also very important. For example, calcium tends to precipitate and forms stones if the urine is too alkaline, uric acid forms stones if the urine is too acid. Cystine stones have only one cause and that is a rare disease called cystinuria in which there is over-excretion in the urine of cystine and some other amino acids. Calcium stones are much the commonest and are twice as common in men as in women. The commonest cause is a condition called idiopathic hypercalciuria. This simply means too much calcium in the urine due to a constitutional defect rather than due to some other disease such as hyperparathyroidism or sarcoidosis. The main points in the management of renal calculi are as follows.

• Give powerful analgesics such as meperidine or morphine for the ureteric colic. No one should have to suffer pain of this severity without this help being given straight away.

• Make sure that the stones are passed. If they are not passed they should be removed in some way by a urologist. There are now some very sophisticated ways being developed to remove stones without open surgery.

• Once the stone is gone it is essential to find out why the patient formed the stone in the first place. All the metabolic abnormalities are capable of being corrected to make sure the patient does not form stones again.

Urologists are extremely skilled in finding ways to remove stones and standards tend to be very high. Regrettably nurses and doctors have not generally been so effective in promptly relieving the pain of ureteric colic or in conscientiously following up to investigate the cause afterwards. This latter process has to be done very carefully with timed urine collections to study excretion rates of various substances. We can all play an important role in reminding patients of the importance of having this done. If the underlying metabolic cause is not identified and corrected the patient will be back with another stone.

4

Renal Failure

Robert Uldall

Always keep a urine sample in a suspected case of renal failure. This is the most important step one can take towards making a diagnosis.

When kidney function is impaired to such an extent that the health of the individual is affected, renal failure can be said to be present. It is useful at the outset to classify the three main types of renal failure because each type has entirely different implications for prognosis and management. The three categories are:

- acute renal failure,
- chronic renal failure,
- end-stage renal failure (terminal).

Acute renal failure is usually of sudden or rapid onset, coming within a few hours or days and it is nearly always recoverable. The average duration is about two weeks, and during this time renal function is nearly always sufficiently reduced that the affected patient has to come into hospital. Although recovery may occasionally occur spontaneously without the need for medical intervention it is more usual to have to intervene to save the patient's life, often by means of a period of temporary dialysis. Unfortunately the mortality rate in acute renal failure is still depressingly high but death, if it occurs, is usually due to the underlying condition which led to the renal failure rather than to the renal failure itself. A small proportion of the total group of patients with acute renal failure remain in renal failure which then becomes end-stage or terminal renal failure.

The second main category, chronic renal failure, means renal damage or impairment which is usually slow and often, though not always, progressive. The kidneys are sufficiently damaged that health is affected but most patients can continue to function fairly well outside hospital. This is because failure is incomplete and patients can manage to live active and useful lives even though they have only a small proportion of their original renal function. Most of the kidney diseases mentioned in the last chapter can cause chronic renal failure and in many cases the degree of damage may remain stable, without progressing appreciably for a number of years. Such patients benefit from careful out-patient supervision; and a number of simple measures may greatly improve their health without actually repairing the kidney damage. Exciting new advances in knowledge of the mechanisms at work in chronic renal failure seem to indicate that careful dietary management of these patients may help to preserve their residual renal function. Hence there is a great resurgence of interest in the active management of chronic renal failure, in contrast to the somewhat pessimistic and passive attitude we had to this condition in the past. However, in spite of all the active measures that can be applied to try to preserve renal function in chronic renal failure, many of the diseases which cause it are in themselves inherently and inexorably progressive. Hence a large proportion of patients with chronic renal failure ultimately progress to end-stage or terminal renal failure.

End-stage renal failure, as the name implies, means that the kidneys are unable any longer to keep the patient alive, even with the best conservative measures that can be provided either in or out of hospital. These patients provide the bulk of the work which is presently being done by kidney centers all over the world. The only ways to preserve life are dialysis and/or kidney transplantantion. End-stage renal failure is also correctly called terminal renal failure. However, many people object to this word because 'terminal' in the minds of the public seems to imply death—rather like terminal cancer; and for most patients in the affluent countries of the western world end-stage renal failure is just another disability which has to be coped with, rather like learning to use an artificial limb to help you to walk after an amputation.

The words chronic and end-stage are often used interchangeably; this is incorrect. One hears, for example, of chronic renal failure being treated by dialysis, whereas a patient with chronic renal failure by definition does not need dialysis, since in this condition renal damage is only partial. What can happen occasionally is that a patient with chronic renal failure may develop a superimposed acute insult to his kidneys resulting in temporary complete failure—acute on chronic. This may lead to the need for dialysis for a few days or even weeks but the acute component of the damage is usually reversible and the patient then goes back to his previous independent state of managing quite well to live with his chronic renal failure.

So the word 'chronic' should not be used for patients with end-stage renal failure, nor to describe their dialysis, which should be described as regular or long-term dialysis.

Acute renal failure

The management of acute renal failure is exceedingly demanding but also tremendously worthwhile and gratifying to everybody if the patient survives. This is because once the renal failure has recovered the patient may be completely independent of all medical help thereafter. The kidneys are about the only vital organs in the body which can fail completely for a significant period of time and yet recover to function normally for the rest of the patient's life. An equivalent period of total failure of the heart, lungs or liver cannot be survived because for these other organs there is, as yet, no adequate artificial substitute. Morover, the kidneys are particularly vulnerable to temporary damage and also remarkably capable of recovery to normal function if given time for healing to occur.

The peculiar vulnerability of the kidneys to acute damage has several causes of which the following are undoubtedly the most important.

Although the kidneys under resting conditions receive a very large blood flow, about 25% of the cardiac output, in keeping with their function of continuously purifying the blood, they do not need this amount of blood for their nutrition. Under conditions of strenuous exercise they can manage with much less blood, which is diverted to exercising limbs. Similarly under conditions of blood volume depletion resulting from hemorrhage, dehydration, extensive burns, etc., a process of renal vasoconstriction directs blood to more essential areas such as the brain. As long as this vasoconstriction is not too severe or prolonged the only penalty suffered by the individual is temporary reduction in renal perfusion and function. Renal function will return as soon as blood volume and full renal perfusion are restored. We have all observed the fact that we tend to produce only a small volume of concentrated urine during a prolonged period of physical exertion. Normal urine volumes return when we go back to a resting state. This is the physiological counterpart of that which takes place during a period of temporary shock. If, however, hypotension and low renal perfusion last too long, ischemic damage will be sustained by the most vulnerable part of the nephron, that is the proximal tubules which are metabolically very active with large requirements for oxygen. When blood volume and renal perfusion are restored it is found that the tubules have suffered temporary acute ischemic damage, a condition wrongly called acute tubular necrosis. The reason this is a bad term is that the tubules are not necrotic as such, only temporarily damaged. On renal biopsy they can be seen to be thin and dilated and separated by interstitial edema (see Fig. 4.1) The condition is more appropriately called acute ischemic nephropathy. But the term acute tubular necrosis (ATN for short) has become so firmly implanted by tradition that it will probably continue to be used for a long time yet.

The other main reason why kidneys are so vulnerable to acute damage is that they are the main route whereby toxic substances are removed from the body. During the removal of such substances, by excretion through the tubules, they are concentrated, sometimes as much as thirty times. So the concentration at the end of the nephron is thirty times higher than that in the blood. This is the second main mechanism of acute renal damage. Substances which are slightly toxic in the body become highly toxic when they have been concentrated in the luminal fluid of the renal tubules to a many times greater concentration. For example, the breakdown products of damaged skeletal muscle, which include the golden-brown pigment myoglobulin, are toxic to the renal tubules and may cause temporary acute renal failure. The same applies to many other poisonous substances such as carbon tetrachloride and inorganic mercury. These latter substances are also toxic to the liver; but the liver usually recovers on its own within a few days. The kidneys

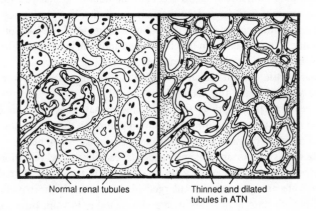

Normal renal tubules   Thinned and dilated
                              tubules in ATN

Fig. 4.1. The left hand panel shows the appearance of normal renal tubules. On the right are seen the thinned and dilated tubules typical of ATN.

usually remain shut down for two weeks or so and during this period
the patient would die without dialysis. Certain antibiotics such as the
aminoglycosides, gentamicin for example, will cause renal tubular damage
if the blood level goes too high. This is why renal impairment predisposes to more renal damage.

Temporary excretory failure will lead to a higher blood level which
then becomes toxic. The majority of cases of acute renal failure derive
from one of these two mechanisms.

Recognition of acute renal failure

In most patients with acute renal failure the condition is recognized by
the development of oliguria. Oliguria is defined as a fall in urine volume
to less than 400 ml a day. In a patient who is on closed bladder drainage
this translates to less than 20 ml per hour and persisting hour after
hour. This would then be called oliguric acute renal failure. However,
not all patients with acute renal failure have oliguria. Patients with acute
ischemic nephropathy, described above, are most often oliguric but may
have normal or even increased urine volumes. This is because a few
remaining nephrons are still excreting large volumes of dilute urine even
though the majority are shut down. This is rather analogous to the
situation in chronic renal failure, except that in acute non-oliguric renal
failure the majority of nephrons are temporarily non-functioning whereas
in chronic renal failure the majority of the nephrons are permanently
destroyed.

The point about non-oliguric acute renal failure is that you will miss
the diagnosis if you depend only on urine volumes for your assessment.
Diagnosis in this case depends on finding a rising level of blood urea and
creatinine. The lesson from this is that you must measure blood levels in
any patient who might be at risk of developing acute renal damage
because of the clinical situation. Otherwise in non-oliguric acute renal
failure you may miss the diagnosis completely.

The third possibility is that the patient may present with anuria.
Anuria means literally no urine at all coming through the bladder catheter.
A patient may be passing no urine at all because of a bladder outlet
obstruction such as an enlarged prostate causing acute retention. But
acute retention should quickly be recognized by the medical staff who
will palpate and percuss the enlarged bladder, even if the patient does
not complain bitterly of a full bladder and inability to void. Insertion of a
catheter will settle the matter. Anuria can only be diagnosed with certainty
after bladder catheterization.

What is the importance of anuria as opposed to oliguria? The importance is that if you confidently diagnose anuria it can only be caused by one of two things, complete obstruction of both ureters or complete devascularization of both kidneys. All the other causes of acute intrinsic renal damage causing acute renal failure are accompanied by some urine output. Theoretically you could have a mixture of the two, e.g. one kidney long since non-functioning due to renal artery embolus and then complete obstruction of the contralateral ureter leading to acute renal failure; but this is unlikely.

If you do diagnose anuria you have a duty to find out urgently whether the problem is ureteric obstruction or loss of blood supply to the kidneys. The point is that both these conditions are potentially remediable. The clinical situation may give you a clue. If the patient has a large malignant growth in the pelvis, bilateral ureteric compression is the most likely diagnosis. On the other hand if the patient has a long history of renovascular hypertension it is possible that both renal arteries have become blocked, one after the other. In this case the diagnosis can be confirmed by a renal scan and arteriograms, and, contrary to what you might think, the kidneys are probably still capable of being saved. A collateral circulation thrugh ureteric and capsular vessels may well be keeping the kidneys alive—or at least one of them. A surgical by-pass graft can restore the blood supply.

Bilateral ureteric obstruction will be diagnosed by retrograde ureteric catheterization, and it may be possible to relieve the obstruction. A word should be said here about relieving obstruction of the ureters in cases of inoperable cancer. Temporary relief of obstruction by means of a ureteric catheter or even by means of an indwelling stent (protruding into the renal pelvis at one end and into the bladder at the other end) is perfectly legitimate to prevent the patient's early demise from the complications of acute renal failure. But permanent relief of obstruction by a urinary diversion operation is totally unjustified. This is because the patient will survive the uremia to die a much more painful death later when the cancer invades the bones and nerves of the pelvis. Death from uremia in pelvic cancer is a relatively painless way to die.

Enough about anuria. Let us go back to the more common problem of the patient with oliguria.

When faced with an oliguric patient with uremia the differential diagnosis is:
- pre-renal uremia,
- renal (intrinsic to the kidneys) uremia,
- post-renal uremia.

Pre-renal uremia

This means oliguria due to inadequate blood volume and therefore low renal perfusion.

Table 4.1. Causes of acute renal failure.

Pre-renal
Shock
Hemorrhage
Dehydration
Burns
Low plasma oncotic pressure (children)

Post-renal
Malignant compression of ureters
Retroperitoneal fibrosis
Bilateral ureteric stone
Bilateral ureteric blood clot
Blocked ureter from necrotic papilla
Unilateral ureteric obstruction—non-functioning kidney on other side

Intrinsic renal
Acute ischemic nephropathy (ATN)
    post-traumatic
    skeletal muscle injury
    aortic aneurysm surgery
    obstetric hemorrhage
    Gram-negative septicemia
    surgery in presence of obstructive jaundice
    myocardial infarction
    acute hemorrhagic pancreatitis
Acute post-streptococcal glomerulonephritis
Rapidly progressive glomerulonephritis
Acute allergic interstitial nephritis
Fulminating pyelonephritis
Acute uric acid nephropathy
Acute nephrotoxicity
    drugs
    poisons
    X-ray contrast media in diabetics and patients with multiple myeloma

---

The common causes are blood loss due to trauma, surgery and spontaneous bleeding from the gastro-intestinal tract, and dehydration due to diarrhea and vomiting or extensive burns. Intravascular volume depletion can also occur as a result of loss of intravascular water into some other tissue compartment such as the interstitial space. For example a small child may have massive generalized edema, 'anasarca' and a greatly reduced intravascular volume due to proteinuria causing loss of colloid osmotic pressure. Water has gone from the blood compartment into the tissues. In all these patients the urine output and renal function should rapidly return if the appropriate fluid is replaced. The patient in shock from hemorrhage will respond to blood transfusion. The dehydrated patient with cholera will respond to large volumes of water and electrolytes. The small child with nephrotic syndrome will benefit from administration of intravenous albumin.

However, these same conditions which cause pre-renal uremia are also well-known causes of acute ischemic nephropathy and established acute intrinsic renal failure. How can one be sure which condition one is dealing with? One answer is to try replacing what is needed and see what happens to the urine output. The trouble with that approach is that you may overdo it. What if the patient has established acute renal failure and we have just administered a large volume of fluid which the patient cannot excrete? Fortunately there are some very helpful tests to guide us. Save a sample of urine for biochemical and microscopic examination. The patient with oliguria due to volume depletion has a concentrated urine with a high specific gravity (1028 or higher) and a high osmolality (800 mosm/kg or more). The urine sodium will be very low (less than 10 mmol/l) indicating active tubular reabsorption of sodium. The urine urea will be high (greater than 40 mmol/l). Furthermore, there should be no protein in the urine and no casts.

In contrast to this, the patient with established ATN will have a low urine osmolality (less than 400 mosm/kg), a high urine sodium (greater than 70 mmol/l) and a low urine urea (less than 20 mmol/l). The patient with ATN will also have protein in the urine and characteristically on microscopy we should see the hallmark of ATN, pigmented granular casts (often called heme-granular casts). If the results of examining the urine are not as clear-cut as this and there is some doubt whether the patient will be helped by volume replacement we can use the central venous pressure to guide us and we can watch the patient closely for any signs of fluid overload, such as a raised jugular venous pressure, and fine crepitations at the bases of the lungs.

It is also quite legitimate to use a diagnostic trial of intravenous mannitol, 25 g given over about 20 minutes, while we watch the output into the urine drainage bag. We may also wish to use a large intravenous dose of furosemide (frusemide) 500−1000 mg. Furosemide is very non-toxic and very safe. If there is no response to this even after adequate volume replacement we can assume that there is established acute renal failure.

At the same time that we are dealing with pre-renal factors and making sure that the patient does not have pre-renal uremia, we should also be thinking of the possibility of a post-renal cause. We have said that complete anuria implies no blood flow to the kidneys or bilateral ureteric obstruction. Unfortunately the absence of anuria does not rule out ureteric obstruction. Ureteric obstruction may cause oliguria and may even be associated with a normal urine volume. So if there is any chance that obstruction may be present it has to be excluded. Diagnostic ultrasound may be helpful by demonstrating a dilated renal pelvis or a dilated ureter or both. But if one is still in doubt one has no choice but to carry out cystoscopy and retrograge ureteric catheterization. Acute relief of the obstruction, if this can be by-passed with a catheter, will also deal with the renal failure in the majority of cases by simply allowing the kidneys to drain.

It should be mentioned here that long-standing obstruction may lead to a state of polyuria when the obstruction is relieved. Though this is uncommon it may be seen after long-standing prostatic obstruction. A catheter is placed in the bladder and the patient passes 9–10 litres of urine per day. If fluid and electrolytes are not replaced the patient will very quickly become dehydrated. This is thought to be a kind of nephrogenic diabetes insipidus, caused by long-standing back pressure on the lower part of the nephron. The good news is that it always recovers eventually, though it may take several weeks.

Prevention of acute renal failure

Since the majority of cases of ATN are caused by shock, blood volume depletion or prolonged hypotension, the best way to prevent ATN is to prevent shock. In practice this is done by prompt and adequate transfusion of blood and other appropriate fluids. In fact the incidence of many forms of renal failure, particularly the surgical and obstetric groups, has declined rapidly since the need for adequate transfusion has become widely known. Raising the blood pressure by the use of vasopressor compounds, which act by producing vasoconstriction, is no substitute for transfusion. These compounds are usually positively harmful since they also cause renal vasoconstriction. The actual level of the blood pressure is not nearly so important as the state of perfusion of the peripheral parts. If the hands and feet are warm, it is likely that the kidneys are also being adequately perfused. If the hands and feet are cold and clammy, the kidneys are likely to be in danger. These observations can be made on any seriously ill patient within a few seconds and are extremely valuable.

If blood is not immediately available for volume replacement, reconstituted dried plasma is probably the best substitute. It is likely that plasma protein solution will be more generally available in future. This has the important advantage that it is known to be free of hepatitis virus. For this reason it is likely to take the place of reconstituted dried plasma. Great caution should be exercised in the use of artificial dextrans. Low molecular weight dextrans such as rheomacrodex are not recommended for the treatment of shock because they themselves have been shown to cause osmotic damage to the renal tubules, so-called osmotic nephrosis. Certainly they should not be given to patients who are oliguric; and if they are administered, blood samples for crossmatching should be taken first, since dextrans are inclined to interfere with cross-matching techniques.

A special and rather mysterious form of ATN is that caused by operations on patients with obstructive jaundice. Acute renal failure may occur post-operatively even when there has been no shock or hypotension. It has been shown now that this can nearly always be prevented by the use of mannitol infused intravenously during the anesthetic—so much so that this has become standard practice among anesthetists at this type of operation.

Renal damage from nephrotoxic substances can sometimes be prevented or reduced by prompt use of an antidote (e.g. BAL for mercuric chloride poisoning) or exchange transfusion to remove the poison (as in arsine poisoning).

An important obligation of medical and nursing staff in this field should be to prevent renal damage from overdoses of drugs. Drugs which are nephrotoxic in high serum concentrations must therefore be given very cautiously and with reduced frequency in patients with impaired renal function especially if their main route of excretion is by the kidneys. The main antibiotics which cause renal damage are polymyxin, kanamycin and gentamicin. Neomycin is so nephrotoxic that it is rarely given intramuscularly.

Tetracycline is now known to be highly catabolic in its effects and is probably nephrotoxic to some extent. It may precipitate acute renal failure if administered in normal doses to patients with chronic renal impairment. The only tetracycline which is free of these disadvantages is Vibramycin (doxycycline). This can be given in a normal dose of 100 mg daily for an adult.

Nitrofurantoin (Furadantin) should be avoided in patients with renal impairment since it may cause polyneuritis if blood levels rise too high.

Cephalosporins, especially cephaloridine, are nephrotoxic when given in conjunction with Lasix (furosemide) and this combination should not be used.

Carbenicillin, which is used for the treatment of *Pseudomonas* infections, must be given in reduced dosage in patients with acute renal failure who are on dialysis. If given in full dosage it may cause a severe and dangerous bleeding condition from the mouth and gastro-intestinal tract. One should always observe carefully for signs of oozing from the buccal mucosa if a patient with acute renal failure is on carbenicillin.

It is a good rule to check renal function by a blood urea or creatinine estimation before any of these drugs are used. The long-term effects of mixed analgesic ingestion have been described in Chapter 3. Sclerosing agents used to inject varicose veins inevitably leak into the general circulation to some extent and may cause renal damage if the stated dose is exceeded. Finally, intravenous X-ray contrast media should be avoided in patients with myelomatosis because they may precipitate acute renal failure due to widespread cast obstruction of the tubules. It is equally important to avoid any form of dehydration in patients with multiple myeloma for the same reason. Some people believe that the dehydration is more harmful than the contrast medium. The same warning applies to carrying out any X-ray examination in a diabetic if it involves use of contrast medium. Diabetics who already have some chronic renal impairment are especially susceptible to further acute renal damage; this may be only partially recoverable. The rule should be to avoid contrast media in diabetics wherever possible but, if it is necessary to use them, always make sure the patient remains well hydrated throughout. The patient must be told that the study is a calculated risk and informed consent must be obtained.

Diagnosis of other causes of acute renal failure

If there is any doubt about the cause of acute renal failure, after excluding pre-renal and post-renal causes, we have to look more carefully at the kidneys themselves. For example, there may be no history or special features to suggest acute ischemic nephropathy. The patient may simply be in renal failure with no obvious explanation. An assessment of renal size at this point is very important. If the kidneys are normal or only slightly reduced in size, we have to assume that the kidney disease is potentially recoverable. If, on the other hand, the kidneys are less than 7 cm in length on both sides, we know that this is some end-stage process and there is no point in looking further. Even if you are curious to know what the disease was that destroyed the kidneys, a biopsy at this stage probably will not help you, because it will show only scar tissue. In the late stages all renal parenchymal disease looks the same. If the patient has normal sized kidneys as shown by the plain abdominal X-ray or the ultrasound examination, a biopsy should be the next step. However, a patient in acute renal failure, who needs a biopsy for diagnosis, must have dialysis first. The reasons are as follows. Uremia predisposes to bleeding and if the patient bleeds after the renal biopsy, in the form of a large peri-renal hematoma, dialysis then becomes more urgent because of the blood clot leading to tissue breakdown and a further rapid rise in blood urea. Peritoneal dialysis is impossible in the presence of a large retroperitoneal hematoma because all the dialysate will be drawn by the colloid osmotic pressure into the hematoma space. Hemodialysis is dangerous because of the heparin which is likely to set off or aggravate the bleeding.

Therefore, we should never put ourselves in the position of having to dialyse a patient who has just bled after a renal biopsy. The patient should be thoroughly dialysed before the biopsy. Bleeding will then be less likely, and, even if it occurs, dialysis is not likely to be required again, at least for a few days. Renal biopsy for unexplained acute renal failure is normally best performed with diagnostic ultrasound to guide the operator to the safe spot at the lower pole of the kidney. An intravenous urogram is unlikely to be helpful to localize the kidney in this type of case because with impaired renal function there will not be enough contrast medium to allow the kidneys to be seen clearly.

The biopsy will be performed as soon as possible after a thorough dialysis; and the slides showing the light microscopy should be available within 24 hours. A number of the well-known causes of acute renal failure can now be treated with an excellent prospect for a successful outcome. Examples are steroid therapy for acute allergic interstitial nephritis, and immunosuppressive therapy with plasma exchange for Goodpasture's syndrome. Most patients with rapidly progressive glomerulonephritis also respond to treatment nowadays if it is started early enough.

Other conditions such as acute hypercalcemic renal failure and acute uric acid nephropathy, the diagnosis of which will probably be made on clinical and biochemical information, will usually respond very well to dialysis.

Management of acute renal faillure

Once a patient has been firmly diagnosed as having ATN we can anticipate on average a 14-day period of oliguria. During and for some time after this period he will be in a highly vulnerable state. Acute renal failure is accepted as being the special province of the renal physician. On being consulted he will probably want the patient to be transferred immediately to his care. To delay referral and transfer to a special unit may be to risk the patient's life. If we can remind ourselves of the main functions of the kidneys described in Chapter 1 we will soon appreciate the problems caused by acute loss of those functions. The various problems and how they can be dealt with will now be considered in turn.

Water

Even if hydration is normal at the onset of ATN, failure to excrete water will rapidly lead to overhydration with heart failure, pulmonary congestion, or cerebral edema unless water is judiciously restricted. An average man loses 700−800 ml of water in 24 hours by insensible losses from the skin and the lungs. His endogenous production of water in normal metabolic processes in the body is 200−300 ml/24 hours. The net loss excluding any urine is therefore about 500 ml/24 hours. The loss will be proportionately greater if fever causes excessive sweating. Other losses such as from a nasogastric tube or from diarrhea must also be taken into account. Under normal circumstances, and if no extra losses exist, the daily fluid allowance should be 500 ml plus the volume of the previous day's urine output. Hydration should be controlled by an accurately kept intake and output chart and checked by daily weighing—preferably at the same time each day.

Nitrogenous waste products

With the onset of ATN the rate of rise of blood urea will depend on the rate of urea production from tissue breakdown, infection, starvation and other factors. If there is no infection or injury, blood urea may rise quite slowly, perhaps only 5−15 mmol/l (14−42 mg/dl) per day. In severe multiple injuries such as road traffic accidents there will be a high catabolic rate with a correspondingly rapid rise in blood urea, up to 50 mmol/l (140 mg/dl) per day. A high calorie diet has a protein-sparing effect and it has also been shown that a small amount of first-class protein is preferable to no protein at all. The modern trend is to keep the patient as well nourished as possible and to use dialysis early and frequently to control the uremia. The choice of whether to use peritoneal dialysis or hemodialysis is discussed more fully in the next chapter. In general, one tends to use peritoneal dialysis in uncomplicated acute renal failure with a low catabolic rate. Hemodialysis, being more efficient, is always used when the catabolic rate is high, and in some cases dialysis may be necessary every day. If it is anticipated that hemodialysis will be necessary, the patient should be transferred to a special center with appropriate facilities as soon as possible. This will allow the staff time to assess the patient and carry out essential procedures such as the placing of a shunt in an arm or leg to obtain access to the circulation. No matter where the patient is treated or by what dialysis method, blood must be obtained for estimation of urea and electrolytes and preferably also serum creatinine every day. In seriously ill patients more frequent estimations may be necessary.

Electrolytes

You will remember from Chapter 1 that sodium is the main cation controlling the volume of the extracellular fluid. Sodium overloading tends to precipitate hypertension, heart failure and pulmonary edema. Sodium deficiency causes hypotension and peripheral circulatory failure. During ATN the patient is unable either to excrete or conserve sodium so that his intake must be carefully controlled. Abnormal losses from the gastro-intestinal tract must be replaced but if there are no such losses sodium intake should be restricted to a minimum. It is possible to provide a nourishing diet containing no more than 20–30 mmol sodium per day. If sodium excess is threatening the patient, the only way to remove it is by dialysis. Sodium deficiency can be corrected by dietary intake if there is no urgency or by intravenous saline infusion if speed is essential.

Serum potassium rises progressively during ATN unless there are abnormal potassium losses from diarrhea, nasogastric suction or vomiting. Hyperkalemia used to be a frequent cause of death before the advent of dialysis and other methods for controlling it. Any level above 6 mmol/l is dangerous, though cardiac arrest seldom occurs at levels below 7.5 mmol/l. The greater the tissue damage the faster will be the rise in serum potassium. A low potassium diet and frequent dialysis are usually adequate to control serum potassium, but in an emergency the following methods may be used.

• 10 ml of a 10% solution of calcium gluconate given intravenously will not change the serum potassium level but will tend to counteract the toxic effects of potassium on the heart.

• Insulin given in combination with glucose intravenously makes potassium go into the cells. 20 units of soluble insulin and 50 g glucose are commonly used.

• If, as is often the case in ATN, the patient has a degree of metabolic acidosis, intravenous infusion of alkali in the form of sodium bicarbonate rapidly lowers serum potassium by correcting the acidosis and making potassium enter the cells. The medical staff can work out the right dose by a glance at the serum electrolytes. Sodium bicarbonate 8.4% solution is useful because it contains 1 mmol bicarbonate per ml.

• These first three methods of dealing with hyperkalemia are very efficient but also very temporary. They merely buy time until something else can be done. If, at this point, dialysis still has to be postponed for some reason, use should be made of cation exchange resins. These are substances which, when placed in the gastro-intestinal tract, exchange another cation for potassium. The most effective by far is the sodium containing resin called Kayexalate (in Britain, Resonium A). It can be given in a dose of 15 g three or four times a day by mouth or 40 g rectally every four hours. It is a powder which has to be made into a thin paste with water. Nauseated patients may not tolerate it by mouth (it has an unpleasant taste) and it should never be given orally to feeble or seriously ill patients who may vomit and inhale it into the lungs. It is extremely effective and safe when given rectally as a high retention enema in a creamy consistency. The rectum should be irrigated with saline after four hours before the next dose is given. This is important. If the old resin is not removed it will harden like a block of cement. In one patient this led to rupture of the colon with fatal results. The effects of Kayexalate are quite long-lasting and serum potassium can be kept down for a considerable time by this method.

• Dialysis is the main method used during acute renal failure for lowering serum potassium. Both peritoneal dialysis and hemodialysis are very efficient in this respect.

Magnesium is not normally a problem during acute renal failure unless soluble magnesium salts are administered in error (see p.31). Certain conditions such as prolonged gastro-intestinal losses and severe burns may cause hypomagnesemia. Under these circumstances soluble magnesium salts may have to be infused intravenously.

Acid—base balance

Patients with acute renal failure are usually acidotic unless they have lost a lot of gastric hydrochloric acid by vomiting. Acidosis may lead to hyperventilation, it aggravates hyperkalemia, and it predisposes to cardiac arrythmias. Intravenous infusion of sodium bicarbonate will control the acidosis but one has to be careful not to overload the patient with sodium. Dialysis corrects the acidosis and this is usually sufficient provided it is done frequently enough.

Infection

For reasons which are not fully understood, uremia predisposes to infection. Patients with acute renal failure are very liable to develop infections of various kinds. The common infections are those of the skin, mouth, salivary glands, urinary tract and lungs. Septicemia is also quite common. The methods which should be adopted for dealing with infection are as follows.

- Frequent dialysis for optimal control of uremia.
- Culture of all infected or potentially infected sites, e.g. blood culture if the patient develops fever, sputum culture at the earliest sign of chest infection, swabs of any infected skin lesions. Throat swabs and urine cultures should be done routinely even if there is no clinical evidence of infection. Obtaining these cultures is frequently a responsibility of the nursing staff.
- Good oral hygiene and good skin hygiene. Bladder catheters should never be left in unless there is a compelling reason. Accurate recording of urine output is not a justification for long-term use of a catheter.
- Barrier nursing in pressurized, clean-air cubicles is desirable in some cases and this facility is certainly useful if it is available.
- Prompt and adequate antibiotic therapy as soon as infection is recognized. Bacterial sensitivities may dictate a change in treatment when the cultures become available. Medical staff will also have to modify the dose of those antibiotics whose accumulation in renal failure may cause toxic effects.

With prompt and thorough treatment it should be possible to eradicate the majority of infections. It should not be forgotten that while infections are active they will increase uremia by increasing tissue breakdown and urea production.

Bleeding

Uremia causes a bleeding tendency because of its effects on platelets. Though total numbers of platelets may be normal or quite adequate there is a qualitative defect of platelets which makes them less efficient in stopping bleeding. The defect disappears when uremia is corrected. With the modern trend towards early and frequent dialysis, bleeding has become less of a problem.

Anemia

At the onset of acute renal failure a normal person has a normal hemo-globin unless there has been an acute blood loss. Anemia gradually develops and progresses as long as the uremia lasts. The anemia then disappears when the renal failure recovers. This anemia is more of a problem in chronic renal failure, and will be discussed in more detail later. Its main causes are mentioned on pp.304−310. If the hemoglobin becomes too low there is no alternative to blood transfusion.

Epilepsy

Uremia predisposes to major seizures and there is a further risk of epilepsy as a result of the dialysis disequilibrium syndrome (see p.276). It is therefore quite common to place patients with acute renal failure on anticonvulsant therapy throughout their illness. This can be withdrawn during convalescence. Phenobarbitone is a useful drug as also is sodium phenytoin. These can be given orally, or by intravenous injection if the oral route is unreliable because the patient is too ill. A small practical point is to avoid giving sodium phenytoin through the rubber diaphragm of an intravenous infusion line. It will solidify and block the infusion. It is poorly absorbed when given intramuscularly.

Pericarditis

This may occur in acute renal failure but is commoner in chronic renal failure (see p.117).

The diuretic phase

About 10−14 days after the onset of ATN most patients begin to show an increase in urine output. This is gradual at first but later increases rapidly. At first the urine is dilute with a low urea content so that blood urea will continue to rise after dialysis. Then after a few days the blood urea will begin to level off and fall spontaneously. Renal function gradually increases and it may be several months or up to a year before it returns completely to normal. A minority of patients are left with a legacy of permanent though usually slight renal impairment. During the early diuretic phase there may be an excessive loss of sodium and potassium and the electrolytes have to be watched carefully. It is common to have to give oral potassium supplements at this time. Fluid intake is calculated on the same basis as before with appropriate increases to keep pace with urine output. Once the patient is ambulant and free of uremia and infection he can be discharged from hospital to receive further medical surveillance as an out-patient. The patient who has been on hemodialysis will have his shunt (or his subclavian catheter) removed before he leaves. These procedures are described fully in Chapter 7.

Chronic renal failure

Chronic renal failure really means irreversible destruction of kidney tissue of severe degree. It is usually caused by one of the main kidney diseases described in the last chapter but other rare conditions crop up from time to time. A minor degree of impairment of renal function causes no symptoms and no disability. It is only when the majority of the functioning nephrons have been destroyed that the blood urea begins to rise and other abnormalities appear which cause symptoms. One of the first things to happen is a loss of ability to concentrate the urine. The damaged kidneys tend to produce a large volume of dilute urine. One of the first symptoms is inability to sleep right through the night without getting up to pass urine. Thirst and polyuria then develop during the day. Uremia tends to be associated with anemia, and anemia makes the patient feel tired and lethargic. The patient may consult his doctor and be given iron for the anemia but this will produce no benefit. Lack of response to iron may lead to investigation, when the true cause will be found. Headaches are a common early symptom because chronic renal failure is so often associated with hypertension. The combination of hypertension and a bleeding tendency caused by uremia may lead to repeated epistaxis. Alternatively spontaneous bruising may be noticed, or multiple bruises from apparently trivial trauma. Some degree of fluid retention may appear as ankle edema or puffy eyes. As renal failure advances the majority of patients develop anorexia as well as nausea and vomiting. This may lead to dehydration which will further aggravate the renal impairment. In an advanced case of severe uremia very troublesome generalized itching of the skin may add to the patient's discomfort. The exact mechanism of this is not known. It is not associated with any rash except that which is caused by scratching. It is a potent cause of insomnia in uremic patients and it usually disappears quite soon if uremia is relieved, for example by diet or dialysis. Some chronically uremic patients develop distressing diarrhea which is due to uremic colitis. It is difficult to treat successfully without relieving the uremia, but codeine phosphate 30 mg three times daily by mouth may be helpful.

The clinical signs in chronic renal failure may be very few. The commonest are pallor caused by the uremia and a characteristic muddy or earthy pigmentation of the skin which looks rather like faded suntan or old parchment. Hypertension, edema and bruising have been mentioned. Occasionally hyperventilation may be noticed and this will probably be due to the metabolic acidosis of severe renal impairment. Urine examination may reveal proteinuria and a fixed urine specific gravity in the region of 1010. The diagnosis is made by checking the blood urea and creatinine and distinguishing the condition from acute renal failure. The history may provide some clues here but this can be notoriously misleading. Chronic renal failure will be confirmed if X-rays show that the kidneys are small and contracted. Other points suggesting chronic renal failure are anemia and a low serum calcium. At the onset of *acute* renal failure patients are not normally anemic. The cause of the low serum calcium in chronic renal failure is partly poor absorption of calcium from the gut and partly inadequate phosphate excretion with high serum phosphate and a reciprocally low serum calcium.

Once chronic renal failure has been diagnosed we have a duty to elucidate the underlying cause if this is possible by such tests as IVU and renal biopsy. It is important to exclude any treatable condition such as obstruction or infection or uncontrolled hypertension. Correct treatment of the renal lesion even at a late stage may prevent further deterioration. We must also assess the severity of the renal impairment by creatinine clearances. One or two carefully obtained estimations will serve as a baseline from which to judge future progress.

Management of chronic renal failure

Management of chronic renal failure can be considered under the following headings:

1 Specific treatment of the renal lesion to arrest the disease process.

2 Diet to prevent damage from the hyperfiltration process.

3 Control of hypertension.

4 Avoidance of nephrotoxic drugs.

5 Control of additional nephrotoxic factors.

6 Dietary control of uremia to control uremic symptoms.

7 Manipulation of fluid and electrolytes to compensate for defective renal regulation.

8 Treatment of complications.

9 Preparation of the patient and family for a life with end-stage renal failure.

10 Terminal care for the patient who is unable to receive or does not want dialysis.

Since the publication of the second edition of *Renal Nursing* in 1977 there has been a radical change in the way we approach the management of chronic renal failure. It used to be thought that the only virtue of protein restriction in chronic renal failure was for the purpose of controlling uremic symptoms. It was generally believed that lowering the blood urea in the early stages of chronic renal impairment made no difference to the rate of progress of nephron damage which depended only on the rate of progress of the intrinsic disease, whatever that was. It was known that superimposed hypertension would aggravate the renal damage and it has been an article of faith for many years that the most important therapeutic intervention one could make in any case of chronic glomerulonephritis was meticulous control of the blood pressure. A protein restricted diet has for years been reserved for the late stages of chronic renal failure when uremia started to cause symptoms. We all taught our patients that there was no particular merit in dietary management at an earlier stage. Now, as a result of very convincing independent studies and trials both in animals and humans, a new policy has emerged, the most articulate proponent of which is Dr Brenner in the United States.

Let us consider each of these approaches in turn.

1 Specific treatment of the renal lesion to arrest the disease process

This has already been dealt with in Chapter 3. Examples are antibiotic treatment to deal promptly with any urinary infection in chronic pyelonephritis and eradication of chronic infection to prevent progression of secondary amyloidosis. Unfortunately most causes of chronic renal failure do not, as yet, have any very effective specific treatment. For example, chronic glomerulonephritis and polycystic kidney disease will continue to damage the kidneys regardless of what we do.

2 Diet to prevent damage from the hyperfiltration process

The new evidence, which is too numerous to list, is now widely accepted and is beginning to be put into practice by the world nephrological community. What this evidence suggests is that once there is a reduction in the amount of functioning renal tissue, for whatever reason, the filtration load of each nephron is going to be greater. In other words the remaining kidney tissue will have more work to do. This extra work load probably does not become important until the amount of residual healthy tissue is down to less than half normal. At that point the more work the nephrons have to do the more they will suffer slowly progressive damage. Thus, as more nephrons are destroyed, the remaining population has to carry a yet greater load, and the rate of damage will accelerate. It thus becomes a vicious circle. The proponents of this theory would have us believe that once a patient's kidney disease gets to a certain critical point the damage will be self-perpetuating and progressive at an accelerating rate, even if the original disease, which caused the damage in the first place, has become inactive. This has become known as the hyperfiltration theory; and the damage resulting from the extra work is mainly sustained by the glomeruli. They now develop a progressive sclerosis.

The theory also states, with a mass of highly convincing evidence to support it, that one can reduce the damage, even if one cannot stop it completely, by reducing the load the glomeruli have to filter. This can be done by judicious implementation of protein-restricted diets in the early stages of chronic renal impairment long before uremic symptoms appear. By doing this it seems that one can protect the glomeruli from the damage caused by hyperfiltration and cause the chronic renal failure to stabilize. This does not, of course, mean that by diet we can prevent all future cases of end-stage renal failure. Many forms of chronic kidney disease remain active throughout their course and will destroy all the nephrons, independently of any superadded hyperfiltration factor. Nevertheless it seems entirely possible that renal function could be preserved much longer in the majority of patients with chronic renal failure if correct dietary management were instituted early enough. How early is it necessary to do this? At what level of renal function is it wise to start dietary restriction? And, having started it, how much protein should we allow and at what level should we be trying to maintain the blood urea? The short answer to these questions is that nobody really knows.

Most of us, however, are sufficiently impressed by this new information that we are now advocating a protein restricted diet for our patients once the glomerular filtration rate gets down to half of normal or when the serum creatinine level gets up to twice normal for that patient. At this point we institute a diet containing 0.4−0.6 grams of protein per kilogram of body weight per day. This degree of protein restriction should provide adequate nutrition if most of the protein is in the form of high quality protein containing a balanced combination of the essential amino acids. This will be mainly in the form of meat and eggs. It means that from now on dietitians are going to have a very important role, even more important than before, in the health care team; and we will have to be continually preoccupied with a discussion of diet whenever we see these patients for review.

The next few years can be expected to clarify the impact of this change in policy.

3 Control of hypertension

The need for meticulous control of hypertension in patients with chronic renal failure has become more and more evident in the last few years, and it is fortunate that during the same period we have become blessed with an excellent selection of anti-hypertensive drugs. It should now be possible to control blood pressure in everyone without exception provided that the patient is willing to cooperate. Even what was formerly considered to be refractory hypertension should respond to the correct combination of strategies. These may include weight loss, stopping smoking, reducing alcohol, restricting salt, and the right combination of drugs. Time must be spent talking to patients and explaining that they are likely to feel worse when their blood pressure is brought down from a high to a normal level. They may feel weak, lethargic and drowsy, but if they stick with it they will get used to a lower level of blood pressure and in the long run they will benefit. Part of the secret is to get the patient involved and make him responsible. More and more we are teaching patients to take their own blood pressure lying and standing and keep a record to show us when they come to see us. Side-effects such as the effect on sexual performance should be discussed openly and with understanding. It is not enough just to tell patients imperiously to take this or that drug. Patients should know the names and dose strengths of each medication and be told what side-effects to watch out for. If patients are taken completely into our confidence and made to feel an important part of the team the results are likely to be good.

4 Avoidance of nephrotoxic drugs

Patients and their family doctors must be made aware of which drugs may be dangerous. For example all tetracyclines except doxycycline (Vibramycin) should be avoided. Nitrofurantoin is dangerous in chronic renal failure because it may cause polyneuritis. Aminoglycosides are also dangerous and if they have to be used the doses should be very carefully controlled by monitoring blood levels.

5 Control of additional nephrotoxic factors

For a long time it has been known that phosphate is harmful in patients with chronic renal failure if the level is allowed to go too high. It seems that hyperphosphatemia is a nephrotoxic influence and steps should be taken to keep the level normal. Low phosphate diets and drugs which bind phosphate in the gut may both have to be used. See p.314 on control of hyperphosphatemia in dialysis patients.

Serum calcium tends to be low in chronic renal failure. Osteomalacia can be prevented by giving vitamin D (see p.311). However, one should be very careful to avoid letting the serum calcium go too high becaue hypercalcemia damages the kidney tubules. The only way to prevent hypercalcemia is to monitor the serum calcium regularly.

Hyperuricemia is a common feature of all patients with renal failure and we know that gout can cause interstitial renal damage as well as uric acid calculi. Does this mean that we should put all patients with chronic renal failure on allopurinol to prevent the rise in serum uric acid which would otherwise occur? We do not know, but most people agree that we should at least control the very high levels. As time goes by we will no doubt identify the various nephrotoxic influences more clearly.

6 Dietary control of uremic symptoms

As renal failure advances patients may start to develop symptoms of uremia in spite of their protein restriction. With very severe renal impairment it is sometimes possible to keep the patient ambulant and comparatively free of symptoms on only 18–20 g of dietary protein in a specially designed diet devised by Giordano and Giovannetti. This has come to be known as the Giovannetti diet and it contains almost equal amounts of all essential amino acids in the form of the first class animal proteins (mainly as eggs and meat) with the exception of methionine which has to be given as a supplement in tablet form—about 500 mg three times a day. The patient is unable to eat ordinary bread because of the protein content of the flour. Instead special 'Giovannetti flour' must be used to make 'Giovannetti bread'. The unappetizing nature of this bread is one of the main disadvantages of the diet. The diet should have a high calorie content in the form of carbohydrates and fat and useful additions are supplementary glucose or fructose in Hycal (from Beecham) or Caloreen (from Scientific Hospital Supplies Limited) respectively. Unfortunately only the most determined patients with great moral fiber are able to tolerate the diet for any length of time. If the diet is taken conscientiously there is no doubt that the blood urea can be kept at acceptable levels and there is evidence that urea is actually utilized in the synthesis of proteins. Uremic symptoms will disappear and the hemoglobin may rise so that strength and energy may improve. A serious disadvantage of the diet is the nature of the symptoms which develop when terminal renal failure finally supervenes. Patients develop a distressing generalized bleeding tendency and strange mental symptoms resembling an acute anxiety state. During the last few days before death the patient may have troublesome hallucinations and terrifying nightmares. For these various reasons the Giovannetti diet has gone somewhat out of favor among most physicians in this field. Instead there is a tendency to give a more liberal diet and start dialysis at an earlier stage—before the patient's general condition has deteriorated too far.

7 Manipulation of fluid and electrolytes

Dietary sodium should always be considered separately from protein. Some patients with chronic renal failure, especially those with predominantly tubular damage, lose large amounts of sodium in the urine and they may need a liberal salt intake. Others with predominantly glomerular damage tend to be hypertensive with a low urinary salt loss and salt will need to be restricted. Moderately severe salt restriction is represented by a diet containing 30 mmol sodium per day. It is very hard to construct a diet containing less than 20 mmol sodium per day and this tends to be very uninteresting. The necessity for such severe sodium restriction can often be avoided by giving big doses of sodium-losing diuretics such as furosemide (Lasix). Appendix 1 on p.394 gives the sodium and potassium contents of various foods.

Potassium retention is not usually a problem in chronic renal failure until the very late stages. Foods containing a lot of potassium such as citrus fruits and meat extracts may have to be avoided. The powerful diuretics such as furosemide may help by provoking urinary potassium loss. Occasionally oral ingestion of ion exchange resins on a regular basis may have to be considered but they are not well tolerated for prolonged periods of time.

Fluid intake in chronic renal failure should generally be liberal. In the early stages most patients have polyuria and will drink a lot because they are thirsty. Intercurrent illness may lead to dehydration since water cannot be conserved. There is more danger from dehydration at this stage than from overhydration. As renal failure advances urine output may gradually decrease. A patient may have to reduce his intake to avoid fluid retention, which in turn can be detected by daily weighing. A weight gain exceeding 0.5 kg per day must be due to fluid rather than dry weight. Acidosis can be corrected by administration of sodium bicarbonate or potassium citrate. The choice depends on which of the two cations, sodium or potassium, is most appropriate or least undesirable.

8 Complications of chronic renal failure

Anemia

There is no really satisfactory treatment for the anemia of chronic renal failure. Iron, vitamin B_{12} and folic acid are all without benefit unless the patient happens to be deficient in one or more of these factors. Blood transfusions confer temporary benefit and should no longer carry a risk of transmitting hepatitis B since all blood should be screened for hepatitis B (as well as for AIDS) before it is released to the patient. It used to be thought that blood transfusions might have an adverse effect on future renal transplantation; but now it is generally agreed that blood transfusions reduce the frequency and severity of graft rejection episodes, hence substantially improving transplant results.

Anemia in the pre-dialysis patient can probably be improved by conservative dietary methods for reducing uremia to a minimum.

Polyneuritis

Long-standing uremia sometimes leads to the development of a symmetrical peripheral neuritis mainly affecting the feet and legs. Pins and needles and loss of sensation are later followed by loss of power with foot-drop. Loss of vibration sense is often the earliest sign and nerve conduction studies are useful in detecting the early case. The conditon may deteriorate acutely when dialysis is first started but usually gradually improves thereafter if thorough and frequent dialysis is continued. Patients also improve after renal transplantation. The onset of polyneuritis in a patient with chronic renal failure is an indication to start dialysis as soon as possible in order to avoid further deterioration.

Pericarditis

The normal heart is covered by a pericardial sac, smooth lubricated membranes which surround the heart and allow it to move efficiently with minimum friction. When these membranes become inflamed they become sticky and no longer slide smoothly over the heart's surface. The friction of the surfaces is painful and is felt as a continuous pain in the front of the chest. Auscultation with a stethoscope reveals a scratching sound like sandpaper in both systole and diastole. There are a number of causes of pericarditis of which chronic renal failure is one. When pericarditis occurs in chronic renal failure it is due to the uremia—the more severe the uremia the more pericarditis is likely to occur. In the old days when dialysis was not available for end-stage renal failure, it was noted by one observer that death followed within an average of ten days from the time that pericarditis was first detected, yet the onset of pericarditis is not strictly related to the level of blood urea. The actual level of blood urea at which patients develop pericarditis is very variable. When pericarditis does become evident it is always a sign that something must be done urgently unless it has been decided to let the patient die of uremia. Dialysis must be started at once in patients who have not yet been dialysed, and, in those who are already on regular long-term dialysis, it is a sign that the present treatment is inadequate. Dialysis must be improved. Actually it is very rare to encounter uremic pericarditis in any patient on regular long-term dialysis nowadays because dialysis is generally of such a high standard. However, if one does encounter a case, what should be done? The scratching sound, the pericardial friction rub, will be the diagnostic clue, but nearly always there will be increased pericardial fluid, and this is best confirmed by an echocardiogram. Often when the fluid increases the friction rub disappears but this is not always so. A loud rub may be audible even in the presence of a large pericardial effusion. The echocardiogram can be done regularly (every one or two days) to see whether the effusion is getting bigger or smaller.

The first essential of treatment is early and frequent dialysis. This by itself may deal with the problem. If, however, the effusion becomes large it will compress the heart since the sac is not infinitely distensible. Compression of the heart by fluid is called cardiac tamponade. It interferes with normal pumping and will lead to a drop in cardiac output which will be seen as a fall in blood pressure. Tapping the fluid through the chest wall relieves the pressure and immediately improves cardiac output, but usually the fluid will re-accumulate. Each time it does so it tends to become more hemorrhagic, so that one may end up with a lot of thick clot in the pericardial cavity which is impossible to remove by needle aspiration. Eventually it may be necessary to remove this surgically by making a pericardial window.

Because of this tendency for the effusion to become hemorrhagic it is traditional to use as little heparin as possible during dialysis for pericarditis.

Non-steroidal anti-inflammatory drugs such as indomethacin have been advocated and are commonly used to reduce the inflammation of uremic pericarditis but their efficacy has not been proven by controlled clinical trials.

A rare complication of uremic pericarditis, which may occur many months after recurrent severe attacks, is constrictive pericarditis. This is a thickening and fibrotic contraction of the pericardial sac which grips the heart and prevents normal contraction. It leads to chronic congestive heart failure. Some of these patients have been successfully treated by surgical removal of the thickened membranes, an operation called pericardectomy.

Renal osteodystrophy

The exact mechanism of bone disease which occurs in some patients with chronic renal failure is not fully understood. Impaired calcium absorption in uremia is certainly a factor. The metabolic acidosis which accompanies chronic renal failure especially in tubulo-interstitial disorders such as pyelonephritis is perhaps important also because calcium tends to dissolve out of bone in an acid environment. We now know that some patients are more at risk of bone disease than others. Significant independent risk factors are youth, the female sex, tubulo-interstitial types of nephropathy, and long duration of uremia. Whatever the cause, the main symptoms are bone pain, mainly in the spine and the long bones of the legs. The condition may present as rickets in children and osteomalacia in adults. Both groups may also have a degree of hyperparathyroidism. This is secondary to the renal failure and is therefore called secondary hyperparathyroidism. If severe it may result in pathological fractures. Although the mechanism of renal bone disease is not fully understood (at least by this author) it fortunately responds in nearly all cases to treatment with oral vitamin D. The dose is regulated by the serum calcium which, as has already been said, must not be allowed to go too high.

It is well recognized that the osteomalacia of renal bone disease is aggravated by regular consumption of barbiturates and other anticonvulsants. These drugs should therefore be stopped completely unless they are absolutely essential for the control of epilepsy.

Uremic carbohydrate intolerance

Patients with long-standing and severe chronic uremia may develop a diabetic tendency, manifested by hyperglycemia, glycosuria and a diabetic glucose tolerance curve. Investigation has shown that this is due to reduced sensitivity to insulin even though insulin secretion may be increased. It is unusual for such patients to require insulin injections since the diabetes is more chemical than symptomatic. The diabetic tendency disappears as soon as the patient receives regular and adequate dialysis. It appears that some dialysable factor is causing the diabetes.

We should remember that glycosuria in a patient with chronic renal failure does not necessarily imply carbohydrate intolerance or diabetes. Many patients with near normal renal function may have moderate tubular damage sufficient to prevent normal tubular reabsorption of glucose. This condition of low renal threshold for glucose or glucose leak is also seen in some women during pregnancy when the glucose tolerance test is completely normal.

Gynecomastia

Some men with chronic renal failure develop a troublesome and rather painful enlargement of the breasts. The cause for this is not clear. It is a nuisance but not a danger and is usually only temporary. It may be on one or both sides.

Infections

Uremia predisposes to infection. Urinary infection is particularly common even when the primary condition is not pyelonephritis. For this reason urine cultures should be taken routinely from all patients with chronic renal failure when they attend out-patient clinics. A neglected urinary infection is particularly dangerous in someone who already has a slender reserve of functioning renal tissue.

Pruritus

A generalized and troublesome itching of the skin is common in the late stages of chronic renal failure. It is usually a sign that dialysis should be started soon. However, pruritus is discussed fully in Chapter 8, p.317.

9 Preparation of the patient and the family for a life with end-stage renal failure

When it becomes clear that a patient is heading inevitably towards renal failure it is important that the patient's physician should start some discussion of the subject. It makes it much easier if the patient and family are prepared as well as possible for what is to come. In western Europe and North America the ministries of health and their equivalents have accepted responsibility, at least in theory, for treating all the patients who need treatment. Medical and nursing staff therefore have an obligation to accept everyone who wishes to be treated. At various times, and in various countries, it has not always been easy to take everyone who needs help. Facilities have been overcrowded at times to the point of crisis. But it is not the job of medical and nursing teams to ration treatment in order to avoid embarrassing governments. The doctor and the nurse must be the advocate for the patient. If facilities are inadequate they must somehow be found.

It has been shown repeatedly that almost everyone who wants treatment for end-stage renal failure is capable of benefiting from it. No arbitrary criteria, such as the presence of ischemic heart disease, diabetes, blindness, old age or schizophrenia, should be used to exclude patients from treatment. If the patient's quality of life is such that he or she is anxious to continue to live, it is up to us to find a way. In our program we now draw the line at a patient in an advanced state of dementia in a nursing home. Furthermore we never try to force people to accept treatment if they genuinely do not want it. Patients should be told about what options exist and should be given the chance to meet and talk to patients who are already on dialysis programs.

Many large renal centers have a renal nursing coordinator who finds time to meet the patients and their families, to explain what life on dialysis means, to answer questions and to try to deal with the patient's anxiety.

At this point, while the patient is still relatively healthy, the hepatitis B antigen should be checked. If it is negative the patient should be advised to undergo hepatitis B vaccination (see p.295). There is a greater chance of inducing protective immunity if vaccination is started before the patient is in advanced uremia.

If it is decided that hemodialysis is the preferred method of treatment, arrangements should be made for the patient to have an arteriovenous fistula constructed. If home dialysis is planned we should be taking a look at the patient's home to see what alterations may be required.

If there is a possibility of a kidney transplant from a living related donor, potential donors should be interviewed. Often it is possible to have the donor ready to give the kidney by the time the patient reaches end-stage renal failure. See p.338 for selection and investigation of living related kidney donors.

Terminal care in patients with renal failure

Terminal care for patients with renal failure may be required under three main sets of circumstances. The first is that in which our best efforts have been made to treat a patient with acute renal failure, but there are one or more lethal complications which are preventing recovery. This happens most often in desperately ill patients in intensive care units. Often there are several different medical teams involved. Perhaps the patient started off having a routine cholecystectomy, but things went wrong. Peritonitis and Gram-negative septicemia led to acute tubular necrosis. Inhalation pneumonia led to respiratory failure and the need for a ventilator. Now the patient has multiple intra-abdominal abscesses and the surgeon does not think that another major operation can be survived. Perhaps up until now every complication has been potentially reversible but we know that the patient cannot survive unless the infection is drained. If we are not very careful we will all be trying earnestly to deal with our own failing system but no one is looking at the whole picture. It is very important in this type of case for one doctor to be in charge. He or she will obtain expert help and opinions from the others but must not allow the whole affair to drag on indefinitely. There usually comes a time when a decision must be made to stop. We are no longer realistically saving a life but instead we are prolonging a death. The renal team must not be put in a position of having to dialyse a patient day after day when there is no hope of recovery and some of the other teams have already given up. Either everyone works together or everyone should decide jointly to stop and let the patient die in peace. This is where a wise physician in charge will call a conference of involved teams and make a decision. One hopes that the family has been met with on a daily basis and the various complications patiently explained. Relatives will cope with incredible stress and disaster if the doctor appears to know his job and takes the trouble to keep them informed.

The patient may or may not be conscious enough for us to communicate with him, but the nurse involved in treating him is often an excellent judge of what the patient can feel. Small discomforts are important.

The second type of case is that in which a patient wishes to die of uremia rather than go on dialysis. This is an unusual situation in our experience and one which makes us feel uncomfortable and inadequate. Everything must be done to keep the patient comfortable and make the last few days as tolerable as possible. Visiting privileges for relatives should be as liberal as is compatible with efficient nursing care. There is a terrible tendency to avoid such patients when we make our rounds in the hospital because we do not like to be reminded of our failure to help. The fact is that we can help by respecting the patient's wishes and visiting often. The patient should not be left alone unless he expressly wishes to be alone. We should worry about details such as the pressure areas and the state of hydration. Does the patient have a dry mouth and what can be done about it? Let us not talk in front of the patient as if he is not there. He can probably hear what we are saying even if he seems to be asleep. Is he having nightmares and does he need more morphine? Many hospitals have highly professional palliative care teams who can be of enormous help in situations like this. Does the patient want to talk to the minister or the priest? Is there any particular member of the family he wants to see again? Fortunately death, when it comes, is usually peaceful due to cardiac arrest from hyperkalemia.

The last scenario with which we may be confronted is the patient who has been living with end-stage renal failure too long and is finally tired of it.

During the last twenty years of dealing with renal failure I have encountered this on about three occasions. Each time the patient has approached me deliberately and seriously and asked to have his or her dialysis stopped. On each occasion it was a carefully thought out decision reached after prolonged thought and deliberation. The greatest fear that patients have on these occasions is that their wishes will not be respected, that the doctor will want to change their minds. On each occasion I have spent time talking to the patient and come to the conclusion that the patient's wishes should be respected. I have not looked on it as an act of suicide—simply a desire to stop having one's life prolonged by extraordinary means when it has ceased to be enjoyable. There may at such times be opposition from the patient's offspring. But the doctor's duty is first to the patient. Such patients want to know what will happen. Will I feel ill? Will it be painful? Will you continue to look after me? How long will I live once I stop dialysis?

In my experience and in the experience of others I have talked to such patients usually continue to feel well but die suddenly of hypokalemia about a week after the last dialysis. The last week can be spent quite happily with family and friends, an opportunity to meet and chat for the last time. This can be done equally as well in the hospital or at home and the patient should decide where he or she wants to be. Again one has a duty to protect the patient from the discomfort of excessive fluid intake which might cause dyspnea due to pulmonary congestion. Detailed attention should be paid to preventing physical discomfort or alleviating it by analgesics or sedations.

We will not be doing too badly if we 'cure sometimes, relieve often, and comfort always'.

5

Some Introductory Remarks about Dialysis

Robert Uldall and Eileen Young

In Chapter 1 we learned that when two aqueous solutions are separated by a semipermeable membrane, the composition of any dissolved substances tends to equalize on the two sides of the membrane. Thus, if glucose is added to one compartment but not to the other, it will, after it has dissolved, diffuse through the membrane until the concentrations are equal on both sides. Any molecule that is small enough to pass through the pores of the membrane will always travel from the area of high concentration to the area of low concentration. Water, on the other hand, because of the principle of osmotic pressure, will always tend to flow from the area of low osmotic pressure to the area of high osmotic pressure. This phenomenon brings about equality of composition and concentration on the two sides of the membrane and they are really the principles underlying dialysis.

Dialysis really means the process of altering the composition of a solution by composing a solution of different composition and then placing the two solutions on opposite sides of a semipermeable membrane. Dialysis is employed in numerous industrial and chemical processes but for the purposes of our discussion we will confine ourselves to renal dialysis, now performed in almost every country in the world as an imperfect yet lifesaving substitute for absent or inadequate renal function.

As every nurse knows, there are two methods of dialysis employed clinically in the treatment of patients, namely peritoneal dialysis and hemodialysis. In peritoneal dialysis we use the peritoneum itself as a semipermeable membrane and the process takes place inside the body. The peritoneum is a thin cellular layer which covers all the intra-abdominal organs. It usually has a surface area of between one and two square metres and it is richly supplied with capillary blood. The carefully composed physiological solution which is poured into the peritoneal cavity is called the dialysate.

In hemodialysis, on the other hand, dialysis takes place outside the body in what we call an extracorporeal circulation called a dialyser, consisting of two compartments, one for the blood and one for the dialysate. The two compartments are separated by a man-made semi-permeable membrane, the first of which to be used successfully (by Dr Kolff in Holland in 1945) was cellophane. Many different membranes have been used since then, and they are still being developed—also many different configurations of dialyser. It is at the level of the peritoneum in a patient on peritoneal dialysis and in the dialyser in a patient on hemodialysis that the blood is changed in composition by being exposed to dialysate, separated only by a thin membrane across which diffusion occurs.

There is nothing magical about the dialysate; and its composition can be anything we want it to be, realizing that, whatever composition (or mixture of chemicals) we put in the dialysate, the blood will approximate towards it. For example, if the plasma potassium is dangerously high and threatening to bring about cardiac arrest, we can lower the plasma potassium by dialysing with a dialysate containing potassium in low concentrations. Potassium will then cross the membrane from the area of high concentration (the blood) to the area of low concentration (the dialysate) and the plasma potassium level will be lowered. In the same way the concentration of other plasma electrolytes can be lowered or raised in order to correct an excess or a deficit. Remember that we are only dialysing the plasma of the blood. We cannot directly dialyse the intracellular fluid or the interstitial fluid. Their composition will change by a form of natural dialysis inside the body. The interstitial fluid will equilibrate with the intravascular (blood) space by a form of dialysis across the capillary wall, and the intracellular composition will change because of changes in the interstitial fluid. Thus, by dialysing the blood plasma we can change the composition of all the fluid compartments of the body. These changes are not instantaneous. It takes time for equilibration to occur, just as it takes time to perform the artificial dialysis.

At this point let us list some of the similarities between peritoneal and hemodialysis and then some of the most important differences before going on to read the individual chapters on each method.

Similarities between the two types of dialysis

1 In both methods the dialysate is composed in order to correct metabolic abnormalities in the blood. Unwanted substances are removed by and deficient substances are acquired from the dialysate. For example, unwanted end-products of nitrogen metabolism such as urea and creatinine are removed, serum potassium is lowered if it is high, and serum calcium is raised if, as is usually the case in renal failure, it is low.

2 The dialysate must be warmed to body temperature. Cold dialysate is not only very uncomfortable for the patient but also causes hypothermia. Hot dialysate, in the case of peritoneal dialysis, will cause pain and damage to the peritoneal cavity, and in the case of hemodialysis it will destroy (hemolyse) the red blood cells.

3 In both types of dialysis infection must be prevented. In peritoneal dialysis the dialysate must be sterile since it is entering the peritoneal cavity. In hemodialysis the whole inside of the extracorporeal blood pathway must be sterile to prevent septicemia. The dialysate in hemodialysis does not have to be sterile since bacteria are too large to cross the pores in the membrane. Heavy bacterial growth in the dialysate is, however, undesirable. Amongst other things it may make the dialysate more acid.

4 Both types of dialysis require an access route. In peritoneal dialysis a catheter carries the dialysate into the peritoneal cavity and out again after equilibration has occurred. In hemodialysis there must be some method for gaining repeated entry to the circulation for removal and return of blood. These access methods are crucially important. They must always remain patent to provide good flow, yet they must never allow entry of infection.

Differences between peritoneal and hemodialysis

1 Peritoneal dialysis is a simple method employing simple equipment. It can be performed by any nurse and doctor in any hospital once a few simple techniques have been learned.

Hemodialysis on the other hand uses complicated equipment, advanced engineering and electronic technology. It is a machine-orientated discipline and requires highly specialized training on the part of both doctors and nurses. The capital equipment is very expensive and needs highly trained and specialized technical staff to service and maintain it.

2 The dialysate for peritoneal dialysis is usually supplied commercially in sterile plastic bags and has been formulated according to an agreed

prescription at the request of the medical staff. Dialysate for hemodialysis is composed on the spot in the dialysis unit by proportioning a commercially prepared concentrate of chemicals with a large volume of pure water. The responsibility for purifying the water must be taken by the dialysis unit. The machines will proportion the concentrate with the water to give the correct final composition. The machine does this by keeping the final dialysate within a narrow range of electrical conductivity. If the conductivity is correct the composition will be correct, since electrical conductivity is linearly related to the concentration of the ionic electrolytes in solution. It is not feasible to buy the dialysate for hemodialysis already proportioned because the volumes required are too large. For example, one patient on dialysis usually requires 500 ml of dialysate per minute or 30 litres per hour or 120 litres for a four hour treatment. If there are ten patients on dialysis at any time in a dialysis unit we may use 1200 litres of dialysate in the course of a morning. Obviously this is an impossibly large amount to have delivered commercially. Hence, one of the most important functions of a hemodialysis unit is the proportioning of dialysis concentrate to give us the desired composition of our final dialysate. There is now an increasing tendency to vary the composition according to the special needs of the patient. Individual machines are available to do this.

3 Peritoneal dialysis is slow and gentle, bringing about gradual changes in body chemistry. It may be done intermittently, but increasing numbers of patients are having peritoneal dialysis continuously, even while they go about their daily lives, as you will learn in the next chapter. Hemodialysis is extremely efficient and tends to be performed intermittently for short periods of time. The time taken to achieve a particular change in blood composition has become progressively shorter since the treatment was first used. This speeding up of the process is now only limited by what the body will tolerate. This, in turn, depends on the rate at which equilibration occurs with the other fluid compartments of the body.

4 Most patients with renal failure tend to accumulate water in their bodies because they are passing little or no urine but continue to receive water in food and drink and sometimes intravenous infusions. Thus, one of the functions of dialysis must be to remove the excess water by arranging for it to pass from the blood to the dialysate. In peritoneal dialysis this can *only* be done by using the principle of osmotic pressure— that is, to arrange for the osmotic pressure of the dialysate to be higher than the osmotic pressure of the blood. Water will then cross the peritoneal membrane from the blood to the dialysate. In practice this is usually done by raising the glucose concentration of the dialysate. Osmotic

removal of water can also be used in hemodialysis but in hemodialysis we have another method. We use the principle of hydrostatic pressure. By raising the pressure in the blood compartment and/or by arranging a negative pressure in the dialysate compartment we can produce a 'trans-membrane pressure' of several hundred millimetres of mercury. The higher the transmembrane pressure the greater will be the removal of water. In fact with modern hemodialysis this method is so efficient that one can, if one chooses to do so, manage without any glucose in the dialysate at all.

5 Peritoneal dialysis can be performed without any systemic anticoagulation. Hemodialysis, because it involves passing the patient's blood through an extracorporeal circuit, requires the use of heparin to prevent the blood from clotting. This may be undesirable and even dangerous if the patient is already bleeding or is undergoing surgery. Methods are being developed for conducting hemodialysis without the use of heparin but at the time of writing these methods are not yet widely available. Thus, peritoneal dialysis is safer in a patient who is actively bleeding.

6 Peritoneal dialysis is usually the treatment of choice for uncomplicated acute renal failure but it is technically not possible in certain conditions. For example, peritoneal dialysis cannot be performed in the presence of a large retroperitoneal hematoma since the dialysate will be drawn by osmotic pressure across the peritoneum of the posterior abdominal wall into the hematoma space which will become progressively larger. Peritoneal dialysis is not really feasible in the presence of recent abdominal surgery since the dialysate will leak through the wound and out of drainage sites. It can be done if there is no alternative but it is not desirable. Peritonitis or any intraperitoneal infection is also usually a contra-indication. Peritoneal dialysis may also be impossible in the presence of multiple intra-abdominal adhesions since the dialysate becomes loculated and fails to drain easily in and out of the abdomen. Peritoneal dialysis may also be inadequate in patients who are highly catabolic due to multiple injuries, bleeding and infection. The rate of rise of blood urea is too fast for this form of dialysis to keep pace. Large intra-abdominal masses such as polycystic kidneys or a gravid uterus may so fill the abdomen that the patient cannot accommodate the dialysate. Hence, patients with large polycystic kidneys and women who develop renal failure in the late stages of pregnancy may need hemodialysis. Peritoneal dialysis is easy to perform in children and babies simply by using smaller, shorter catheters and smaller volumes of dialysate. Hemodialysis in babies and small children requires special scaled-down equipment and specialized training for its safe performance.

However, peritoneal dialysis and hemodialysis should never have to compete with one another. Rather they should complement one another. Neither method is 'better' than the other. Both methods have their advantages and disadvantages and may appropriately be used at different times in the same patient. The following two chapters will go into these methods more fully.

Selecting the method of treatment

How should the dialysis method be selected for individual patients? Each hospital or institution will have its own policies on this and to some extent the choice will be dictated by the availability of facilities.

Selecting the dialysis method for patients with acute renal failure is usually a strictly medical decision. Peritoneal dialysis is usually the treatment of choice for uncomplicated cases of acute renal failure. Hemodialysis is used if, for some reason, peritoneal dialysis is contra-indicated. The decision must be made quickly when the patient has been fully assessed by the doctors on duty. Usually there is not much time to waste. Once the decision has been made the nursing team will be approached since their help will be needed.

Making the decision about dialysis methods in a patient with end-stage renal failure (ESRF) is generally a more leisurely process since there is usually plenty of warning that end-stage renal failure is approaching. Medical, social, domestic and occupational factors will need to be taken into account. In our hospital, as in many others all over the world, we have a Renal Nursing Coordinator who meets all patients who are approaching ESRF, preferably with the key members of their families. She will discuss the problem with the patient's nephrologist and will usually spend time showing the patient and a close family member the different dialysis facilities and what is involved with each method. Most centers look first at the possibility of a transplant from a close living relative, a brother, sister or parent. If this is feasible—the prospective donor has a compatible ABO blood group and is also completely healthy and completely willing after being told all the facts—then it is usual to plan a living donor transplant to be performed within a few weeks. The patient will then usually be placed on hemodialysis to achieve the best degree of rehabilitation and preparedness in the shortest possible time. Such a patient will not occupy a hemodialysis place for very long and it is usually not worth contemplating self-care dialysis training or home dialysis training.

If a patient is a suitable recipient for a kidney transplant and does not have a potential donor in the family, but happens to be blood group A, it is unlikely that such a patient will have to wait long for a cadaver kidney. There always seem to be plenty of donors for Group A recipients. In this case a short period on hemodialysis may again be all that is needed. However, for all other patients with ESRF a carefully considered choice has to be made.

Ideally the patient should be encouraged to have some say in the matter. If all methods are available it is appropriate to let the patient choose or at least state a preference. Sometimes the decision will be obvious. For example, a highly active motor mechanic who spends all day crawling about under cars and getting oil on his hands is not a good candidate for CAPD. Such a patient should be on hemodialysis, preferably at home if he has a wife or girlfriend to help him, or on a self-care program in a dialysis unit where he will perform his own treatment in the evening or overnight so as to have his daytime hours completely free for his gainful occupation. On the other hand, an elderly lady who stays mainly at home but lives a long way from a dialysis center is an ideal CAPD patient. One of the best ways to provide information to the patient and family, to assist them in making a choice, is to introduce them to a patient already on dialysis who is coping successfully with treatment and also leading an active and happy life. This kind of example is a wonderful encouragement when the problems seem overwhelming. Always the aim should be to try to avoid assigning patients to the in-center, fully staffed hemodialysis unit because this is the place where all the patients end up who are unable to go anywhere else. The hospital hemodialysis center is nearly always fully occupied and overflowing. Ways must be found to take the pressure off it. In the present state of inadequate or barely adequate facilities for management of end-stage renal failure which exist all over the world, every attempt must be made to make every patient as independent of the hospital as possible, each according to his or her own ability.

Figure 5.1 is a diagrammatic scheme of the possible options currently available for patients reaching end-stage renal failure. Rectangles with solid lines have been drawn around those programs and facilities which should always, if possible, be regarded as temporary stages in patient rehabilitation. Patients spend time there on the way to a more long-term or permanent form of treatment. The long-term forms of treatment which allow independence from the hospital center are shown surrounded by interrupted lines. These are the different forms of home dialysis and renal transplantation and theoretically they are indefinitely expandable. Our aim should be to create an ever increasing population of completely

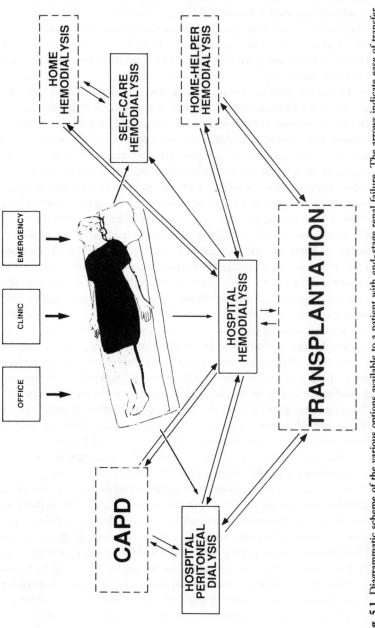

Fig. 5.1. Diagrammatic scheme of the various options available to a patient with end-stage renal failure. The arrows indicate ease of transfer from one program to another.

successful transplant recipients who only require minimal outpatient supervision at infrequent intervals.

The next best thing is home dialysis, whichever type is more suitable for the patient. It is entirely legitimate for patients to continue on home dialysis indefinitely if they wish, or they may use home dialysis as a temporary step on the way to renal transplantation. If home hemodialysis is not possible because of lack of a spouse or partner, self-care dialysis outside normal working hours, either in the hospital or a satellite dialysis facility, is the next best alternative. For this kind of program only minimal nursing supervision is required to help patients in the event of an emergency. Finally there are a few highly selected elderly patients for whom peritoneal dialysis is not possible and transplantation has been ruled out, and who live so far from the hospital center that in-center hemodialysis is not really feasible. To make such patients travel long distances to the hospital three times a week may be quite inhumane. For this small and highly select group the only reasonable solution is to employ a 'home hemodialysis helper'. This would usually be a trained hemodialysis nurse who happens to live close to the patient. She will go into the patient's home three times a week and carry out the dialysis. She should be paid and supervised by the parent dialysis center and keep in touch at regular intervals by telephone. Home helpers are usually married women who want to work part-time and have flexible hours.

So far there has been considerable reluctance on the part of ministries of health in various countries to accept responsibility for funding home helper programs. In our opinion they form an essential part of humane and comprehensive health care and as such they should be supported. They form a tiny fraction of health care costs and it is unlikely that the system will be abused. Usually the financial savings from the cost of providing transport will be close to the cost of paying the nurse.

One more point should be made about this comprehensive and integrated organization for looking after patients with end-stage renal failure. At any time a patient may run into a problem which requires a change, either temporarily or permanently, to a different method of treatment. For example a patient on CAPD may develop a fungal peritonitis requiring removal of the PD catheter to clear up the infection. Hemodialysis will be needed for about a month before the catheter can be reinserted. A home hemodialysis patient may have to come into the hospital for dialysis for two weeks in order to allow the spouse to take a much needed holiday. In other words, there has to be complete mobility to allow patients to be transferred between one modality of treatment and another. For this to occur there has to be complete cooperation between the medical and nursing personnel of the different programs. We all need to help each other. We do this by maximum cooperation and intelligent and considerate communication. Only in this way will our patients receive the best standard of care it is possible to offer.

Training patients for self-care

It has long been noticeable that the healthiest long-term dialysis patients tend to be those who carry out their own treatment. This may be partly because those who are naturally vigorous and independent are also the patients most capable of learning self-care. However, it is also clear that the feeling of achievement and sense of independence gained by mastering the techniques of self-dialysis seem to induce a degree of physical and psychological well-being far beyond that which can be explained by any improvement in the control of uremia. We frequently observe frightened and discontented patients receiving full and devoted nursing care, who blossom into self-assured, positive and confident individuals once they are dialysing themselves. It seems that the mere act of learning self-care has a positive health-giving effect.

Part of this must be that patients in charge of their own treatment have a more responsible attitude to their own welfare. For example, if a patient knows that if he gains three or four kilograms in weight between one hemodialysis treatment and the next he will have to remove this fluid during the dialysis, it may make him considerably more careful about how much fluid he drinks. Removing large amounts of fluid during dialysis may be difficult and uncomfortable. It would be better not to gain that much water in the first place.

In the early days of home hemodialysis some centers concentrated their efforts on training the spouse to dialyse the patient who was regarded as too ill to carry out his or her own treatment. This encouraged the patient to remain helpless and passive while the spouse, who as often as not had to play the role of bread winner, was forced to shoulder the extra load of learning to be a dialysis nurse. This policy tended to throw an intolerable strain on the healthy partner who soon began to resent the one-sided nature of the whole arrangement. It soon became apparent that the right strategy was to say to the patient 'We are sorry you have this problem but you must accept it as *your* problem. We will teach you how to look after yourself.' It is wise to involve the spouse and partner as little as possible and get the patient to do as much as possible unassisted.

This applies to peritoneal dialysis which can be done entirely alone and unassisted and almost as much to hemodialysis in which the partner need only be there to cope with difficulties or emergencies.

The worst scenario is that in which a domineering and cantankerous husband (also the patient) lies back giving orders to his long-suffering and obedient wife while she tries to carry out his dialysis for him in a way which pleases him. This is the nightmare of a husband teaching his wife to drive, only a hundred times more so—a sure recipe for marriage breakdown or more likely a failure of home dialysis and a return to the center for treatment.

Home dialysis training is both an art and a science. It tends to be done by specialized teams of nurses under the guidance of one nursing team leader. The most successful formula seems to be to assign one nurse to one patient for the whole period of the training and preferably in a single room with no distractions. Training for continuous ambulatory peritoneal dialysis (CAPD) may take from one to three weeks while training for hemodialysis may take three to six weeks by virtue of the increased technical complexity of the method and the greater opportunity for causing sudden death in the event of a mistake.

Both groups of patients, once trained and sent home, will require periodic supervision, regular medical check-ups and, in the case of hemodialysis patients, technical back-up in the event of machine failures.

6

Peritoneal Dialysis

Ramesh Khanna, Sharon Izatt,
Betty Kelman and Dimitrios Oreopoulos

Introduction

Peritoneal dialysis has an undisputed role in the treatment of acute renal failure. Despite the problem of infection, its many advantages, such as simplicity and avoidance of specialized personnel and equipment, have made it the treatment of choice for patients with uncomplicated acute renal failure in most hopitals. However, peritoneal dialysis has gone through several phases. During the 1960s because of the frequency of complications, nephrologists preferred hemodialysis to peritoneal dialysis as a long-term kidney replacement treatment. However, in the 1970s as safe access to the peritoneal cavity became available, peritoneal dialysis technique improved and continuous ambulatory peritoneal · dialysis (CAPD) was introduced. With these innovations, peritoneal dialysis became as important as hemodialysis in the treatment of end-stage renal failure.

Basic principles

During peritoneal dialysis physiological solution (the dialysate) is infused into the peritoneal cavity, which is lined by a membrane called the peritoneum—from the Greek *peritonaion* meaning to stretch around. This serous membrane is composed of simple squamous mesothelium lined by connective tissue. The peritoneal membrane is continuous and is comprised of the parietal peritoneum, which lines the cavity, and the

135

visceral peritoneum which encloses the abdominal organs. The space
between these two layers is the peritoneal cavity (Fig. 6.1). All the
abdominal organs are extraperitoneal, but are surrounded by peritoneum
and suspended from the posterior abdominal wall by a double fold of
peritoneum—the mesentery, which carries the blood vessels supplying
the suspended organs. The peritoneal connective tissue contains many

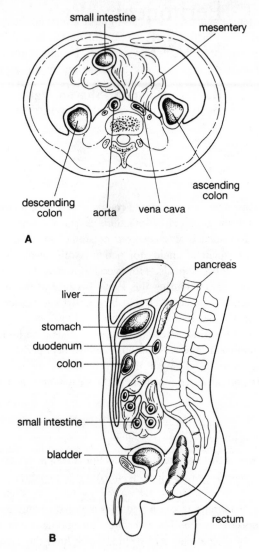

Fig. 6.1. Cross (A) and sagittal (B) sections showing the relationship of peritoneal
membrane to internal organs.

macrophages, which ingest any micro-organisms that may enter the peritoneal cavity. In addition the connective tissue of the greater omentum may contain significant quantities of stored fat. Under normal conditions, the peritoneal cavity contains a small amount of fluid, about 100 ml. This space can be enlarged by the instillation of fluid. Most normal adults can tolerate without discomfort two or more litres of fluid instilled acutely into their peritoneal cavity.

The peritoneal membrane consists of three layers: (a) the mesothelium with its basement membrane (Fig. 6.2); (b) the peritoneal interstitium; and (c) the capillary endothelium with its basement membrane and pericytes. The various solutes, which dialyse out of the capillaries into the dialysis solution have to cross all three layers.

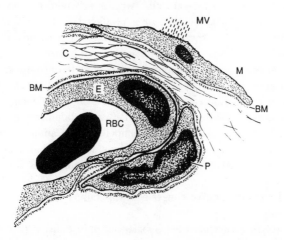

Fig. 6.2. Diagram showing the layers of the peritoneum. M=mesothelial cell, MV= microvilli, BM=basement membrane, C=collagen, E=endothelial cell, P=pericyte, RBC=red blood cell.

The peritoneal membrane has a surface area of approximately one square metre but the area that actively participates in dialysis is significantly smaller—2 to 4% of the total peritoneal area. During peritoneal dialysis solutes move across the peritoneum by diffusion or by ultrafiltration—convective transport of water and solutes. The diffusion of a solute depends on the difference between its concentration in blood and that in the dialysate, while the convective movement, which follows the removal of water by ultrafiltration, is a result of the osmotic difference between blood and the dialysate.

Because of the small effective peritoneal surface available for dialysis, both urea and creatinine clearances are about one-quarter to one-sixth of the values obtained by hemodialysis, even with high dialysate flow rates. These clearances are achieved with a dialysate flow rate of three to four litres per hour. Higher flow rates produce only small increases in peritoneal clearances and, beyond six litres per hour, there is practically no further increase. The clearance of middle-sized and large molecules by peritoneal dialysis is significantly higher than during hemodialysis because the peritoneal membrane has a larger pore size.

Indications for and contra-indications to peritoneal dialysis

Indications

The general indications for peritoneal dialysis are the same as for hemodialysis. Except for hypercatabolic patients in whom peritoneal dialysis cannot remove the amount of urea produced each day and in those recovering from extensive abdominal operations, peritoneal dialysis can be considered in most patients with acute renal failure. Even in hypercatabolic patients, the contra-indication is relative because we can find out whether peritoneal dialysis can keep up with the rate of catabolism only by trying it. Furthermore when hemodialysis is not feasible some physicians have employed peritoneal dialysis soon after an abdominal operation with success. Peritoneal dialysis has a compelling indication when systemic anticoagulation, necessary for hemodialysis, is contra-indicated; or when vascular access is difficult. Other common indications for peritoneal dialysis are:
- Fluid retention and/or congestive heart failure that does not respond to diuresis.
- Electrolyte and acid−base imbalances unresponsive to conservative therapy.
- Drug intoxications, especially with compounds which have a high degree of tissue or protein binding.
- Renal replacement therapy for end-stage kidney disease.
- Acute pancreatitis, especially the hemorrhagic form.
- Acute peritonitis secondary to perforation of a viscus, treated with continuous high-flow technique.
- Lactic acidosis, preferably using bicarbonate dialysate.
- In patients in whom vascular access would be difficult such as very small children and elderly persons with a diffuse arteriosclerosis or diabetes mellitus.
- Patients with accidental hypothermia—here one uses solutions that have been warmed to 37°C. This technique rewarms the body rapidly, smoothly and without complications.

● Intraperitoneal chemotherapy for intra-abdominal malignancy.

Occasionally it is necessary to start peritoneal dialysis immediately when the patient is suffering from severe hyperkalemia or has been poisoned with a dialysable agent. In other cases of acute renal failure, the clinician has two options: the prophylactic use of peritoneal dialysis before the uremic syndrome is established, or its initiation only after some objective criteria are met, for example, blood urea over 30−35 mmol/l (blood urea 90−105 mg/dl), electrolyte disorders, severe metabolic acidosis or overhydration.

Contra-indications

Recent intra-abdominal, retroperitoneal or 'gut' surgery with abdominal drains or diaphragmatic tears

In these circumstances peritoneal dialysis may produce excessive over-distension of the abdominal cavity which would cause leakage into the subcutaneous tissue or externally. If possible, peritoneal dialysis should be delayed until the incision has begun to heal, generally about two to three days unless the patient is critically ill, is hypercatabolic, or is receiving steroids. The presence of paralytic ileus may interfere with the drainage of fluid and increase the risk of bowel perforation during catheter implantation. If peritoneal dialysis has to be undertaken in the presence of ileus or previous abdominal operation, it is best to implant the catheter surgically.

Respiratory insufficiency

Distension of the abdomen with dialysate may interfere with respiration in patients with chronic obstructive lung disease. Therefore, one must be cautious about undertaking dialysis in such patients. Dialysis fluid volume is adjusted to the patient's respiratory capacity rather than to his subjective tolerance and it is advisable to monitor the blood gases during dialysis.

Peritoneal dialysis schedules

Intermittent peritoneal dialysis (acute or long-term)

Here two litres of dialysis solution are infused into the peritoneal cavity, allowed to equilibrate for 10−20 minutes, and then drained out by gravity. These cycles of inflow, equilibration and outflow are repeated until one achieves the desired clinical and biochemical improvement. For therapy of acute renal failure, or as a maintenance treatment for end-stage renal disease, patients require at least $40-48$ (2×20) hours per week. This was the only method of peritoneal dialysis before the advent of CAPD in 1978.

Minor variations of intermittent peritoneal dialysis, such as continuous flow peritoneal dialysis, rapid intermittent peritoneal dialysis, or lavage and intermittent recirculation peritoneal dialysis, have been introduced but none of these modifications has shown sufficient advantage to replace the standard technique.

Continuous ambulatory peritoneal dialysis (CAPD)

In 1976 the development by Popovich and Moncrief of the concept of CAPD led to a resurgence of interest in peritoneal dialysis. This technique employs the continuous (24 hours a day, 7 days a week) presence of dialysis solution for equilibration in the peritoneal cavity. The solution in the cavity is drained out and replaced three or four times a day (details of this method are given later in this chapter).

Continuous cyclic peritoneal dialysis

This technique is a modification of CAPD; the patients use an automatic cycler to exchange 6 to 8 litres every night over 9 to 10 hours. At the end of dialysis, 2 litres of the solution is left in the peritoneal cavity until the following night when the patient again connects himself to the machine.

Peritoneal dialysis solutions

Sterile peritoneal dialysis solution is now marketed in plastic bags in volumes of 500, 1000, 1500, 2000, 3000 and 5000 ml. It is available in various forms—hypotonic (0.5% dextrose), slightly hypertonic (1.5% dextrose) or very hypertonic (2.5% and 4.25% dextrose). The 1.5% dextrose solution has nearly the same total osmolar solute concentration as plasma and produces minimal ultrafiltration (fluid removal). The hypertonic solution is a hyperosmolar solution, which induces various degrees of ultrafiltration from $300-1000$ ml per cycle depending on duration of dwell time. In 1974 nephrologists agreed upon a common formula for dialysate and since then this formula has been used in most countries with only minor modifications. Table 6.1 shows the composition

Table 6.1 Composition of currently used Dianeal solution

Sodium	132 mmol/l
Chloride	101.5 mmol/l
Calcium	3 or 3.5 mmol/l
Magnesium	0.5 or 1.5 mmol/l
Lactate	35 mmol/l
Osmolality	347 up to 486 mosm/l
pH	5.2
Dextrose	0.5, 1.5, 2.5 or 4.5 g/dl

of currently used dialysis solution. In France acetate has been used quite widely in place of lactate but many authorities are concerned that this may cause a form of sclerosing peritonitis leading to formation of adhesions. Lactate is now generally accepted as being superior for conversion in the body to bicarbonate in order to correct the metabolic acidosis. If the patient already has lactic acidosis, a bicarbonate containing dialysate can be used.

A potassium-free solution is used in the dialysis of most renal failure patients, because potassium clears relatively slowly through the peritoneal membrane. Thus, even in the presence of hyperkalemia, a potassium-free dialysate would not induce excessively rapid potassium loss. However, if a patient is receiving digitalis, potassium should be added to the dialysis solution especially during the initial dialysis, to avoid too sudden changes in serum potassium which might lead to myocardial irritability and a potentially fatal arrhythmia.

Peritoneal Access

Stylet catheter

This catheter is used for patients who require peritoneal dialysis for only a short period (Fig. 6.3). It is a semi-rigid plastic catheter with a central metal stylet (trocar) for piercing the abdominal wall. Its distal end has a number of small perforations to assist drainage. If these small perforations become blocked with blood clots or fibrin, fluid would still be able to enter through the central large hole at the end of the catheter but its drainage may be blocked. When assisting in the acute insertion of a catheter, the nurse should prepare the patient both physically and psychologically. The former may include fleet enemas to empty the rectum and descending colon, a patch-shave about 2.5 cm below the umbilicus, and cleansing of the skin with a povidone-iodine scrub. The patient should

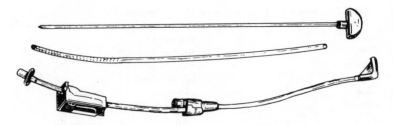

Fig. 6.3. Showing the acute dialysis catheter (TROCATH) with its steel stylet and the tube for connecting it to the giving set.

be instructed to empty his bladder before the procedure. Emptying the bowel and bladder will reduce the risk of perforation during catheter insertion. In an unconscious patient, if doubt exists about the bladder, it may be justified to insert a bladder catheter.

The patient should be given a simple explanation of the procedure and assured that he will receive efficient local anesthesia. He is told that many people are aware only of a sense of pressure on insertion of the catheter. The patient is given an opportunity to practice distending his abdomen by 'blowing out'—a step required during catheter insertion. A similar effect can be achieved when the nurse places one hand on the patient's forehead and asks him to push up strongly against her hand. The doctor should make sure the bladder and rectum are empty.

A pre-medication with diazepam 5 mg orally or intramuscularly is helpful but heavy sedation should be avoided in order to retain the patient's cooperation.

Next, the nurse should assemble the equipment. To expedite this, a sterile pack containing all necessary equipment is stored in the central supply department and sent out as needed.

Before the procedure the nurse should mask, wash her hands with povidone-iodine solution and set up and flush the Y administration tubing to remove the air. A 1.5% solution with 500 units of heparin per litre is used to initiate dialysis. When the doctor arrives, preparations are completed while he scrubs. The patient is placed in a supine position with one pillow for head support. The gown pack, gloves and tray are opened and necessary additions made to the tray.

Once catheter insertion is begun, the nurse's principal function is to manage the dialysis, assess returns and provide emotional support to the patient.

The stylet catheter is inserted at the bedside using the following technique.

1 Shave the hair from the lower abdomen and pubic area. Clean the skin with povidone.

2 Everybody in the room should wear a mask.

3 If the patient is conscious, describe the procedure and demonstrate the Valsalva maneuver. Have the patient practice deep abdominal inspiration and expiration, bearing down at the end of deep inspiration to achieve maximum abdominal distention.

4 The best site for insertion is the midline 2−3 cm below the umbilicus.

5 Infiltrate the skin with 2% Xylocaine.

6 The skin incision should be small (2−3 mm) so that the catheter can pass through easily and be held firmly to minimize mobility.

7 If the skin bleeds profusely, maintain firm pressure for 3−5 minutes before proceeding.

8 With the stylet in place, the catheter is forced through the abdominal wall by a short thrust or with rotating motion while the patient bears down firmly and distends his abdomen maximally. See Fig. 6.4.

9 As the peritoneal cavity is entered, the loss of resistance is recognized as a 'pop'. At this point, withdraw the trocar completely, otherwise further advance will be difficult and the catheter may not enter the small pelvis.

10 Directing its tip toward the tip of the coccyx, advance the catheter deep into the small pelvis. At this stage, the patient will experience a sense of pressure in the rectum. See Fig. 6.5.

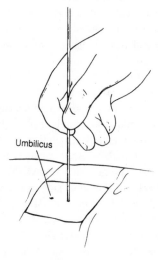

Umbilicus

Fig. 6.4. Insertion of the acute stylet catheter.

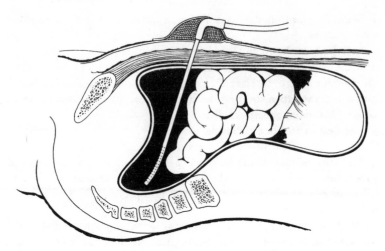

Fig. 6.5. Showing the position of the stylet catheter in the pelvis.

11 If the catheter encounters resistance or if the patient complains of pain, stop the advance in this direction and try another direction.

12 After two or three satisfactory exchanges with a good inflow and outflow, secure the catheter firmly to the skin by the metal disc provided with the catheter.

13 For the initial few exchanges, avoid using hypertonic dialysate especially if the patient is acutely dyspneic. Such patients breathe with the abdominal muscles predominantly and the ultrafiltration induced by a hypertonic solution will further distend the abdomen and thus decrease the efficiency of the abdominal muscles. If the patient develops 'one-way obstruction' (i.e. free inflow but not outflow), retention of dialysate in the peritoneal cavity would be disastrous for the acutely dyspneic patient.

Once the acute catheter is in position and a satisfactory flow has been established, a dry abdominal dressing is applied (Fig. 6.6). A 10×10 cm gauze, placed under the metal disc, stabilizes the catheter and minimizes abrasions from the metal edges. Approximately four 10×10 gauzes are cut to fit around the catheter and placed over the metal disc. Two abdominal pads are placed on either side of the acute catheter. A larger abdominal pad, laid over the entire dressing, is held in place by paper or silk tape rather than pressure tape. A light dressing allows early detection of leaking from the catheter site. Damp dressings are replaced immediately because they are uncomfortable and a potential source of bacterial growth. The dressing is changed at least daily. Frequent dressing

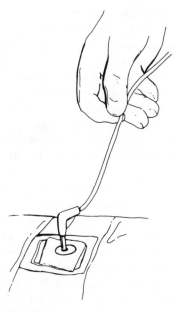

Fig. 6.6. Acute stylet catheter attached to the connecting tube. Metal disc around the catheter to stop it from slipping into the abdomen.

changes may indicate the need for catheter replacement. Masks are worn and a three-minute scrub done before the dressing change.

Stylet catheter insertion may be associated with complications. About 7−10% of patients have inflow and outflow pain due to: (a) pressure of the catheter tip on the internal organs, (b) acid dialysis solution (pH 5.5), (c) hypertonic solution, (d) overdistension of a small abdomen due to excessive fluid or ultrafiltration, (e) entrapment of omentum in the catheter lumen. Shoulder or costal margin pain, a frequent complication, is usually due to accumulation of air under the diaphragm.

Nearly one half of patients will have blood-stained exchanges after catheter insertion. This bleeding (usually minor) comes from the small vessels in the abdominal wall. After a few exchanges such bleeding usually subsides unless a major vessel has been damaged during insertion or the patient has a bleeding disorder. Occasionally, a transfusion of fresh blood may be necessary. If significant, the bleeding may obstruct the catheter; in this event, one can add 1000 units of heparin to each litre of dialysate to minimize the risk of clotting.

The most frustrating complication of acute catheter placement is dialysate leak. The risk of such leakage from the exit site is increased by frequent manipulations of the catheter to improve drainage but is minimized by securing the catheter to the skin with the aid of the metal disc. The risk of leakage is higher in elderly or chronically ill patients, and in multiparous women with lax abdominal walls. The raised intraabdominal pressure produced by large polycystic kidney(s) may induce an external leak. Fluid may extravasate into the abdominal wall, particularly in those who have had an abdominal operation or multiple catheter insertions. Usually such extravasations result from tears in the peritoneum or represent infusion of dialysate into the potential space between the layers of abdominal wall. Acute hydrothorax may result from a traumatic or a congenital defect in the diaphragm. In such cases, peritoneal dialysis is discontinued and hemodialysis is instituted.

Inadequate drainage, which is frequent during acute dialysis, may be due to one or more of the following: loss of the siphon effect, one-way obstruction, and incorrect placement of the catheter. One-way (outflow) obstruction may be due to fibrin or blood clots in the catheter blocking the terminal holes, especially when dialysis is complicated by major hemorrhage or peritonitis. Poor outflow may also reflect extrinsic pressure from adjacent organs such as a sigmoid colon full of feces. Occasionally, drainage is poor when the catheter penetrates the extraperitoneal space; in such a situation, continued infusion produces further dissection, the fluid becomes trapped and is no longer available for drainage. Loculation of fluid, another cause of poor drainage, is encountered in patients who have had previous intra-abdominal operations or peritonitis. Such loculation not only diminishes the surface area available for dialysis but may greatly reduce ultrafiltration capacity.

Published reports of organs perforated or lacerated during stylet catheter insertion include bowel, bladder, liver, a polycystic kidney, aorta, mesenteric artery and hernial sac. Such perforation is more likely in the presence of abdominal distension due to paralytic ileus or bowel obstruction, or in those who are unconscious, cachectic or heavily sedated. Clinical evidence of bowel perforation includes sudden sharp or severe abdominal pain followed by watery diarrhea, and poor drainage of dialysate, which may be cloudy, foul-smelling or mixed with fecal material. In most patients the perforation seals off completely in about 12 hours but in some cases surgical intervention may be necessary. If surgical intervention is planned it is better to leave the catheter in place till the patient goes to the operating room since the catheter will lead the surgeon to the site of the perforation.

In patients receiving short-term peritoneal dialysis for acute renal failure, the catheter can be replaced between treatments by a short plastic plug called a Deane's prosthesis. This keeps the catheter track open and facilitates replacing the catheter for the next dialysis. See Fig. 6.7.

In patients with acute renal failure treated with peritoneal dialysis, the incidence of peritonitis depends on the type of peritoneal access and the duration of each dialysis. The diagnosis and treatment of peritonitis is discussed in the section dealing with CAPD.

Bedside technique for insertion of Tenckhoff catheter

Because of the frequent complications seen with stylet catheter insertion, a Tenckhoff catheter (Fig. 6.8) may be preferred for peritoneal access, even for acute dialysis. The following procedure applies for catheter insertion for both acute and long-term use. The Tenckhoff catheter can be implanted at the bedside using a special trocar or in the operating room under direct vision.

At the bedside the Tenckhoff catheter is inserted as follows. First the patient is examined to exclude those conditions that promote complications during dialysis. For example, before implanting a permanent catheter one must eradicate active peritonitis from previous acute dialysis. Similarly, if the patient had a Deane's prosthesis it must be removed at least 24 hours before insertion of the permanent catheter. Infected abdominal incisions and stomas predispose to peritonitis during any peritoneal dialysis. Therefore, catheter insertion should be delayed until these defects have healed. Poor wound healing associated with abdominal scars, a lax abdominal wall from old age, multiple pregnancies or steroid treatment may

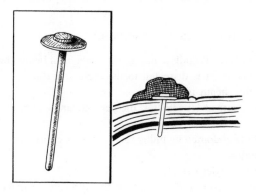

Fig. 6.7. Deane's prosthesis, insertion.

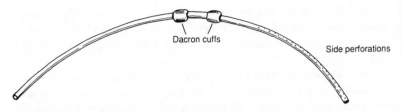

Fig. 6.8. Tenckhoff permanent peritoneal catheter.

predispose to leakage. In patients with these conditions dialysis should be delayed for 24 to 48 hours after catheter insertion, and the initial exchange volume should be small, e.g. 500−1000 ml per exchange. When present, hernias can be repaired at the time of catheter insertion and, if the patient's condition permits, dialysis should be delayed for a week to allow the wound to heal. It may be desirable to support such patients with hemodialysis through a subclavian catheter until satisfactory healing takes place. Carriers of hepatitis B antigen should be isolated from other patients on dialysis, and all necessary precautions observed in handling their blood and dialysate.

Preparation of the patient before permanent catheter insertion

1 Shave and prepare the abdomen.
2 Give a cleansing enema the night before catheter insertion.
3 Give a prophylactic single dose of antibiotics (tobramycin, 1.7 mg/kg of body weight iv; cephalothin, 1 g iv) half an hour before the procedure.

Steps in bedside catheter insertion

- A 2−3 cm vertical midline incision is made 3 cm below the umbilicus.
- Subcutaneous fat is dissected to the rectus sheath.
- The rectus sheath is slit open.
- Using an acute stylet catheter, the peritoneum is entered as described previously.
- Distend the abdomen by filling the peritoneal cavity with 2−3 litres of dialysis solution.
- Remove the stylet catheter.
- Through the same hole, introduce the specially designed trocar into the peritoneal cavity while the patient is bearing down.

• Introduce through the trocar a single-cuff Tenckhoff catheter stiffened by a soft obturator.

• Once the tip is in the peritoneal cavity, tilt the trocar about 45° to direct the tip toward the coccyx.

• Advance the catheter gently until the patient reports a sense of pressure over the rectal area.

• Withdraw the obturator and test catheter patency by draining off 200–300 ml of dialysate.

• Separate the trocar into its two longitudinal halves and withdraw them.

• Bring the catheter out of the skin through a 2–3 inch subcutaneous tunnel which is directed towards the head. Close the subcutaneous tissue with catgut and the skin with a running Mersilene suture.

Surgical implantation of the permanent catheter

Surgical implantation involves the following steps. A short transverse lateral incision is made over the rectus muscle. The rectus sheath is divided transversely and the muscle split longitudinally. Through a small incision in the posterior sheath and peritoneum, the cannula is implanted in the pelvis, and peritoneum is closed around it. The muscle is placed over the Dacron cuff. The catheter is angled to come out through the anterior rectus sheath through a hole, separate from the transverse incision in the anterior rectus sheath. This gives the catheter a more caudal direction and helps keep it in the pelvis. Then, through a short tunnel directed towards the head, the catheter is brought out superior to the transverse skin incision. See Fig. 6.9.

'Break-in' technique

Following catheter insertion 500–1000 ml of dialysate is infused and drained off immediately to assess catheter function (Fig. 6.10). Slow inflow may indicate improper positioning or partial obstruction by blood-clots. Clots can be flushed out by dialysate infused under pressure; malpositioning requires manipulations of the catheter until drainage becomes adequate. The nurse assesses the effluent with respect to its color, clarity, volume and rate of flow. Although it is normal for the fluid to be pinkish to red after insertion, a volume of bright red drainage greater than the instilled fluid, accompanied by a fall in blood pressure and tachycardia may signal the perforation of a major blood vessel. Bowel perforation is identified by the presence of cloudy effluent, occasionally

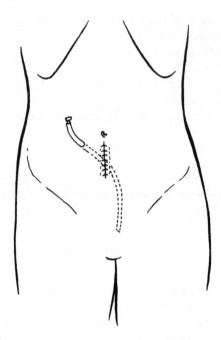

Fig. 6.9. Tenckhoff catheter in place after surgical implantation.

containing fecal material with or without abdominal pain. Bladder perforation is characterized by a low volume of drainage through the catheter, bladder spasms and increased dilute 'urinary' output. In the patient with ascites, the dialysate is drained away slowly to avoid the complications of rapid loss of ascitic fluid. During each exchange one should drain away 100 to 500 ml in addition to the infused volume. When drainage has reached the prescribed volume, it is stopped even though it has a good flow rate, and the next exchange started. This approach permits a gradual reduction in the ascites.

To maintain aseptic technique the nurse should wear a mask and wash her hands well before adding medications and changing the bags. Medications given intraperitoneally may include heparin, KCl, Xylocaine, antibiotics and insulin. Unless otherwise indicated by the doctor, these may be mixed in the same bag. Heparin, 500 units per litre, is given routinely to prevent obstruction of the catheter by blood clots or fibrin. The remaining medications are given according to the individual patient's requirement. Thus KCl is added if the patient's potassium level is below 3.0 mmol/l or if he is starting a second day of continuous dialysis.

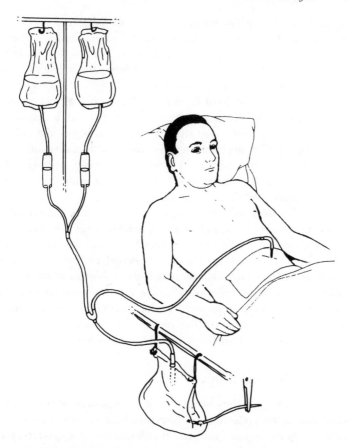

Fig. 6.10. Showing the tubing set and bags during manual peritoneal dialysis.

Also, if the patient is receiving digitalis, has a serum potassium less than 5.0 mmol/l and is receiving dialysis for the first time, 3 mmol KCl/l should be added to the dialysate to minimize the effect of rapid shifts in potassium. To alleviate abdominal discomfort one may add Xylocaine without epinephrine—5–10 ml of 1% or 2% solution per litre of dialysate. However, one must determine the cause of the abdominal pain before such use because indiscriminate suppression of abdominal pain with Xylocaine may mask the onset of an intra-abdominal complication.

Antibiotics such as cephalothin and tobramycin may be ordered prophylactically to prevent peritonitis. Diabetics are given regular insulin intraperitoneally to offset the extra glucose load absorbed from the dialysate. Here the capillary blood sugar is monitored every four hours to assess individual insulin requirements. Intraperitoneal insulin is discontinued two hours before the end of dialysis to avoid post-dialysis hypoglycemia. During dialysis, in addition to the intraperitoneal insulin, the diabetic continues his subcutaneous dose.

The first dialysis is delayed for at least 24 hours in high-risk patients. For those on steroids, diabetics, multiparous women, etc., it is delayed for several days. During this period and until dialysis is begun, the catheter is irrigated every 12 hours on the first day and daily thereafter with 10 ml of heparinized (2000 U heparin + 8 ml sterile saline) solution. After irrigation, the catheter lumen is filled with 3000 units of undiluted heparin solution (1000 U/ml) and the external tip is covered with a sterile cap. To avoid incisional leakage, every patient is maintained on intermittent peritoneal dialysis (IPD) with small volumes (500 ml the first time and 1000 ml thereafter) twice a week for at least two weeks before commencing CAPD training. During this period and between dialysis, the catheter is filled with 3000 units of heparin solution as before.

Dialysis may be started soon after the catheter insertion except in those high-risk patients mentioned earlier. CAPD is postponed for at least two weeks to minimize the risk of dialysate leak. During the interval, the patient is maintained on IPD or hemodialysis.

Records for manual dialysis

The term, 'exchange', refers to the total of inflow, dwell and outflow. For manual dialysis we prefer using 3 litre bags because they minimize the number of bag changes and medication additions. In the dialysis recorded in the chart shown in Fig. 6.11 each bag provides three exchanges, each of one litre. With this first bag the fluid can be instilled and drained rapidly. This 'flushing' permits an early assessment of catheter function and tends to flush out clots which may have formed during catheter insertion.

One cannot assume that a 3 litre bag contains 3 litres of dialysate. For example, with Travenol solutions there is always an extra 40 ml per litre. Thus each 3 liter bag contains 3120 ml.

In the example shown in Fig. 6.11 the first litre was infused over five minutes beginning at 10:00 and drained immediately at 10:05. In recording this exchange, the time of starting the inflow, recorded in column 2, corresponds to the check in column 7, and the time noted for the start of draining out corresponds to the check mark in column 8.

After one full bag has entered the abdomen and all three exchanges

(Numbers — refer to columns in written section)

Patient's name: ....

Ideal Weight ......60 Kg......

1	2	3	4	5	6	7	8	9	10	11
		NUMBER OF EX-CHANGE	STRENGTH OF SOLUTION	LOT NUMBER OF SOLUTION	MEDIC-ATION	AMOUNT OF SOLUTION		CUMU-LATIVE FLUID BALANCE	WEIGHT HOUR	REMARKS
DATE	HOUR					IN-STILLED	DRAINED			SIGNATURE, POSITION
Nov.20 1984	1000	1				3120 ✓			63.6	returns slightly
	1005						✓			pink; draining
	1015	2	1·5%	AP206P3	1500	✓				well
	1020				units Heparin		✓			
	1030	3				✓				
	1035						3000 ✓	+120		+120 E. Kelman RN
	1045	4				3120 ✓				returns clear
	1100						✓			
	1110	5	4·25%	AP200R6	1500	✓				tubing kinked
	1125				units Heparin		✓			poor outflow
	1155	6				✓				
	1210						3300 ✓	−60		−180 E. Kelman RN
	1225	7				3120 ✓				
	1235						✓			
	1245	8	4·25%	AP200R6	1500	✓				
	1300				units Heparin		✓			
	1310	9				✓				
	1325						3450 ✓	−390		−330 E. Kelman RN
	1335	10				3120				
	1350									
	1405	11	1·5%	AP206P3	1500					
	1420				units Heparin					
	1430	12								
	1445	12					3100	−370		+20 E. Kelman RN

Fig. 6.11. Manual dialysis record sheet.

have been drained out the total drainage is measured in a graduated cylinder and recorded in column 8. The difference between these two volumes is entered in the 'Remarks' column and then transferred to column 9. The positive balance of 120 ml after three exchanges means that this volume has been retained by the patient.

Exchanges 4, 5 and 6 are allowed longer dwell times, exchange number 5 taking altogether 45 minutes presumably because of the outflow problems recorded in column 11. But by the end of six exchanges we are beginning to remove fluid from the patient as shown by the negative cumulative balance (-60 ml) recorded in column 9. After nine exchanges the negative balance has increased to -390 ml. The aim of gradual fluid removal from the patient is therefore being achieved. The time required for the different phases of the exchanges shows that the catheter is patent and the fluid balance is satisfactory.

The remaining columns on the dialysis record sheet show information concerning dialysate composition and additives and information about the patient.

Column 4 shows the strength and composition of the solution. Recording the lot number in column 5 provides a reference if this is needed to investigate dialysate-associated complications. Column 6 records medications administered intraperitoneally and these are signed off in column 11 by the nurse responsible. The patient's weight is recorded in column 10. The weight and vital signs are recorded every four hours unless otherwise ordered. The nurse writes comments related to the dialysis in the remarks column. Ideal (or dry) weight is that which the doctor believes reflects the patient's normal hydration. As long as the patient's weight is more than 1 kg above the ideal one should use hypertonic solutions—2.5% or 4.25%. However, frequent hypertonic exchanges in close succession remove water rapidly. They may be painful and may result in hypotension. For this reason body weight should be brought back to the ideal slowly over a two to three day period.

Certain duties, such as procedures which involve interrupting the system should be reserved for specially trained dialysis staff. This rule ensures that all connections, disconnections, tubing changes and irrigation procedures are done by those who use these skills daily. The non-dialysis nurses employed during acute dialysis often are drawn from the hospital's 'float' staff; they receive a two-day orientation which reviews renal nursing and dialysis procedures, and they are given an opportunity to perform manual peritoneal dialysis under supervision in the dialysis unit.

Nursing requirements for termination of dialysis

The termination of acute dialysis may employ one of three approaches: the acute catheter may be (a) removed, (b) left *in situ*, or (c) removed and replaced by the Deane's prosthesis. Reinsertion is necessary with the first approach whereas the other two options provide access for later dialysis. If the catheter is left in, the old tubing set is replaced before starting dialysis. This approach often leaves the patients afraid to move and sets the stage for clotting of the catheter.

When a catheter is removed, its tip is sent for culture and sensitivities and the exit hole is covered with a small airstrip bandage. If the patient has been drained fully before catheter removal, the site rarely leaks and should seal itself within 24 hours.

Replacement by a Deane's prosthesis avoids the need for a new incision for a new catheter. However the device is often difficult to insert because the patient tends to tense his abdominal muscles. It is unwise to force the device against such resistance. In preparation for insertion of this prosthesis, the nurse reassures the patient and encourages a state of relaxation. The catheter site is cleansed with povidone-iodine and alcohol before removal of the original catheter. As with all dialysis procedures, the nurse should mask, scrub, glove and maintain aseptic technique. The patient is masked, asked to take a deep breath as the catheter is removed and directed to exhale as the prosthesis is inserted. Two small bandages and a small airstrip holds the prosthesis in place. It should be changed weekly until the attending physician makes a decision about the patient's further dialysis requirements.

The prosthesis should be removed at least 24 hours before the surgical insertion of a permanent catheter. On removal, a swab from the tip of the stem portion is sent for culture and sensitivity.

Complications of acute peritoneal dialysis

The introduction of dialysis solution into the abdominal cavity induces many changes in systemic hemodynamics. Most of the medical complications (Table 6.2) encountered during acute peritoneal dialysis are related to the rapidity with which these changes are brought about.

Hypovolemia of varying severity is common during acute peritoneal dialysis, particularly in those subjected to repeated peritoneal dialysis. Usually this complication, which develops when large volumes of fluid are removed too rapidly, can be prevented by anticipating it and by

Table 6.2. Complications of acute peritoneal dialysis

Medical complications
- hypovolemia
- fluid overload, heart failure and pulmonary edema
- arrhythmia and hypokalemia
- ischemic cardiac events

Pulmonary complications

Neurological complications
- disequilibrium syndrome
- convulsions
- mental confusion

Metabolic complications
- hyperglycemia
- hypoglycemia
- hypernatremia

attending to it promptly. Tachyarrhythmias are frequent during dialysis, especially in patients with underlying heart disease or in those receiving digitalis. Those with ischemic heart disease tolerate hemodynamic fluctuations poorly, hence rapid ultrafiltration, accompanied by a sudden fall in blood pressure, may precipitate angina and, in some, frank myocardial infarction.

Basal atelectasis, acute purulent bronchitis, pneumonia and pleural effusions have been reported as a direct consequence of peritoneal dialysis. Repeated upward displacement of the diaphragm following overdistension with dialysate may induce basal atelectasis. During peritoneal dialysis the PO_2 of arterial blood falls by 3 to 26 mm Hg when the abdomen is distended with two litres of dialysate and returns to its basal level when the fluid is drained out. A special danger is vomiting and inhalation of gastric contents, which may be fatal; also sudden right-sided pleural effusion.

The term 'disequilibrium syndrome' has been applied to a group of symptoms and signs observed chiefly in hemodialysed patients during the first dialysis. The cerebral edema underlying this syndrome reflects an osmotic gradient set up between CSF and blood after the rapid removal of urea and other solutes from the extracellular compartment, which is not followed by equally rapid changes in CSF. The patient complains of headache, may vomit and proceeds to hypertension, convulsions and coma—the last may be fatal. This syndrome is rare after peritoneal dialysis probably because of the relatively slow transfer of urea across the peritoneal membrane compared with the rapid movement during hemo-dialysis.

Hyperglycemia and hypoglycemia are frequent during dialysis, especially in diabetics. Hypoglycemia is always the result of the administration of excessive amounts of insulin especially if insulin is given in the dialysate throughout the procedure. Mild degrees of hypernatremia are common following ultrafiltration using hypertonic solutions; at those times, more water than sodium is lost from plasma and extracellular fluid.

Patients on peritoneal dialysis may develop either respiratory or metabolic alkalosis. The former may develop during the initial stages of dialysis when hyperventilation, due to a low spinal fluid pH, may continue to reduce P_{CO_2} while serum bicarbonate increases as the body generates bicarbonate to correct the extracellular acidosis. Since the bicarbonate ion diffuses slowly across the blood–brain barrier, cerebral fluid pH does not change promptly and the respiratory center (responding to the acid pH) continues to direct hyperventilation, further reducing P_{CO_2}. This tendency may be slight during dialysis because lactate conversion to bicarbonate in the liver occurs slowly enough to permit the cerebral fluid pH to adjust. In view of this cycle of events, one should not infuse bicarbonate to achieve rapid correction of acidosis. In any event, no harmful effects have been attributed to temporary respiratory alkalosis.

Metabolic alkalosis occasionally may develop slowly in patients on peritoneal dialysis, especially if they receive significant amounts of 7% dextrose solution. These solutions are banned throughout North America.

Long-term peritoneal dialysis

In maintenance therapy to sustain life, patients with end-stage renal disease now have a choice between intermittent peritoneal dialysis (IPD) or continuous peritoneal dialysis (CAPD or CCPD). In the early 70s nephrologists did not recommend long-term treatment either in hospital or at home, because it involved repeated abdominal-wall puncture, an uncomfortable stiff plastic catheter, and the risk of recurrent peritonitis. Furthermore, equipment had not yet been developed which permitted patients to carry out their own treatment.

This state of affairs was changed by two developments: firstly, a soft peritoneal catheter made of silicone rubber allowed unsupervised home dialysis. It could be left in the peritoneal cavity for long periods without being changed. There are now a number of variations on this original Tenckhoff catheter. Our main alternative is the Toronto Western Hospital catheter developed by Oreopoulos in collaboration with the late Gabor Zellerman. This catheter, illustrated in Fig. 6.12 has a number of soft silastic discs mounted on it at intervals. This modification helps to prevent migration of the catheter out of the pelvis, thus ensuring good outflow during the drainage phase.

Next the introduction of continuous ambulatory peritoneal dialysis (CAPD) in 1977 revolutionized long-term peritoneal dialysis. Its many advantages included a simple operation, freedom from mechanical equipment and electrical supplies, promotion of home dialysis, compatibility with travel and an overall reduction in cost. In addition to its social advantages, CAPD has many medical advantages: an increase in the weekly clearances of small and middle molecules, few dietary and fluid restrictions, and decreased incidence of thirst, anemia and hypertension. Because of these benefits, about 30 000 patients throughout the world were receiving treatment with CAPD by the end of 1986.

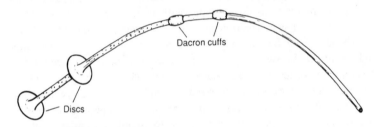

Fig. 6.12. Toronto Western Hospital catheter with discs.

Long-term intermittent peritoneal dialysis

This form of peritoneal dialysis (IPD) was widely used before CAPD became popular. Patients were dialysed for 40 hours per week—either 2 × 20 hours in hospital, or 4 × 10 overnight hours at home, with a flow rate of 3−4 l/h. The peritonitis rate was 0.3% in hospital. However, in many patients the long-term results were poor, especially in those who were anuric and required more than 60 hours per week to maintain adequate biochemical control. Many were unable to continue and had to be transferred to hemodialysis. To date, the longest period of maintenance on long-term IPD has been eight years.

Long-term IPD is now reserved for those who have to be treated in hospital, for example those who are unwilling or unable to perform CAPD at home, the blind and the very old. In addition, those waiting to be trained for CAPD are maintained on IPD. These patients require a permanent peritoneal catheter and access to a peritoneal dialysis machine. Peritoneal access for IPD is achieved through a permanent peritoneal catheter.

Peritoneal dialysis machines

Dr Boen introduced the first automated machine, which consisted of a cycler which circulated dialysate in a 40 litre container, presterilized by heat. Later on, Tenckhoff introduced a device which sterilized distilled water by heat and added a concentrated solution of solute to produce the dialysate. Although these were closed systems, neither gained wide acceptance. In contrast, in recent years, the automatic peritoneal cycler, designed by Lasker, and later the reverse osmosis PD machine, designed by Tenckhoff, have come into wide use. However, despite its advantages the use of the latter has declined sharply because of the complicated design and frequent failures.

Of the various cyclers on the market, most are based on the principles of the Lasker machine (American Medical Products Cycler); this is the one used most frequently at the Toronto Western Hospital.

The Lasker cycler (AMP) (Fig. 6.13)

This is composed of two components—the heater and the cycler. It operates by gravity and the flow of the dialysis solution is controlled by a clamping device, which determines inflow and outflow of the dialysate. Six to eight bags are hung above the level of the heater to allow fluid to flow by gravity from the bags to the heater. The dialysate volume in the heater can be preset according to the space allowed for the heater bag and this depends on the patient's requirements. Generally, new patients begin with one litre volumes, which gradually are increased to two litres over a two-week period. Smaller volumes, such as 500 ml, may be used in special circumstances such as very small or obese patients who risk incisional leak with larger volumes. The cycler has two timers, and a clamping system with two bars, which control the flow of the dialysis solution. The timers control the 'fill' and 'drain' cycles. During the 'drain' cycle, the solution flows from the bags to the heater and from the patient into a weighing bag at one side of the cycler. The bag, which hangs from a scale, is placed at a level lower than the patient's bed so that the fluid can drain easily into the bag by syphoning. A scale inside the cycler measures the volume drained out and compares it with the volume infused. If the volume drained from the patient is greater than

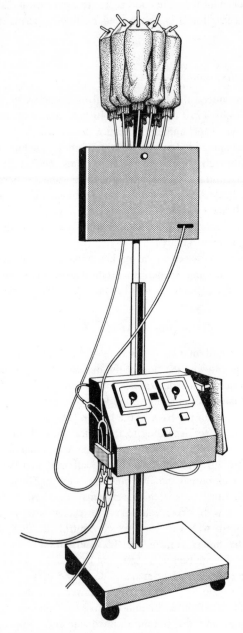

Fig. 6.13. Lasker peritoneal cycles.

the predetermined level the timer automatically switches to the 'fill' cycle. During the 'fill' cycle, warm dialysate is infused from the heater bag into the patient where it 'dwells' for the prescribed time, while simultaneously the fluid from the weighing bag empties into a floor drain.

The cycler is equipped with various alarms, which give an early warning of malfunction. Thus, a drain alarm sounds if the outflow is deficient. Inadequate drainage may reflect poor catheter function or simply kinking of the tubing due to the patient's position. If this occurs, the drain phase is reset manually to allow another few minutes of drainage and the patient's abdomen is checked for the accumulation of fluid. In the event of heater malfunction, a temperature alarm prevents the inflow of overheated dialysate. Overheated solution produces significant pain and probably damages the peritoneal membrane. Recent models have an alarm, which goes on if the weigh bag does not empty properly. Others have an alarm that detects a cloudy effluent.

Even though the cycler is relatively safe and easy to operate, each time it is used for peritoneal dialysis the nurse must go through a safety check of the tubing and alarm systems. Once the patient is connected, the machine should be checked every four hours.

In preparing the cycler for dialysis, the nurse follows the unit's guidelines concerning rate of exchange. Currently our policy is as follows:
• Three litres an hour for those patients on long-term intermittent peritoneal dialysis, i.e. two litres every 40 minutes, which is equivalent to a fill (+ dwell) time of 28 minutes, and a drain time of 12 minutes.
• For patients on short-term intermittent peritoneal dialysis in preparation for CAPD training, the flow rate is only two litres an hour—a fill (+ dwell) time of 48 minutes, and drain time 12 minutes.

The patient is weighed every four hours and, based on the changes in weight, the nurse chooses the osmolality of the solutions. During the initial dialyses, it may be necessary to check the weight more frequently to establish the individual patient's pattern of fluid loss and thus avoid unexpected dehydration. It is interesting that the ultrafiltration rate is higher during the night than during the day.

When medications are given to patients on the cycler, they are injected into one bag. All the heparin is injected into one bag and all the potassium chloride (if it is needed) is injected into another. Since all bags empty simultaneously the medicated solutions will be evenly mixed with the remaining bags as the dialysate enters the heating bag. During dialysis drug doses can be changed easily by replacing the medicated bags. Also, adding the total amount of one medication to one bag minimizes the number of breaks in the system and maintains a relatively closed system.

Usually an eight or ten prong tubing is used to reduce the number of spike connections made during a 20-hour treatment. We prefer a five-pronged tubing with three litre bags (or eight-pronged tubing with two litre bags) for diabetic patients to permit us to adjust the dose of intra-peritoneal insulin according to the blood sugar values which are obtained after every 15 to 16 litres infused. Thus, each time this number of bags has been added and emptied we recalculate the insulin requirements. More frequent glucose estimations are done for unstable patients.

Patients have few complaints about the cycler and this machine provides efficient and safe delivery of dialysate. Rarely a patient who drains in less than the preset time may complain of abdominal discomfort at the end of the cycle. However this is corrected by individualizing the drain time. Also, a patient may overfill if the tubings in the control system were installed incorrectly. This is avoided if the nurse adheres to the predialysis safety checks.

As with all machines, the new patient will express fears and concerns, which should be discussed openly. The various alarms and machine functions are described in detail before dialysis to reduce these fears to a minimum. Appendix 2, p.408, contains detailed instructions for starting and terminating a dialysis in a patient on long-term IPD.

Continuous ambulatory peritoneal dialysis (CAPD)

Indications and selection criteria

In the early years of CAPD the selection criteria were arbitrary and it was used mostly for those unable to perform intermittent peritoneal dialysis (IPD) or hemodialysis. This alternative mode was chosen for one or more of the following reasons: poor biochemical control with high pre-dialysis serum creatinine; anemia (hemoglobin 5 g/dl in a patient who was not anephric); need for repeated blood transfusions; poorly controlled hypertension; excessive fluid gain between dialysis; progression of metabolic and neurologic complications; and those who had no train-able partner to assist with home IPD.

During the past six years, a large experience has supported the following specific indications and contra-indications for CAPD.

Indications for CAPD

- Promotion of home dialysis.
- Older patients with complicating cardiovascular disease.
- Children with small body size and poor vascular access.
- Diabetics with end-stage renal disease.
- Uncontrollable hypertension during dialysis.
- Malignant hypertension with renal failure.
- Severe anemia requiring multiple blood transfusions.
- Pretransplant maintenance dialysis.
- Acute renal failure.

Contra-indications to CAPD. Poor peritoneal clearance is an absolute contra-indication to CAPD. Relative contra-indications include:
- Vertebral disease with backache.
- Abdominal hernias.
- Presence of a colostomy or ileostomy.
- Concurrent immunosuppressive treatment.
- Chronic obstructive lung disease.
- Poorly motivated and/or depressed patients.

Standard Toronto Western Hospital technique for CAPD

These are the principal features of the technique: two-litre plastic bags containing dialysate are connected to the permanent peritoneal catheter by a short plastic tube with appropriate connectors at each end. After inflow, the empty bag, still attached to the connection tube, is rolled up in a cloth waist purse and carried under the clothing. At the end of the diffusion period, the dialysate is drained into the same bag and the connection tubing is removed from the older bag and connected to a new one, using an aseptic technique. After one or two months the connection tube is changed under sterile conditions by the patient or by a nurse.

Most patients will require four bags per day; the timing of the exchanges is tailored to the patient's convenience. A significant group of patients (25−35%) can be maintained on three bags (6 litres per day) if, on 8 litres per day, they have a serum creatinine of less than 900−1000 μmol/l (10−11.5 mg/dl). On the other hand, those (5−10%) who, on four bags (8 litres per day), have a serum creatinine over 17−18 mg/dl will require five bags (10 litres) per day. Finally, 30−35% of the patients will tolerate 3 litre exchanges. A 3×3 litres/day program involves fewer exchanges, a lower infection rate, and a larger daily volume, giving a better solute clearance and better ultrafiltration than the 2×4 litres/day scheme.

Guidelines for choice of peritoneal dialysis solution

These are general guidelines only. The rate of fluid removal varies from patient to patient. The choice of dextrose concentrations is based on desired dry and present weight, lying and standing blood pressure, and the presence or absence of edema and congestion. Other factors considered in this choice are the presence of diarrhea, vomiting, anorexia or increased fluid intake. Finally, one should take into account the patient's intake and output, and his total fluid balance.

At the Toronto Western Hospital we observe the following guidelines:
• If the patient's weight is more than 0.5 kg below his dry weight use 0.5%.
• If patient's weight is at dry weight ($\pm$ 0.5 kg) use 1.5%.
• If patient's weight is between 0.5 to 1 kg above dry weight use 2.5%.
• If patient's weight is greater than 1 kg above dry weight use 4.25%.

Dry heat is the only acceptable method of warming solutions. Water baths should *not* be used because of the danger of bacterial contamination. If a warm bag is unavailable, use a bag at room temperature. A hot dialysis solution should never be used. Recently, some people have recommended warming of the solution in microwave ovens as a rapid and safe method.

If the patient is receiving hypotensive medications or coronary vasodilators, use hypertonic solutions with great caution.

Small individuals, those with large cystic kidneys, those with active peritonitis, and those with hernias may require volumes less than two litres.

Short and long-term effects of CAPD

Because CAPD is a continuous process, this treatment does not produce the fluctuating 'pre−post' biochemical and hemodynamic changes characteristic of intermittent forms of dialysis. With regard to clearance of various sized molecules, CAPD is less effective than hemodialysis in removing small-sized molecules. Peritoneal clearance increases with hypertonic solutions, not only because of the ultrafiltration volume, but also because of the solvent-drag effect. Because of increased protein losses with this treatment (6−12 g/day), most CAPD patients have hypoproteinemia and some may be in negative nitrogen balance, especially during episodes of peritonitis when protein losses increase.

CAPD removes a significant amount of sodium (100−200 mmol/day) especially if hypertonic solutions are used. Similarly, it achieves excellent control of serum potassium in most patients. About 10% of these patients may develop hypokalemia, and may require oral potassium supplements. Hypokalemia is particularly frequent in those patients who also receive large doses of diuretics. Potassium should not be added to the bag because this invades the sterile system. Also, such addition does not raise the serum potassium substantially. When hyperkalemia appears, as it may in about 5−10% of patients, potassium should be restricted and a cation exchange resin given by mouth.

During CAPD, improvement in anemia is striking, and in some patients the hemoglobin may reach normal or even supernormal levels. The mechanism of this improvement is unknown but it may represent removal of toxic substances, which have suppressed the bone marrow's response to erythropoietin.

Hypertension, which is common in patients starting dialysis, can usually be controlled if the patient is maintained close to dry weight at all times. The control of hypertension with CAPD is superior to that with IPD. Most patients, even those with malignant hypertension, become normotensive after one to two months on CAPD and some may become hypotensive. The blood pressure returns to normal at a time when body weight is increasing, probably as a result of sodium depletion. If the patient becomes hypotensive, the blood pressure will usually return to normal if the oral sodium intake is increased while the body weight is kept stable by dialysis.

CAPD removes some parathyroid hormone fractions (PTH), but does not reduce the plasma level of parathyroid hormone. This decreases only when its secretion is suppressed by an increase in serum calcium. Osteitis fibrosa persists despite treatment with 1,25-dihydroxy vitamin D. If the physician wishes to decrease the serum PTH and stimulate healing of the osteitis fibrosa, the serum calcium must be maintained at slightly hypercalcemic levels (2.6−2.75 mmol/l) (10.5−11 mg/dl). Hypercalcemia in the presence of uncontrolled serum phosphate levels will lead to soft-tissue calcification and kidney stones. By itself CAPD does not keep the serum phosphate at normal levels. Hence these patients require small amounts of phosphate binders. When the serum phosphorus is 1.5 mmol/l (6 mg/dl) or higher, the patient must avoid vitamin D or its metabolites to minimize soft-tissue calcification.

Nerve-conduction velocities do not decrease during either hemodialysis or peritoneal dialysis, except in those who are underdialysed or severely malnourished. Studies in patients on CAPD for periods of three to five years have shown no deterioration in nerve conduction velocities.

Pericarditis is always a risk in any patient undergoing long-term dialysis. It presents with chest pain, a pericardial friction rub, low-grade temperature, and mild leukocytosis. Patients on peritoneal dialysis who have pericarditis tend not to develop tamponade. Generally, pericarditis without tamponade responds to conservative management, namely increased dialysis, salt restriction, and strict control of fluid intake. Incidence of pericarditis among patients on CAPD is extremely low (4–5%), and, when it occurs, it usually develops in a noncompliant patient who has not done enough dialysis.

Complications of CAPD

Peritonitis. Peritonitis, the most frequent complication of CAPD, is classified according to the causative organism or the route of invasion. Since the introduction of the Toronto Western Hospital technique, the addition of the Luer-Lock adapter between the catheter and tubing, and the institution of monthly tubing changes, the incidence of peritonitis has decreased to about one episode every 10 to 12 patient months.

Most of the peritonitis in CAPD patients (about 70%) is due to normal skin flora, i.e. *Staphylococcus epidermidis* and *Staph. aureus.* Usually *Staph. epidermis* peritonitis is mild and has a good prognosis. In contrast, *Staph. aureus* peritonitis has a tendency to hypotension, severe course and abscess formation. *Streptococcus viridans* produces a severe peritonitis with marked constitutional symptoms. However it can be controlled with antibiotics and has a good prognosis.

Twenty per cent of peritonitis is caused by Gram-negative organisms, which presumably originate from the bowel. Such infection may be due to a single organism or to mixed pathogens in various combinations with a fungus or Bacteroides. Although the isolation of enteric organisms from the dialysate during peritonitis suggests a bowel leak, either a micro or macro perforation, occasionally, in the presence of an abnormal bowel motility, the organism may cross the intact bowel wall. Chronic constipation and diverticulosis both predispose to bowel leakage.

Our experience with fungal peritonitis suggests that the most important step in its management is prompt removal of the peritoneal catheter. These patients may start CAPD again about four weeks after the infection has been controlled. Tuberculous peritonitis, although uncommon, produces prolonged peritonitis. In such cases one would discontinue CAPD and maintain the patient on hemodialysis and antituberculous treatment.

True 'culture-negative' (aseptic) peritonitis, which is uncommon

(2—5%), may be due to chemicals, endotoxins, and various other irritating substances. Eosinophilic peritonitis is an asymptomatic, culture-negative inflammation, which is accompanied by a cloudy dialysate composed of eosinophils. The cause of this entity is unknown and its course is self limiting.

A patient suspected of having peritonitis should be examined in the unit which has accepted responsibility for his or her management. Patients who live far from the unit should be examined by a doctor who is familiar with CAPD and its complications. Peritonitis has two types of presentation. Most patients have minor symptoms, but 25 to 30% are extremely ill. Patients with peritonitis due to *Staph. aureus* or *Strep. viridans*, and those with fecal peritonitis, present with a severe illness. The longer the peritonitis remains untreated the more severe it becomes.

Dialysate white-cell count is useful in the diagnosis of doubtful cases; a count above $100/mm^2$ indicates peritonitis. The white cell count is also important in the follow-up. An unexpected increase after an initial decrease may indicate recurrence.

When done by an experienced technician, the Gram stain will demonstrate the offending organism in 50—60% of cases. This procedure is particularly valuable in the detection of fungi, which otherwise may take 5—6 days to grow. In the early stages of fecal peritonitis, the Gram stain may show a mixture of Gram-negative and Gram-positive organisms.

Diagnosis depends on:
• the identification of an organism on Gram stain or on culture of peritoneal effluent;
• the presence of cloudy peritoneal effluent containing inflammatory cells; and
• symptoms and signs of peritoneal inflammation.
A firm diagnosis of peritonitis requires at least two of these three.

Treatment. Three exchanges (preferably using 1 litre of 1.5% Dianeal) are instilled and drained as quickly as possible, without the addition of antibiotics. Thereafter exchanges are performed every 3—6 hours. The fourth exchange contains 1.7 mg/kg body weight of tobramycin, 1000 mg of cephalothin, and 1000 units of heparin per litre; each subsequent exchange contains 8 mg of tobramycin/litre, 250 mg of cephalothin/litre, and 1000 units heparin/litre of dialysate. Tobramycin and cephalothin should not be mixed in the same syringe, but can be mixed in the same dialysate bag. This antibiotic regimen is continued until the sensitivities of the causative organism(s) are known. Then, if necessary, appropriate changes can be made (Table 6.3).

Table 6.3. Loading dose of antibiotics in the treatment of peritonitis in CAPD patients

	Loading dose*	Maintenance dose
First-line drugs		
Cephalothin	500	250
Tobramycin	1.7 (mg/kg/bag)	8
Second line drugs		
Ampicillin	500	50
Cloxacillin	1000	100
Ticarcillin	1000	100
Septrin (sulfamethoxazole-trimethoprim)	400/80	25/5
Clindamycin	300	50
Amikacin	125	25
Penicillin	1 000 000 u/litre dialysate	50 000 30 mg (ip)
Vancomycin	1000 mg (iv)	

*In mg/litre dialysate, if not indicated otherwise.

The resolution of peritonitis is monitored by clinical examination, by daily effluent cultures, and by serial effluent white-cell counts. Usually the effluent bacterial cultures become negative after $1-2$ days. If cultures remain positive for more than $4-5$ days, the antibacterial regimen should be changed and catheter removal considered. Treatment is stopped seven days after the first negative culture. Phosphate binders or other constipating drugs should be withheld during the treatment of peritonitis. This treatment protocol may need to be modified for fungal, tuberculous and 'surgical' peritonitis, peritonitis due to multiple organisms, and tunnel abscess or severe exit-site infection. During this period the patient's protein intake should be increased because protein losses increase during peritonitis.

After $2-3$ days of treatment, if the patient is feeling well, he can be treated at home if he has been trained to add antibiotics to the bag. If the patient cannot inject the antibiotics into the solution and if the infection is due to Gram-positive organisms, treatment is continued with oral cephalexin (0.5 g at the time of each exchange) four times a day.

Part of the treatment in certain patients with peritonitis is removal of the permanent peritoneal catheter. The indications for such removal are:
• Persistence of infection for more than $4-5$ days, despite appropriate antibiotics.

- The presence of fungal peritonitis. Usually these patients present with cloudy fluid and, occasionally, without pain. Catheter removal brings a rapid improvement in symptoms and signs within the first 24 hours. Thereafter, the patient is maintained on hemodialysis for about four weeks and then the peritoneal catheter is replaced. During this interval, antifungal agents can be given orally or systemically. However, these agents may not be necessary because, in the absence of the foreign body, the peritoneal defense mechanism can handle the fungus well.
- Severe skin exit infection.
- Tuberculous peritonitis.
- Suspected fecal peritonitis not responding to standard treatment.

After two or three days when the diagnosis of fecal peritonitis is confirmed, in addition to removing the catheter, the patient may require a laparotomy to seal off or resect the leaking bowel.

After peritonitis has been treated and before the patient goes home, a trained nurse reviews the patient's technique to determine whether errors in technique contributed to the peritonitis.

During peritonitis, probably because of an increased blood flow through the peritoneum, peritoneal clearances of large and small molecules increase and glucose absorption also increases. As a result, these patients may develop hypophosphatemia, hypokalemia and hypoproteinemia, and may also have difficulties with ultrafiltration. If peritonitis leads to extensive adhesion formation as may occur after fecal, *Pseudomonas* or *Staph. aureus* peritonitis, the peritoneum may lose its capacity for ultrafiltration and peritoneal dialysis may have to be abandoned.

Complications other than peritonitis. Accidental contamination of the spike during a bag change is managed by changing the tube and giving a 10-day course of oral cephalexin (1 g/day). If this accident is not treated, clinical peritonitis usually develops two or three days after contamination.

Catheter malfunction with one-way obstruction is rare during CAPD, but when it does occur it appears in association with peritonitis. Temporary obstruction may be encountered in some patients who form fibrin; it is not known why some patients form fibrin more frequently than others. Addition of 1000–2000 units of heparin to each bag of dialysate usually controls the tendency (at these concentrations, heparin is not absorbed through the peritoneum).

Infrequently, a bloody effluent may be observed especially in young menstruating females; it may be the result of endometriosis or 'retrograde' bleeding through the Fallopian tube. Invariably, the bleeding stops after a day or two and requires no specific intervention. To prevent blood clots, which may plug the catheter, it may be necessary to add heparin to the dialysate. If the bleeding is persistent and profuse, one may consider administration of estrogens.

Early dialysate leaks are common immediately after surgical insertion of a catheter when the intra-abdominal pressure is increased too soon. Dialysate usually leaks through the incision and exit site. If dialysis is avoided for one to two weeks and the incision and exit site are given enough time to heal, most of the leaks stop spontaneously. If longer periods are required, the patient can be given 'back-up' hemodialysis, using a subclavian line. The first evidence of a leak into the abdominal wall is subcutaneous pitting edema or a bulging in the abdominal wall with or without pain. If dialysis is continued in the presence of a leak, the edema may spread to the genitalia and thighs.

Medical complications of CAPD. In many patients it is difficult to decide whether these complications are the result of CAPD, or of old age *per se*, and it is possible that CAPD may accelerate pre-existing medical complications. In any event some complications clearly can be attributed to CAPD.

The continuously elevated intra-abdominal pressure secondary to constant presence of dialysate in the peritoneal cavity may induce abdominal hernias—incisional, inguinal, diaphragmatic or umbilical. Older patients, whether they have surgical scars or not, are prone to this complication. Women may develop a rectocele or a cystocele, with or without uterine prolapse. Persistently raised intra-abdominal pressure also may aggravate existing hiatus hernia and hemorrhoids.

In patients with vertebral disease, the exaggerated lordosis (adopted while holding the dialysate in the abdomen) tends to aggravate the pain and other symptoms. Such complaints may force the discontinuation of CAPD.

CAPD may aggravate the circulation already compromised by generalized atherosclerosis in the lower extremity and partial occlusions in ileofemoral vessels. Reduced perfusion as a result of hypotension, which is not uncommon during CAPD, can provoke ischemic complications. Such patients may require corrective or palliative surgery to relieve their symptoms. These patients have multiple cardiovascular and cerebrovascular problems, such as recurrent angina, arrhythmias, acute myocardial infarction, transient ischemic attacks, and complete strokes, but as yet no one has defined the contribution of CAPD to their pathogenesis.

Some workers have suggested that the increased incidence of cardiovascular and cerebrovascular complications in CAPD patients is due to accelerated atherosclerosis associated with hypertriglyceridemia and low levels of high-density lipoproteins. Although many patients coming to CAPD are older and hence have complications in heart and brain, it is possible that CAPD may accelerate these complications.

Peritoneal dialysis in special situations

Peritoneal dialysis in diabetics with end-stage kidney disease

Diabetic patients on IPD are advised to continue daily subcutaneous injections of insulin. In addition, depending on the concentration of dextrose infused, insulin may be added to the dialysate bags during intermittent dialysis. The insulin requirement must be individualized by trial and error because of the wide variation between patients. It is advisable to monitor blood sugar during dialysis to determine the exact amount of insulin required for a given patient. Because of the poor long-term results, IPD is not recommended as a long-term home treatment for diabetics with end-stage kidney disease.

Blood sugar control in patients on CAPD

Since its introduction, continuous ambulatory peritoneal dialysis has offered diabetic patients with ESRD better management than other forms of peritoneal dialysis. At the same time, it has controlled blood sugar (by the intraperitoneal administration of insulin) in a way that stimulates the secretion from the normal pancreas. Because our initial experience was encouraging we now use this method extensively in diabetics who require dialysis. In many centers, CAPD has become the preferred mode of dialysis for diabetics.

Blindness in diabetics is not a contra-indication to carrying out CAPD. Many blind diabetics have been trained to carry out their treatment completely unassisted. The incidence of peritonitis in these patients may be as low or lower than in those patients with normal vision. Success depends on having a standard layout in which all the necessary items can be located by touch. The danger of contamination can be reduced by some of the newer methods for automatic connection of the bags with the tubing sets. These methods are designed to make it physically impossible for contamination to occur by accidental touching.

The aim of treatment is to achieve a fasting blood sugar below 140 mg/dl, and one-hour, post-meal (breakfast, lunch and supper) levels below 200 mg/dl at all times. The patient is hospitalized for the initiation of CAPD. All patients are dialysed with four 2-litre exchanges a day. The bags are exchanged during the day, 20 minutes before the major meals, i.e. breakfast, lunch and supper. The fourth exchange is made at around 23:00 hours. At this time, the patient has a snack consisting of a sandwich and a small drink.

Usually dialysis solutions of three different glucose concentrations— 1.5, 2.5 and 4.25 g/dl are available in Canada. The patient is advised to consume a diet providing 20−25 kcal/kg of body weight/day and containing 1.2 to 1.5 g protein/kg of body weight. Using a syringe with a long needle, regular insulin is added to each dialysate bag. The bag is inverted two or three times to aid mixing. The dosage of insulin is proportional to the concentration of glucose in the dialysate which, in turn, is determined by the body weight, edema and blood pressure. During the initial control, blood sugar is measured four times a day, i.e. fasting, and one hour after breakfast, lunch and supper. Fingerprick measurement of blood sugar gives quick results, correlates reasonably well with the venous blood sugar levels, and helps to detect unexpected fluctuations. The finger-prick test is performed 5 to 10 minutes before the fluid is infused intraperitoneally.

On the first day, one-fourth of the previous daily insulin requirement is added to each bag of dialysate; a supplemental dose is added for different concentrations of dialysate glucose (Table 6.4).

On the second day, the dose of insulin added to each bag of dialysate is increased (or decreased) according to the previous day's blood sugar levels. The change in the dose of insulin added to the 23:00-hour bag will be reflected in the fasting blood sugars.

As an additional precaution, patients are trained to check blood sugar levels with the fingerprick method. This test is performed 5 to 10 minutes before each bag exchange and, whenever necessary, the insulin added to the next bag is adjusted according to the guidelines given in Table 6.5. During the CAPD training period, the patient becomes familiar with the data in Table 6.5 and practices the method under observation. It should be emphasized that the fingerprick test is a rough guide only and is used to make changes in the insulin dose in the next bag, including the morning one.

The initial control of glycemia requires three or four days in hospital. After stabilization, the average daily insulin requirement varies from 70 to 200 units per day. During the night, the patient needs 30 to 50% less insulin to achieve a normal fasting blood sugar and avoid hypoglycemia. Infection increases the insulin requirement and, if CAPD is temporarily discontinued for any reason, the resulting hyperglycemia may be regulated

Table 6.4. Supplemental dose of insulin for different concentrations of dialysate glucose

Dialysate glucose strength (%)	Regular insulin (units/litre dialysate)
0.5	0
1.5	1
2.5	2
4.25	3

Table 6.5. Suggested adjustment to the basal dose of insulin added to the dialysate

Fasting blood sugar (mmol/litre)	One-hour post-meal blood sugar (mmol/litre)	Amount of insulin change (units/litre)
2.0–7.0	6.0–9.0	No change
2.0	4.0	−1
2.0	2.0	−2
—	2.0	−3
9.0	12.0	+1
12.0	20.0	+2
20.0	20.0	+3

by continuous intravenous infusion of insulin. This scheme of insulin administration eliminates the need for multiple subcutaneous injections— an advantage which sustains the patient's morale and promotes better compliance.

These patients may show hypoglycemia or hyperglycemia, commonly in association with uremic complications such as nausea, vomiting and infection. It is rare to encounter ketoacidosis or hyperglycemic coma during CAPD.

Renal transplantation in patients receiving peritoneal dialysis

In the mid 70s it was feared that transplanting a patient on peritoneal dialysis might be associated with more infectious complications. Our experience of transplantation has demonstrated no significant differences in patient or graft survival between those receiving hemodialysis, and those on peritoneal dialysis during the pretransplant period. Also similar in the two groups were: causes of death, incidence of wound infection, bacterial sepsis (positive blood culture), pneumonia, cytomegalic virus infection and other infections such as those of the urinary tract, and the pattern and incidence of episodes of rejection during the first year after transplant. Mild episodes of peritonitis were more frequent in the group on peritoneal dialysis, but, as mentioned before, these infections were treated successfully with the conventional protocol.

Peritoneal dialysis can usually be continued successfully in the immediate post-transplant phase if renal function is absent or inadequate. The PD catheter is usually removed after about three months if the kidney is working well. For the living donor transplants with an identical match, in whom excellent function can be anticipated immediately, we usually remove the catheter at the time of transplantation.

7

Hemodialysis

Robert Uldall and Franca Tantalo

In this chapter we will also discuss briefly the related disciplines of hemofiltration, slow continuous ultrafiltration (SCUF) and continuous arteriovenous hemofiltration (CAVH).

During hemodialysis the patient's uremic blood, in order for it to be purified, must be drawn from the patient's vascular system, passed through a sterile and non-toxic extracorporeal circulation, through a dialyser, in which dialysis takes place, and returned in its purified state to the vascular system. The total amount of blood outside the body at any one time is actually rather small, usually only about 200–300 ml, so in order to expose all the patient's blood to the purifying process, it is circulated fairly fast—usually in excess of 200 ml per minute in an adult. While the blood is passing through the dialyser some unwanted substances are removed, certain other desirable substances may be added, and usually a small amount of water is removed, most often by employing the principle of hydrostatic pressure to produce 'ultrafiltration'. Actually certain desirable substances such as water soluble vitamins may also be unavoidably lost or 'dialysed out' but this is not usually serious since they can easily be replaced by oral vitamin supplements.

In order to learn about hemodialysis we first have to learn about the component parts of the extracorporeal circuit. It might be considered logical to start with the dialyser because it is in the dialyser that the exchange of water and chemicals takes place.

The dialyser

The first dialysers to be used in attempts to treat humans with renal failure were made from long cylindrical tubes of celloidin. These served as the blood pathway while the dialysate surrounded them, and was in turn enclosed in a larger glass cylinder. In those days the only anticoagulant available was hirudin, the natural anticoagulant of blood-sucking leeches. Hidurin was obtained by crushing the heads of large numbers of leeches, and was really too toxic to be useful. The first dialysis to be successful in saving a human life was performed by Dr Wilhelm Kolff in Holland in 1945. Kolff used cellophane tubing, which had become commercially available for sausage skins, and heparin which had recently been developed as an anticoagulant. The cellophane tubing was wound around a drum which rotated in a bath of dialysate. See Fig. 7.1.

Once Kolff showed what could be done there followed a series of improvements in design and materials. The next big step forward was the disposable coil dialyser manufactured by Travenol Laboratories; this had cellophane tubing wound concentrically around a plastic mesh (see Fig. 7.2). The dialysate was pumped up through the dialyser so that it flowed between all the layers of cellophane tubing. When they first appeared these dialysers were used in a 100 litre stainless steel tank of dialysis fluid and they revolutionized the treatment of acute renal failure. The

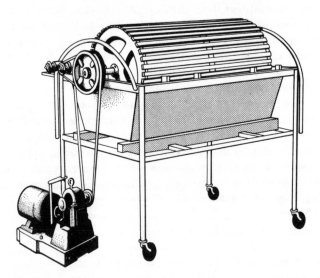

Fig. 7.1. Wilhelm Kolff's first artificial kidney machine, reproduced from an early photograph.

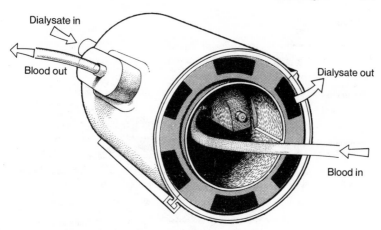

Fig. 7.2. Disposable coil dialyser (positive pressure).

main disadvantage was the high leak rate. When a dialyser leaked, allowing blood to spill into the dialysis fluid, the dialysis had to be stopped and the dialyser had to be changed. Coil dialysers also tended to be distensible so that high pressure generated in the dialyser led to a marked increase in the volume of the extracorporeal circuit.

At the beginning of the 1960s various centers throughout the world began to undertake long-term dialysis for end-stage renal failure. The search was on for ways to make the treatment cheaper—and the dialyser was the most expensive part of the extracorporeal circuit. The most successful and widely used product of this search was the large non-disposable parallel layer disposable dialyser, the best known example of which was the Kiil (see Fig. 7.3). It consisted of three parallel rectangular nylon or polypropylene boards mounted on a tilting trolley. The blood compartments consisted of a pair of cuprophane membranes clamped together between the upper and middle board, and another pair clamped between the middle and lower board (see Fig. 7.4). Blood ports led the blood in at one end and out at the other. Dialysis fluid flowed in the opposite direction between the membranes and the boards. The big advantage was that only the cellophane membranes were discarded at the end of the dialysis, thus saving a great deal of money. Disadvantages were that the boards were bulky and heavy and required a large storage area. They also required skilled personnel to dismantle the boards and build them again for the next dialysis. Sterilization was by means of a 2% formaldehyde solution and this was hard to get rid of completely. This meant that staff were exposed to formaldehyde in the atmosphere and

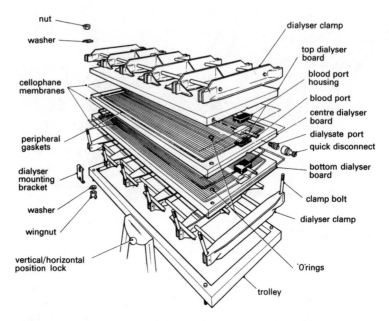

Fig. 7.3. The Kiil dialyser, by courtesy of Watson Marlow Limited.

patients inevitably received small intravenous infusions of formaldehyde at each dialysis. Surprisingly, few ill effects have been attributed to this chronic formaldehyde exposure but one complication seems to be generally acknowledged—that is, the formation of a red cell antibody called anti-N. The incidence of anti-N antibody formation in hemodialysis patients seems to be related to the frequency and duration of exposure to formaldehyde. The same thing has happened on a smaller scale when disposable dialysers have been re-used to save money, using formaldehyde as a sterilizing agent. Fortunately there is very little evidence that anti-N antibody formation interferes with a patient's well-being.

Another more serious danger of non-disposable dialysers such as the Kiil is the potential for pyrogenic reactions. A pyrogenic reaction is brought about when endotoxins from dead bacteria are allowed to come into contact with the bloodstream. The classical way in which this happened was by bacterial growth in the tray used for soaking the cellophane membranes before they were incorporated into the Kiil dialyser. Bacteria would be killed by the formaldehyde but the endotoxins would be left on the membranes. The symptoms of a pyrogenic reaction were dramatic and unpleasant. About half an hour after the start of dialysis the patient

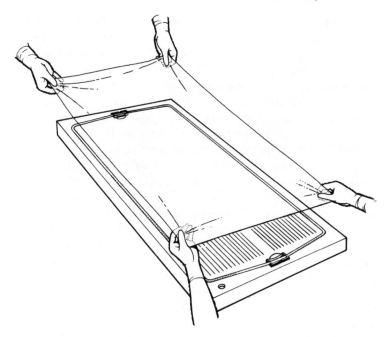

Fig. 7.4. Laying the membrane on the Kiil board.

would develop headache, backache, uncontrollable shivering and a high fever. The correct treatment was to discontinue the dialysis at once and start again with a fresh uncontaminated extracorporeal circuit and dialyser. Often the patient would develop the lesions of herpes simplex on the lips the next day.

Non-disposable dialysers of the Kiil type have largely disappeared now from dialysis centers, not because of pyrogenic reactions which can be avoided by attention to correct methods of building and sterilization, but because they occupy too much space and require too much manpower to look after them. They may still have a place where economy is the overriding consideration and labour is cheap. They are described fully in the second edition of *Renal Nursing* but we will say no more about them here.

Dialysers of various kinds have continued to proliferate and improve and we now have a bewildering variety from which to choose. They are all disposable, intended to be thrown away after one use. However, because money for health care is being rationed all over the world, many centers are re-using disposable dialysers many times. This can be done quite safely as long as the rules are followed—see p.413. The two main types of disposable dialysers are the hollow fiber and the flat plate.

Flat plate dialysers are really a disposable form of the Kiil but they have many layers and they are much smaller than the Kiil (see Fig. 7.5). Hollow fiber dialysers are much the commonest dialyser in use in nearly all countries that carry out a lot of dialysis. The dialysing surface is a hollow capillary tube, about 13 000 of them lying parallel inside a hollow transparent plastic cylinder. The fibers have an internal diameter of about 200−300 μm and a wall thickness ranging from 9−20 μm. They are held at each end by an embedding material which fills in the space between the fibers but leaves their ends open so that blood can flow down the lumens of the fibers. The dialysate washes the outside of the fibers, by being led in and out of the rigid cylinder which contains them (see Fig. 7.6). Hollow fiber dialysers are very compact but have surface areas equivalent to other types. They have a number of advantages: they have a low priming volume, usually less than 100 ml; they have a very low leak rate; their ability to remove fluid by ultrafiltration is very consistent; they have good wash-back characteristics—that means very little residual blood is left in them after dialysis; finally, they can easily be re-used many times.

While dialysers have undergone development and improvement over the last few years, so have the membranes from which they have been made. Most membranes hitherto have only allowed the passage of relatively small molecules up to a molecular weight of about 500 daltons. This limitation certainly applies to the commonly used cellophane and its copper containing modification 'cuprophane'. However, there is now a body of knowledge purporting to show that some of the toxins in uremia are larger than this. The so-called middle molecules, between 500 and 2000, are not well removed by standard dialysers using standard membranes. For removal of these substances thinner membranes with greater permeability are needed.

Dialysis membranes

The first membranes to be used in any quantity were cellophane and its chemically related counterpart containing copper called cuprophane. Cuprophane is still widely used but it has limitations. It is only permeable to small molecules, less than about 500 molecular weight, and it is inclined to precipitate a mild reaction when the patient's blood comes in contact with it. This reaction is thought to be caused by complement activation (an immunological phenomenon) and it is accompanied by a

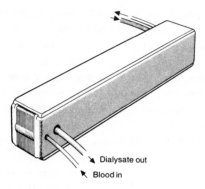

Fig. 7.5. Gambro flat-plate dialyser.

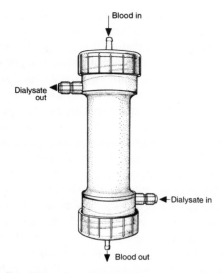

Fig. 7.6. Hollow fiber dialyser (negative pressure).

fall in the numbers of circulating white blood cells. It has been shown that this is due to sequestration of white blood cells in the lungs and it may be accompanied by transient hypoxia. Actually this phenomenon is not usually severe enough to cause adverse symptoms but a number of specially susceptible patients may be quite distressed by it. The commonest complaint on the part of the patient is backache which lasts for a few minutes. Interestingly this reaction does not recur if the dialyser is used for the same patient again, perhaps because the patient's proteins have coated the membrane which can then no longer produce a reaction. Because of these features it has come to be known as the 'first use phenomenon' and is sometimes used as an additional argument in favor of dialyser re-use.

Since the advent of cellophane and cuprophane we have seen the appearance of regenerated cellulose acetate, noted for its high 'ultrafiltration' characteristics (that is its ability to remove large amounts of water for a given transmembrane pressure) and its lack of tendency to cause the first use phenomenon. There are now other exciting new membranes such as polymethylmethacrylate (PMMA) and polyacrylonitrile (PAN). This latter membrane is extremely permeable to water but also to middle molecules and is thought to be very promising for this reason. The high permeability to water can be a disadvantage because it results in an unavoidably high water loss.

We have constructed a table (Table 7.1) in which most of the well-known membranes are listed and their main important characteristics are summarized. It will be noted that cellulose acetate has less tendency to cause clotting and is therefore particularly suitable if one is trying to use a minimum of heparin. Polymethylmethacrylate (PMMA) seemed to combine many of the most desirable features, being very biocompatible (not likely to cause reactions), non-thrombogenic (not encouraging clotting), and not excessively permeable to water. However, further experience has been disappointing. It does cause complement activation, and blood does seem to stick to it, making it very hard to re-use.

Not least among the important characteristics of a dialyser is its efficiency in removing toxic substances from the bloodstream. When we talk about the clearance of a dialyser for a particular substance such as urea or creatinine, we mean the volume of blood which can be completely cleared of that substance by the dialyser in a given time at a specified blood flow rate. For example, a given dialyser may have a urea clearance of 150 ml per minute at a blood flow rate of 200 ml/minute. This means, in effect, that during one minute 200 ml of blood goes through the dialyser but only 150 ml of that blood is completely cleared of urea. The clearance of a dialyser for a particular substance depends on a number of factors which include the thickness of the membrane, the permeability of the membrane, and its effective surface area. For example the effective surface area of a hollow fiber dialyser could be reduced by too close bunching of the fibers so that dialysate cannot freely circulate between them. It has also been shown that increasing the transmembrane pressure to increase the ultrafiltration of water brings about increased solute

Table 7.1. Important properties of the well-known dialysis machines

Membrane	Biocompatibility	Ultrafiltration factor	Small molecule clearance	Middle molecule clearance	Heparin requirement	Re-usability
Cuprophane	Poor	Low	Good	Low	High	Good
Regenerated cellulose	Poor	Low	Good	Low	High	Fair
Cellulose acetate	Good	Medium	Good	Medium	Very low	Very good
Polyacrylonitrile PAN	Excellent	High	Good	High	Medium	Good
Acronitrile and sodium methallyl sulphonate co-polymer AN69	Excellent	High	Good	High	Low	Good
Polymethyl methacrylate	Good	Medium	Good	Medium	High	Poor
Polysulphone	Excellent	High	Good	High	Low	Good

transfer. This is because convection (transport of solute with the solvent) is added to simple diffusion.

In choosing a dialyser for a particular patient one should consider the clinical priorities and decide which dialyser gives the best value for money. Perhaps high clearances for maximal efficiency are the overriding consideration in a large individual in whom you wish to keep dialysis time down to a minimum. Alternatively you may find that a particular dialyser is better tolerated by another patient because it causes a less marked first use reaction. The actual cost of the dialyser may be less important if you have an active and reliable re-use program which allows you to use each dialyser several times. It then becomes a small proportion of the total cost of the treatment.

Production of dialysate

The first artificial kidney machines to be used on a large scale were the 100 litre Travenol tanks in which the dialysate was recirculated through the coil dialyser. After about two hours the dialysate had taken up a considerable amount of toxic solute from the patient and it had to be changed. The spent dialysate was discarded and a fresh batch was made up to allow dialysis to continue for about another two hours. Dialysate made in a batch in this way could be constituted from dry chemicals or from a liquid concentrate of chemicals. The final composition could be checked by chemical analysis of the sodium and potassium levels with a flame photometer in the laboratory. However, if it could be assumed that the proportions of chemicals in the concentrate were correct, one could check the final composition quickly and easily by measuring the electrical conductivity of the dialysate. We know that the electrical conductivity of a solution is related to the number of ionized particles in solution. If the conductivity was correct we knew that the final composition was correct. Small portable conductivity meters became standard equipment for everyone doing a dialysis using a batch system.

Although a batch system is reasonable when conducting one dialysis for one patient with acute renal failure, it is too primitive and time-consuming for simultaneous dialysis of ten or more patients with end-stage renal faillure. For this to be done efficiently the process has to be automated. Modern dialysis machines proportion a commercially prepared liquid concentrate with pure water by a system of continuous conductivity monitoring. The proportions are usually one part of concentrate to 34 parts of water. The proportioning can be done from a central system which supplies a uniform or standardized dialysate by a system of plumbing to all the dialysis stations. This is called a central proportioning system, or central delivery system. But more commonly nowadays each patient has his or her own machine which is proportioning a dialysate which can be customized for the individual patient. This type of 'prescription dialysis' has the advantage that each patient can benefit from a final composition of dialysate which is optimal for his or her case. The machines which do this are called single-patient proportioning machines.

Automatic proportioning is done in two main ways, namely fixed volumetric proportioning and variable proportioning. Fixed proportioning means that concentrate and water are proportioned as one part of concentrate to 34 parts of water. This cannot be varied and is monitored by a conductivity probe which stops the flow of dialysate to the dialyser if the alarm limits of conductivity are exceeded. This alarm condition could occur if the concentrate is of the wrong composition or if one of the proportioning chambers were to develop a leak, or if the supply of concentrate were to run out. A conductivity alarm is a reason to investigate the causes fully and to ensure that the dialysate is now by-passing the dialyser. Conductivity meter adjustments must never be made without prior verification of the correct chemical composition of the dialysate by laboratory estimation.

The variable proportioning systems, operating by mechanical or servo-controlled feedback mechanisms, are self-regulating systems in which a change in conductivity to high or low will result in a change in the relative delivery rates of concentrate and water to keep the conductivity in whatever narrow range you have predetermined. Most modern machines also have pH monitoring so that the machines will go into alarm if the pH varies outside a certain predetermined range.

Before we get into a discussion of the composition of the dialysate, we have to address the problem of the purification of the water.

Purifying the water

In the early 1960s when hemodialysis was adopted as a worldwide treatment, at least for those countries with advanced systems of medical care, not very much was known about the possible toxic effects of contaminants in the water which would be used for making up the dialysing fluid or 'dialysate'. Without thinking too much about it one might be tempted to assume that if water which came out of the taps was fit to drink it would probably also be acceptable for making dialysate which would be on the other side of the semipermeable membrane from the blood. However it is worth remembering that most of us drink only 1–2 litres of water a day. If we absorb undesirable substances from drinking water, we have normal kidneys working 24 hours a day to excrete them. Patients with end-stage renal failure may be dialysed against 30 litres of dialysate per hour, perhaps 150 litres three times a week. If there are low molecular weight toxic solutes in the water there is an enormous potential for them to enter the bloodstream. Once they are in the bloodstream there are no healthy kidneys to excrete them. If this rather simple commonsense logic had been acted on world-wide from the beginning a lot of tragic consequences would have been avoided.

We now know that untreated tap water contains a whole host of potentially dangerous substances, which, if ingested in small amounts are ostensibly harmless, though environmental pressure groups everywhere are constantly pointing to new chemical (mostly organic) compounds which may threaten the health of their communities. If these tap water constituents are not removed from the water used for making dialysate they can cause life-threatening or crippling disease in hemodialysis patients. Three outstanding examples serve to illustrate the point.

The most famous contaminant in water for hemodialysis is aluminum. Deliberately dumped in reservoirs by many different water authorities for purifying drinking water, and also naturally occuring, this element, if not removed from the water for dialysate, can cause a progressive, painful, crippling, vitamin D resistant bone disease—a form of osteomalacia associated with multiple pathological fractures. Aluminum intoxication may also cause a progressive neurological deterioration associated with clumsy movements, slurred speech, involuntary tremor and dementia ending in death. This came to be known as 'dialysis dementia', dialysis encephalopathy, or aluminum encephalopathy. Both these conditions have largely been eradicated since the necessity for water purification was generally recognized (see p.314).

The second classical water impurity is copper. If tap water, purified water or dialysate itself is led through copper pipes (because of the ignorance of those involved in setting up the system) copper will be picked up by the water and cross the dialysis membrane into the patient's blood causing massive hemolysis of the red blood cells and usually fatal intoxication of the patient. Hence the need to avoid any copper parts in the plumbing system for the water or dialysate.

A third classical contaminant is chloramines. These are compounds of chlorine which is widely used by water authorities for its bactericidal properties. Chloramines are powerful hemolytic agents which damage and destroy red blood cells. They must be removed during water purification, usually by adsorption onto carbon filters. Table 7.2 shows a list of some of the more common water contaminants and their main toxic effects. There are undoubtedly many others, and the only safe policy for hemodialysis units is to assume that all tap water is poisonous until fully purified. In the jargon of hemodialysis, the water coming out of the taps in a city or domestic water supply is called the feed water. The final water after purification for dialysis is called the product water.

How should water for dialysis be purified?

There are really two main ways in which dialysis units purify water: deionization and reverse osmosis.

Deionizers were the first instruments to be used on a large scale to purify water for dialysis and they function on the same principle as ion exchange resins used to remove potassium from the gastro-intestinal tract. The cation exchange resin, Kayexalate, exchanges sodium for potassium.

Deionizers remove all ionized particles, both cations and anions, and replace them with hydrogen ions H^+ and hydroxyl ions OH^- which then combine to form water, H_2O. Deionizers are expensive to use if there is a lot of impurity in the feed water and it is dangerous to go on using them after they are exhausted. So a system of checks and warning alarms must be built in to tell the user when it is time to change the tanks. There are two types of deionizers depending on whether the two resins are in different tanks (dual tank) or mixed together in the same tank (mixed bed). The latter type, the mixed bed deionizer, is more expensive but it also produces water of greater purity.

A well recognized danger of deionizers is that they may form small amounts of toxic carcinogenic substances called nitrosamines if the water

Table 7.2. Common contaminants of tap water and their toxic effects

Aluminum	Osteomalacia, dialysis dementia
Copper	Hemolysis and death
Chloramines	Hemolysis
Nitrates	Hemolysis with methemoglobinemia
Fluoride	Bone disease
Nitrosamines*	Potential for causing cancer

*Nitrosamines are not a usual contaminant of feed water but may be formed when certain organic compounds go through a deionizer.

feeding them has not already been through a carbon filter to remove organic nitrogenous compounds. Carbon filters remove impurities by adsorption onto the carbon, much in the same way that activated charcoal will adsorb poisons in the gastro-intestinal tract, so preventing their absorption into the bloodstream. It is therefore common practice to use a carbon filter upstream from the deionizer.

Another potential source of difficulty with deionizers is the tendency for bacterial growth to occur inside them. Microbiological monitoring of the water emerging from the deionizer should be done at regular intervals and the bacterial count should not exceed 200 organisms per ml. The best way to avoid bacterial growth in deionizers is to filter out the organisms before the water reaches it. This can be done by inserting a suitable bacterial filter upstream from the deionizer.

The second main method for water purification is reverse osmosis. The principle is well described by the name. We know that osmotic pressure causes water to move through a semipermeable membrane from the area of low concentration to the area of high concentration. If, however, the hydrostatic pressure is raised sufficiently in the compartment of high concentration the osmotic pressure will be overcome and water will be 'squeezed out' onto the other side of the membrane. In a reverse osmosis machine, water is pumped under pressure through a membrane, often cellulose acetate, and in the process up to 95% of all dissolved solutes are held back.

The process is relatively wasteful of water. Only about 30% of the feed water may be retained while 70% is discarded with the impurities. Nevertheless reverse osmosis has proved itself to be a cheaper and generally more popular means of water purification than deionization if either method alone is used to purify water for dialysis. Many dialysis centers use reverse osmosis as their main method of water purification but insert a deionizer downstream from the RO machine to 'polish' the water to bring it to a very high state of purity before it is used for making dialysate. Deionizers used in this way last for a long time since they receive so little impurity to saturate them.

Whatever method is used for water purification the water quality should be continuously monitored by measuring its electrical resistance. The purer the water, the greater will be its resistance to the passage of an electrical current. The unit of electrical resistance is the ohm and the degree of purity we are aiming for is one megohm (one millionth of an ohm). It is probably unnecessary to have water as pure as this but we must always build into the system a margin of safety. Planning a water purification system for a multiple patient in-center dialysis unit does not solve the problem of what to do for the patient who is to be dialysed in a ward in some geographically separate area of the hospital. In this case one can either fill a batch tank with pure water from the main unit (this concept is largely out-dated since batch systems of dialysate-proportioning have been largely replaced) or the single-patient proportioning machine must have its own portable reverse osmosis machine or its own portable deionizer. The same problem demands a similar solution when a patient regularly carries out hemodialysis at home.

We have recently found that some portable reverse osmosis machines do not adequately remove aluminum and we are coming round to the view that they must be supplemented with portable deionizers. Alternatively a portable deionizer alone can be used.

The day-to-day provision of pure product water for dialysis is usually the responsibility of the chief technologist of the dialysis unit, who will be expected to become an expert on water purification. He will discuss strategy and problems with the medical director. The nurses may play an important role by remaining alert to the possibility that dialysis-related symptoms in their patient could be due to a breakdown in the water purification system.

Composing the dialysate (what should it consist of?)

There is nothing magical or mysterious about the dialysate. It can be anything we want it to be. Furthermore if you visit 50 different dialysis centers and ask to see the composition of the dialysate you may see nearly as many different formulations as the number of centers you visit. There will, of course, be remarkable similarities but the sodium concentration may vary from 130 to 145 mmol/l and the potassium from 0.5 to 3.0 mmol/l. Each center will give good reasons for its own preferred formulation and it is only in recent years that controlled trials have been conducted to test the superiority of one type of composition over another. The truth is that no single formulation will suit all patients and all occasions. What is appropriate in acute renal failure may be quite inappropriate for a stable patient with end-stage renal failure. Gone are the days when a dialysis could be ordered without any thought being given to what the dialysate should contain. Fortunately with the wonderfully versatile machines made available to us by industry, as well as the wide range of different concentrates, we have the opportunity to provide a whole range of different dialysates for different patients. Furthermore, nurses are rightly being asked more and more to help in making decisions about the composition of the dialysate for particular clinical situations and individual patients. We will therefore attempt here to set out what we judge to be sound and sensible reasons for composing the dialysate in the way we do. Once the principles are understood, the decisions are easier and the whole practice of dialysis becomes more interesting.

In any solution of electrolytes the cations must balance the anions so that electrical neutrality is preserved. Let us consider the cations first.

Sodium

The main extracellular cation in the body is sodium, normally present in a concentration of 140 mmol/l. Most patients with renal failure are in positive sodium balance when they come to dialysis. The patient with end-stage renal failure is often completely anuric and losing negligible amounts of salt by sweating. Sodium excess will depend on dietary intake, which should have been restricted. Nevertheless there will be a variable need to remove sodium during dialysis. The lower the dialysate sodium the greater the gradient and therefore the potential for sodium loss into the dialysate. The aim should be to end the dialysis with the patient in a state of mild sodium depletion so as to allow for the unavoidable sodium intake during the interval until the next dialysis. But if you remove sodium too fast you may make the patient hypotensive, especially if you have to remove a lot of water at the same time. So the sodium concentration has to be a compromise and there may be an element of trial and error. Another option on some modern single-patient proportioning machines is to start dialysis with the sodium concentration high (145−150 mmol/l) to maintain blood pressure while water is being removed and then lower the dialysate sodium (138 mmol/l) for the last hour of dialysis so that the patient will not come off dialysis in a sodium overloaded state. In acute renal failure there is usually a more marked sodium overload and it may be necessary to start with a relatively low dialysate sodium concentration, say 130−135 mmol/l. Most dialysis units now carry a number of different concentrates, each with a different formulation, to be used for specific clinical situations.

Mistakes in dialysis fluid composition. It is worth remembering that if the proportioning machine makes a mistake, and the mistake is not detected quickly, the patient's life may be in danger. Any mistake you are capable of imagining, and many others which you cannot, have been made at some time or other. Dialysates have been used in which twice the normal sodium concentration was present (270 mmol/l). When this was not detected the patient developed progressive and ultimately fatal hypernatremia manifesting itself first as hypertension and headache, later as confusion and convulsions and leading to lethal dehydration of the brain cells and brain destruction. Not long ago we saw a less serious case of hypertonic dialysate production occurring in several machines simultaneously due to a fault in the calibration equipment being used to calibrate the conductivity monitors.

Eleven patients were dialysed simultaneously one morning against a sodium concentration of 165 mmol/l. All patients, soon after the onset of dialysis, started to complain of uncontrollable thirst and to ask for drinks of water. Fortunately the head nurse insisted on having the composition of the dialysate checked, and the mistake was discovered. A number of patients who had finished dialysis by this time (their serum sodium levels averaged 155 mmol/l) had to be brought back and dialysed again to bring them back to normal. Uncontrollable water drinking in the presence of such sodium excess would have caused dangerous hypertension and heart failure. Fortunately all escaped with nothing more than a bad scare.

A mistake in the other direction, dialysis against a sodium concentration of 112 mmol/l, will cause severe hyponatremia and water intoxication of the brain. (Notice how the brain is always the most vulnerable organ.) This leads to mental confusion, drowsiness and convulsions. Major seizures on dialysis are always dangerous since they may lead to vomiting and inhalation of stomach contents into the lungs. The resultant cerebral hypoxia could lead to brain damage and even death. The moral from these intentionally frightening stories is that an experienced dialysis nurse will be eternally vigilant and always suspicious that unusual symptoms in a dialysis patient during treatment could be due to an error in dialysate composition. If there is even a remote possibility of a mistake it must be searched for until we are sure everything is correct. An alert, suspicious mind may save lives.

Actually, the quality of proportioning equipment now is so good that mistakes like those described above are very rare. Their very rarity tends to lull us into a state of false security so that we tend not to think of the possibility of errors in dialysis fluid composition. Only the senior, more experienced doctors and nurses are old enough to remember the days when mistakes happened frequently. Now nurses in training have to be reminded constantly that these things still happen.

Potassium

Potassium is the main intracellular cation, being present in cells in a concentration of about 140−150 mmol/l, while the amount in extracellular fluid including plasma is low, 3.5−5.0 mmol/l. Although the concentration is low, the levels are very critical. Hyperkalemia causes cardiac arrest and hypokalemia causes arrhythmias. Both high and low potassium levels cause skeletal muscle weakness. Patients with renal failure requiring dialysis tend to have high plasma potassium levels. This is because of potassium accumulation, which may be aggravated by metabolic acidosis. Hence it is very common to use low potassium concentrations in the dialysate to bring the potassium level down. One has to be careful when a patient is receiving digitalis because a rapid lowering of plasma potassium in the presence of digitalis increases the chance of arrhythmias. It might be wise in this situation to lower the plasma potassium gradually in a stepwise manner by dialysing at first against a dialysate level of 4−5 mmol/l and later changing to a level of 2−3 mmol/l. It may also be sensible to carry out continuous cardiac monitoring during, and for a while after, the dialysis to pick up arrhythmias such as ventricular ectopic beats early.

It is also important to choose the dialysate potassium level carefully if the plasma potassium is normal or low. Patients have died from cardiac arrhythmias induced by dialysing against a low potassium level when the plasma potassium was already low. This is all common sense and usually mistakes will not be made if someone takes the trouble to think about and plan the dialysis. This is a classical example of a case in which an experienced dialysis nurse may be able to help an inexperienced medical resident by getting him to discuss it.

Most patients with end-stage renal failure are dialysed against a less than physiological potassium level to achieve a post-dialysis level slightly below normal, thereby preventing dangerous hyperkalemia from developing before the next dialysis.

Calcium

In renal failure the plasma calcium tends to be low. The aim is to dialyse against a high level so as to finish dialysis with a slightly high level. It will again be subnormal by the next dialysis but in this way the 'median' plasma concentration (i.e. the average concentration throughout the week) will be approximately normal.

Remember that plasma calcium is approximately 50% bound to protein and we only have to concern ourselves with the 50% which is unbound or ionized. The normal level of ionized calcium is about 1.3 mmol/l (5 mg%) but in order to bring the level up to slightly higher than normal we should probably have a dialysate concentration of 1.6 mmol/l (6.5 mg%) or thereabouts. This will be appropriate for most patients with renal failure. But we should not adhere to it slavishly. We once treated a patient with malignant hypercalcemia (serum calcium 4.5 mmol/l or 18 mg%) with a dialysate containing no calcium at all. This brought the serum calcium down very nicely and the patient was much improved as a result.

Magnesium

Magnesium is the other important intracellular cation, being present in cells in a concentration of approximately 50 mmol/l. The normal plasma concentration is 1–2 mmol/l and renal failure does not usually change this very much. We do not usually have to worry too much about the magnesium level in renal failure. Very few patients come to any harm as a result of the magnesium being too high or too low but there are exceptions. One important exception we need to be aware of is the danger of magnesium-containing medications, for example magnesium sulphate in Epsom salts. Magnesium sulphate is soluble and easily absorbed. In renal failure it is not excreted so the blood level will rise. High plasma magnesium levels cause muscular weakness. In this respect it is similar to potassium. We have seen magnesium toxicity to the point of profound muscular weakness in a patient receiving a magnesium-containing laxative. Magnesium-induced muscular weakness has also been described in ten patients on a central system of dialysate delivery who were inadvertently dialysed against a magnesium concentration of 10 mmol/l instead of 1.0 mmol/l. Progressive muscular weakness developed in all the patients, even to the point of inadequate respiratory ventilation until the mistake was discovered. The patients rapidly recovered when they were switched to dialysis with the correct dialysate composition.

Very low magnesium levels can precipitate cardiac arrhythmias, behaving in this way like potassium. Hypomagnesemia is rare in renal failure unless the patient has prolonged fluid losses from the gastrointestinal tract, or receives prolonged parenteral nutrition containing no magnesium.

There is still some discussion about what is the ideal magnesium concentration in dialysate. At one time it was suggested that lowering the concentration to 0.5 mmol/l was good treatment for intractable pruritus in long-term dialysis patients. When we tried this in two patients we found that their pruritus was not relieved but minor cardiac arrhythmias became troublesome. Most dialysis units now use a concentration between 0.75 and 1.5 mmol/l.

Anions in dialysate

To decide upon the anion composition of dialysate it makes sense to look at the anions in plasma. These are chloride (Cl^-), about 100 mmol/l, and bicarbonate (HCO_3^-), 25 mmol/l. There are also some unmeasured anions up to a concentration of about 12 mmol/l. Most patients with renal failure have a metabolic acidosis with a reduced plasma bicarbonate. The plasma chloride level is usually normal. We know that the total cations match the anions because electrical neutrality is always preserved. If the bicarbonate is low and the chloride is normal, there must be extra unmeasured anions in the plasma (more than 12 mmol/l) the so-called 'anion gap'. We need not concern ourselves with these extra unmeasured anions in renal failure except to know that they are there and that they will be removed by dialysis as the bicarbonate level is brought up to normal.

Acetate or bicarbonate

In order to correct the metabolic acidosis we have to bring the plasma bicarbonate up to normal. The most obvious and natural way to do this is to have a higher than physiological level of bicarbonate in the dialysate. Unfortunately if we try to do this by making up a concentrate of chemicals in a small volume of water the bicarbonate will precipitate the calcium. Calcium is relatively insoluble in an alkaline solution. Therefore in order to compose a dialysate containing bicarbonate and calcium we have two alternatives. The first way is to do it by means of the batch method described on p.184. In this method we can add the chemicals separately to a large volume of pure water. For example, we can first dilute all the chemicals, excluding the bicarbonate, in the correct volume of water. Then, as a second step we can add the bicarbonate. The bicarbonate will not precipitate the calcium as long as the calcium is first diluted with water. The second method for producing the dialysate is by an automatic proportioning system using conductivity monitoring but also doing it in two steps. First the liquid concentrate, excluding the bicarbonate, is proportioned with pure water and as a second step the bicarbonate is added as a concentrated solution. Nearly all makers of dialysis machines now have reliable automatic systems for proportioning a bicarbonate-containing dialysate.

Cobe Laboratories have a system which first proportions bicarbonate with pure water and then, as a second step, proportions the dilute bicarbonate solution with the liquid acid concentrate. In their system the ratio of concentrate to water is 1:44. The volume of concentrate is obviously less than that required for a 1:34 proportioning ratio. This results in a corresponding cost saving because the concentrate is less bulky. It makes sense to dilute the bicarbonate with water first, to give a fixed bicarbonate concentration of 35 or 40 mmol/l. The final sodium concentration can be adjusted by the amount of acid concentrate which is added, this being regulated by the final conductivity measurement. With this system the dialysate sodium can be varied between 130 and 160 mmol/l without significantly changing the bicarbonate concentration. In practice, it is unusual to use a dialysate sodium concentration higher than 145 mmol/l.

In the early days before these technical problems of dialysate proportioning had been solved, Dr Charles Mion, a French nephrologist working in Seattle with Dr Scribner, discovered an ingenious alternative to bicarbonate and the problem of calcium precipitation. He showed that if acetate was used instead of bicarbonate in the liquid concentrate there would be no precipitation of calcium. However, during dialysis acetate would cross the membrane into the blood and the body would then convert acetate to bicarbonate, thus correcting the metabolic acidosis. After this important work in 1964 acetate was adopted widely all over the world as the buffer base for hemodialysis. Acetate is still widely used with remarkably few problems but in recent years there has been a swing back to the use of bicarbonate for a number of reasons.

When acetate crosses the semipermeable membrane from the dialysate to the blood it is rapidly converted by most patients to bicarbonate. We know this because blood acetate levels never get very high (the highest level we have seen is 9 mmol/l in a patient being dialysed against a dialysate containing 40 mmol/l) and acetate is virtually always undetectable in the blood by five minutes after the end of dialysis. However, unlike bicarbonate, which is a physiological substance, acetate is an unphysiological substance and it has pharmacological effects until it is metabolized to bicarbonate. The main pharmacological effect of acetate is on the peripheral blood vessels as a vasodilator. In other words it reduces peripheral resistance. Cardiologists would say that it 'reduces the after-load' on the heart. The healthy heart responds to this by an increase in cardiac output so that the blood pressure remains the same. Perfusion of tissues is increased. At first sight these effects would all appear to be quite positive and beneficial. In fact dialysis with acetate has been performed all over the world ever since its introduction by Dr Mion in 1964 and generally it has been extremely successful. It is only in recent years that the routine use of acetate has been challenged simultaneously with the development of reliable equipment to produce a bicarbonate-containing dialysate by the 'three stream' proportioning method.

It has been suggested by some that acetate has a negative effect on left ventricular contraction, a so-called 'negative inotropic' effect. Most authorities do not believe this and our own studies have confirmed that, when acetate acts as a vasodilator, the heart compensates by increasing its output. Nevertheless, as one would expect from its effect on blood vessels, acetate does have a tendency to drop the blood pressure, and this effect seems more pronounced in patients who have not been dialysed against acetate regularly (i.e. patients having their first acetate dialysis and patients who have been having bicarbonate dialysis in the preceding few weeks or months). The hypotensive effect of acetate is also more pronounced in some patients than in others—there is an individual susceptibility. This enhanced effect does not seem to be related to high blood levels. Rather, it would appear to be due to a qualitative intolerance on the part of some patients. We, like others, have found that a small proportion of our patients, probably less than 20%, tend to be upset by acetate and fare better on bicarbonate. Older patients with bad hearts tolerate acetate less well than young patients with normal hearts. In a double-blind controlled trial of the effect of bicarbonate versus acetate dialysis on the incidence of adverse dialysis-related symptoms such as headache, nausea, vomiting, dizziness, and so on, we found that bicarbonate caused significantly fewer adverse symptoms during dialysis than acetate.

It has also been shown by others that these symptoms and effects are greater when highly efficient dialysis is being performed with large surface area dialysers. This is what one would expect because the patient will 'gain' acetate more quickly.

It is noticeable that the correction of metabolic acidosis is not quite so quick or complete with acetate as it is with bicarbonate. This is due not so much to delay in conversion of acetate to bicarbonate in the body but because during acetate dialysis bicarbonate will continue to diffuse from the blood to the dialysate (i.e. from the area of high concentration to the area of low concentration).

Whether we use bicarbonate or acetate for correction of metabolic acidosis the concentration in dialysate should be higher than normal in order to bring the plasma bicarbonate level from below normal to approximately normal by the end of dialysis. In practice the concentration of acetate or bicarbonate is usually 35–40 mmol/l.

In view of this continuing controversy about the relative merits of acetate and bicarbonate, what should our policy be when we actually come to treat patients? Unfortunately there is no completely clear-cut answer. Here are a few suggestions based on our own experience and what we have been able to glean from the literature on the subject.

• Bicarbonate dialysis is more physiological, causes less hemodynamic disturbance, corrects acidosis more reliably, and is probably safer for seriously ill patients with acute renal failure.

• Bicarbonate dialysis is preferable for patients with hypotension and patients with abnormal hearts.

• Acetate dialysis should probably be avoided in patients with liver damage who may have difficulty in converting acetate to bicarbonate.

• Acetate dialysis has been used successfully for many years for stable patients with end-stage renal failure. In the present state of our knowledge there is no reason why it should not continue to be used in this way.

• If the production of bicarbonate dialysate were as easy, reliable, safe and cheap as the production of acetate dialysate, the use of acetate would presumably disappear very quickly. At present, however, acetate dialysate production is still easier and cheaper.

For these reasons acetate will probably continue to be used for some time to come.

Disasters arising from using the wrong concentrate

Acetate dialysis uses only one concentrate, as has been discussed, because all the chemicals can exist in solution without precipitation. Bicarbonate dialysis, because of the precipitation of the calcium by bicarbonate, needs two separate components. The main component (containing all the chemicals except bicarbonate) is called the acid concentrate. This is mixed with product water, and then with concentrated bicarbonate solution, to form the final dialysate.

With the advent of new three stream proportioning systems to produce bicarbonate dialysate, many dialysis units now have a mixture of machines, old and new, as well as a number of different concentrates for acetate and bicarbonate dialysis. To complicate the picture further, some machines proportion concentrates with water in a ratio of 1:44.

The purpose of this preamble is to set the scene for the possible occurrence of a new and possibly fatal dialysis accident caused by using the wrong concentrate. What may happen is this:

Suppose you are intending to carry out an acetate dialysis with a fixed volumetric proportioning machine which is only intended for traditional proportioning of acetate dialysate. By mistake you use an acid concentrate. The conductivity will be too low. The machine will go into alarm and refuse to supply dialysate to the dialyser. This is a safety mechanism. No harm will be done unless you assume, without checking other causes, that something is wrong with the conductivity monitoring, and you decide to override the conductivity alarm. You switch it off and decide to dialyse the patient anyway. The patient will start to be exposed to a dialysate with the wrong sodium concentration, but, much more important than this, the dialysate will contain no base (no alkali). The patient will rapidly lose bicarbonate into the dialysate and within about 15 minutes the blood pH will fall below the level compatible with life. Sadly, we hear that this accident has happened in a handful of centers and patients have died as a result.

The other way this accident may happen is by the use of an acid concentrate in a variable proportioning machine with or without bicarbonate capability when the intention had been to use an acetate concentrate in the acetate mode. The feedback mechanism will bring the conductivity into the correct range and there will be no conductivity alarm. The conductivity monitor on a variable proportioning machine cannot detect the presence of the wrong concentrate. The patient's life now depends on one other monitor—the pH monitor. If this is functioning properly there will be an alarm caused by the abnormally low pH. However, if the machine does not have a pH monitor or the nurse switches the pH monitor off in order to continue dialysis, the patient will die in the same way in about 15 minutes from the effects of profound metabolic acidosis.

A similar but opposite mistake has also occurred when an acetate concentrate was used together with bicarbonate to perform a bicarbonate dialysis. This should also have been prevented by detection of a high pH by the pH monitor. In this case the combined effects of acetate and bicarbonate produced a profound metabolic alkalosis resulting in a major seizure. The patient's life was saved by this clinical event which caused the mistake to be discovered.

What can we learn from these disasters and what can be done to prevent them from happening again? Here are some suggestions.

1 Concentrates are as potent as drugs. To administer the wrong concentrate has as much potential for causing harm as giving the wrong drug, or the wrong dose of drug. The concentrate label should always be read carefully and checked by two people.

2 Never assume that the conductivity monitor on a machine is faulty and never ignore an alarm on the pH monitor. Always assume that a mistake has been made until proved otherwise. Never continue to dialyse when the machine tells you that something is wrong.

3 There is an argument to be made for color coding of acetate and

bicarbonate concentrates as long as this does not encourage dialysis personnel to ignore the labels.

A similar safety mechanism is the introduction of unique male connectors on the concentrate containers which will only mate with the appropriate female connectors on the proportioning machine. This practice has already been introduced by some companies in the dialysis industry.

For our part, we believe that the real answer lies in making everyone aware of the possible dangers. There is no substitute for thorough understanding and constant vigilance.

Glucose

In the early days of hemodialysis the removal of water from the patient to the dialysate was often done mainly by making use of the principle of osmotic pressure. If one added a high concentration of glucose to the dialysate one could greatly increase its osmotic pressure. But the actual fluid removed would also depend on the osmotic pressure of the blood. The plasma osmotic pressure depends on the degree of uremia and also on the level of blood glucose. This in turn will depend on the dialysate glucose concentration and the efficiency of the patient's own endogenous insulin response. If the patient does not easily handle a high glucose load from the dialysate the blood glucose will rise and the osmotic gradient will be relatively less. This will result in less water removal. There may also be a rebound hypoglycemia after dialysis. These difficulties will be compounded in diabetics who will tend to become even more hyperglycemic and require special insulin supplements for dialysis. With the advent of modern negative pressure dialysers and the ability to generate high and controllable transmembrane pressure it has been possible to control water removal very accurately by hydrostatic pressure. We no longer need high glucose concentrations in the dialysate for the purpose of fluid removal. If this is the case, why put any glucose in the dialysate at all?

We believe that the logical thing to do is to have physiological concentrations of glucose in the dialysate, that is 100 mg/dl or 5 mmol/l. This will tend to correct both high and low levels, both in diabetics and in nondiabetics. You know that, if you have a diabetic on dialysis, the dialysis itself will not upset the diabetic control. Instead it will tend to stabilize the diabetes. It will help to prevent severe hypoglycemic attacks as well as very high blood glucose levels. For these reasons all our concentrates contain glucose in a concentration of 5 mmol/l.

Avoidance of hyperglycemia with every dialysis has one more advantage worth mentioning. Repeated glucose infusions have a tendency to raise the level of plasma triglycerides, a problem which has long been recognized in patients on long-term peritoneal dialysis. Although it is doubtful whether this does patients much harm, it is worth knowing that it can be avoided in patients on hemodialysis.

Access to the circulation

In order to perform hemodialysis we must have a way of removing the blood from the body to the artificial circuit outside the body, where it will pass through the dialyser, and then be returned to the body. In an average adult this blood flow rate, out of the body, through the dialyser, and back to the body, should be at least 200 ml/minute for efficient treatment. The need for vascular access for dialysis may be either temporary, as in the case of acute, reversible renal failure lasting one to three weeks, or long-term, as in the case of end-stage renal failure when dialysis may be continued for months or possibly many years.

A third category is the patient requiring only one or at most two dialyses, as for example in the treatment of self-poisoning.

Shunts

The first really big step in the technology of obtaining repeated access to the circulation for hemodialysis was the development by Quinton and Scribner in 1959 of the silastic-teflon shunt. Consisting of flexible silastic tubing and smooth, semi-rigid, tapered teflon vessel tips, this device is placed by a small surgical procedure in an artery and vein. The commonest places to insert it are the radial artery and cephalic vein in the wrist or the posterior tibial artery and long saphenous vein at the ankle (see Fig. 7.7). In the intervals between dialysis the two ends of the shunt are connected together in a loop through which arterial blood flows continuously. At the time of dialysis the shunt is clamped, taken apart and the two separate tubes are joined to the arterial and venous tubing of the extracorporeal circuit.

The main problems of the shunt are that it has a tendency to clot and secondly, because it is a foreign object entering through the skin, it has a tendency to become infected. When it is finally removed because it is no longer needed or because it is no longer functioning, the blood vessels into which it has been inserted will have been destroyed and cannot therefore by used again for vascular access. However, for patients with

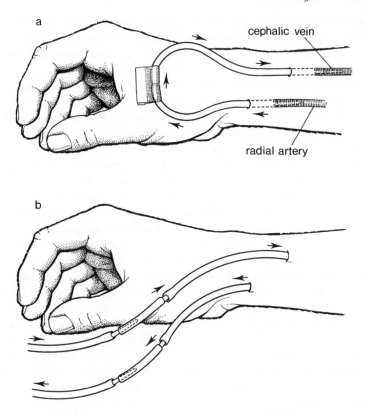

Fig. 7.7. Standard silastic Teflon shunt: (a) loop connected before dialysis, (b) in use during dialysis.

acute renal failure the shunt is only likely to be needed for a few weeks, because if the patient recovers it is unlikely that dialysis will be needed in the future.

In our opinion shunts still have a place in the management of acute renal failure in some patients. They are satisfactory if the patient has good peripheral blood vessels (both arteries and veins) and provided that there is a good blood pressure and adequate cardiac output. Shunts do not work well if the peripheral vessels are inadequate. Elderly arteriopathic patients tend to have diseased and atheromatous arteries. To tie off the posterior tibial artery in such a patient to insert a leg shunt may cause ischemia of the foot. Shunt insertion in the forearm may not be possible because of damage to veins from previous venepunctures or intravenous infusions. Patients in intensive care units not infrequently have an arterial line already in the radial artery.

When the method of temporary vascular access is being considered the medical staff will examine the patient and make a decision. If all the conditions are favorable for insertion of a shunt, one of the doctors will insert it. This is done as a sterile procedure, under local anesthetic, usually at the bedside. If a procedure room or operating room is available and convenient, so much the better. The best way to organize this is to have a sterile tray containing the necessary surgical instruments and the various component parts of the shunt brought to the bedside. Lengths of silastic tubing come in sterile packages and teflon vessel tips, graded in diameter from 13 (large) to 18 (very small) are also supplied commercially. Both artery and vein are cannulated with the largest tip which can be comfortably accommodated without stretching to the point of tearing. The tips are tied into the blood vessels with nonabsorbable silk sutures and will not slip out unless roughly handled. Regular care of the shunt and connections to the arterial and venous tubing of the kidney machine are nursing procedures. Nurses should take the trouble to learn how to handle shunts skillfully. Shunts should never be tugged at, jerked or twisted, and the area of the skin around the site of insertion should be kept scrupulously clean. The skin exit site should be kept covered with a sterile gauze dressing at all times except when being washed or dressed. The two ends of the shunt are joined over a connecting piece which can be provided with a T-junction for blood gas analysis (see Fig. 7.8).

Shunt clotting

Although silastic and teflon are smooth and relatively inert, there is still a tendency for blood clot to form in shunts and to block them in the

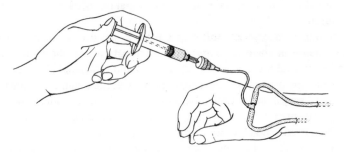

Fig. 7.8. Heparin injection port (heparin T-piece).

intervals between dialysis. Usually the clotting starts in the vein near to where the teflon tip ends. Clotting can be diagnosed by loss of the audible venous bruit and by the appearance of the transparent silastic tubing. The blood in the silastic loop turns dark blue and separates into a thin string of clot and a clear stream of serum. It also feels cold instead of warm. Removal of clot can usually be done easily if it is not delayed for more than a few hours. In most centers hemodialysis nurses are trained to declot shunts. This is a meticulously sterile procedure requiring mask, gown and gloves. It may be possible to aspirate the clot from the arterial side by simple suction with a syringe. Usually it is necessary to use a straight declotting catheter for the venous side, and the same technique may be required for the arterial side. The shunt is then flushed with a dilute heparinized saline warmed to body temperature. Only small volumes are injected, with great care, into the arterial side since sudden injection of large volumes (more than $2-3$ ml) into an artery can cause retrograde passage of clot up into the aorta and thence into a carotid artery with a resultant cerebral embolism. An instrument which has proved to be of value for declotting shunts is the Italian corkscrew (see Fig. 7.9). This comes in various sizes but the most useful size is 1.8 mm diameter. It is introduced into the shunt and screwed into the clot rather like removing a cork from a bottle. Anchor the silastic tubing while withdrawing the clot to avoid pulling on the shunt itself. An occasional complication is fracture of the corkscrew so that part of it is left in the vessel. If this happens there is no alternative but to remove the fractured end by surgical dissection. However, this accident should not happen if the corkscrews are regularly inspected for signs of weakness before use.

Another very useful device for declotting a shunt mechanically is a Fogarty balloon-tipped catheter. The size 3 Fogarty is generally the most useful. The balloon is inflated using a small syringe containing 0.5 ml sterile saline. The catheter is introduced through the shunt tubing and up into the blood vessel with the balloon deflated, and withdrawn with the balloon inflated. Clot can be pulled out in this way. In many centers nurses have been instructed in the use of Fogarty catheters for declotting shunts. As shunts are used less and less, these skills are dying out.

Stubborn clots which resist mechanical declotting may sometimes respond to injection of urokinase solution into the shunt and leaving it clamped for an hour or two. Urokinase is a fibrinolytic agent which dissolves fresh blood clot.

Shunts that clot repeatedly should be X-rayed after injection of radio-opaque contrast medium to identify the point of narrowing. This is

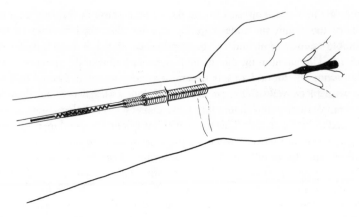

Fig. 7.9. The Italian corkscrew.

frequently just beyond the venous tip. It may be necessary to by-pass this narrowed area by moving the tip a little further up. This is a skilled surgical procedure only performed by experienced medical staff.

Shunt infection

Apart from clotting, the other main complication with shunts is infection. Since the dialysis nurse is most concerned with handling shunts at the start and end of dialysis she must take responsibility for detecting the earliest signs of infection. These are usually discomfort or pain at the site of insertion together with redness, swelling or exudation. You should not wait till you see a fluctuant abscess—by then it is too late. Cultures should be taken from the skin openings in any doubtful case and the medical staff informed immediately, so that appropriate antibiotic therapy can be started if this is thought necessary. Most infections will settle down if treated promptly. An exception is those caused by *Pseudomonas* organisms which are very hard to eradicate without removing the shunt.

Shunt removal

Removal of a shunt which is no longer needed after successful treatment of an episode of acute renal failure should be delayed until one is sure that the patient has entered the diuretic phase and the blood urea and creatinine levels are returning to normal. One should be as confident as possible that the shunt will not be needed again. At this point it is usual to stop the blood flow and let the shunt thrombose by putting a small clamp across the silastic tubing. Once the shunt has been clotted for about three days, it can be removed. This can be done easily and painlessly by infiltrating the vessel insertion sites and the subcutaneous skin tunnels with local anesthetic and then giving a quick hard pull. The shunt with its vessel tip and silk sutures will usually come out in one piece. Bleeding will be minimal and will stop quickly with firm compression. The exit sites quickly heal. If by chance the teflon vessel tip stays behind, it will have to be removed by dissection; but this event, in our experience, is rare.

Arteriovenous fistulas

Silastic-teflon shunts are a satisfactory method of vascular access for a proportion of patients with reversible acute renal failure but, because of the problems of clotting and infection, they have been largely abandoned for patients with end-stage renal failure. In the mid 1960s Brescia and Cimino devised the ingenious concept of the subcutaneous arteriovenous fistula. An artery is joined to a vein under the skin by a skilled surgical procedure so that a fast flow of blood passes up the vein. The vein enlarges and its wall becomes thickened, in keeping with its new role of carrying blood under arterial pressure. It is then possible to insert into the vein thin-walled, wide bore needles, one to remove blood to take it to the extracorporeal circuit, and another to return it higher up the vein, back into the patient's circulation. At the end of dialysis the blood is all returned to the patient and the needles are removed. Pressure has to be applied to the venepuncture sites till the bleeding stops. A band-aid or small dry dressing is usually applied for a few hours. The advantages of the AV fistula are:

- Because there is no foreign body emerging from the skin, but only the patient's own tissues in a subcutaneous position, there should never be any infection.
- Clotting in the fistula is a rare event.
- If there is no clotting and no infection the fistula should be available as an access site for dialysis for as long as it is required. The same fistula may function well for many years.
- Because there is no foreign body emerging from the skin, and the venepunctures heal very quickly, the patient can shower or bathe or swim with impunity. Fistulas do not interfere very much with any normal human activity—at least in the intervals between dialysis.

These advantages are in no way cancelled out by two important responsibilities. These are the necessity for skillful insertion of needles at the time of dialysis, and avoidance of sustained pressure on the fistula or other accidental trauma to it. One of our patients inadvertently caused her fistula to become occluded by thrombosis when she hung her handbag on her wrist while she spent two hours watching a film at the cinema.

Types and position of fistulas

The most consistently successful and useful fistula is an anastomosis made between the radial artery and the cephalic vein in the wrist of the non-dominant arm. This leaves the dominant hand free during dialysis, and for patients who carry out their own dialysis the dominant hand is free for insertion of the patient's own fistula needles.

In the early days the most popular type of anastomosis between the blood vessels was side-to-side, shown in Fig. 7.10. The problem with this type is that it often leads to development of a high blood flow down the distal venous limb with a dilated plexus of veins on the back of the hand and a tendency to venous congestion of the hand. Repeated needling of the proximal venous limb may lead to thrombotic occlusion which will then direct all the blood into the distal venous limb causing further aggravation of the existing problem.

In our opinion the side-to-side fistula is an obsolete operation which should no longer be done. Instead the vein should be anastomosed end-to-side onto the artery, thus allowing all the blood to flow up the arm as in Fig. 7.11.

A legitimate alternative to this operation is the end-to-end fistula shown in Fig. 7.12. This is the operation we favor in our hospital, for two main reasons. Firstly, the operation can be performed by a very simple gluing technique using a special cyano-acrylate tissue adhesive to join the blood vessels. Secondly, when the blood vessels form a continuous curve as shown in Fig. 7.12, it is very easy to remove thrombus if the fistula clots. Declotting can often be done percutaneously, without a surgical operation, by passing a Fogarty catheter in a reverse direction down the vein and round the bend of the anastomosis. A gauge 3 Fogarty catheter can be passed into the vein through a size 15 Angiocath. When the declotting is complete the Fogarty catheter and the Angiocath are both withdrawn through the skin puncture. Simple pressure will stop the bleeding just as if one were removing a fistula needle (see Fig. 7.13).

If the veins of the forearm are inadequate for fistula construction it is possible to use the veins of the upper arm. The cephalic vein running up the lateral aspect of the upper arm can be anastomosed onto the side of

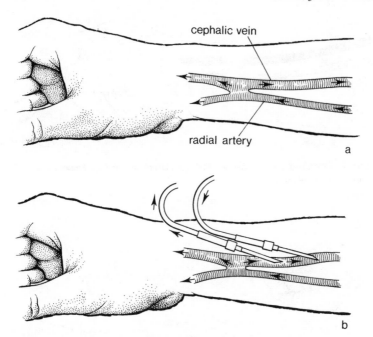

Fig. 7.10. Subcutaneous arteriovenous fistula: (a) anatomy of fistula, (b) needles in place for dialysis.

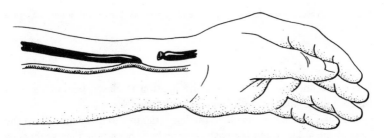

Fig. 7.11. End-to-side AV fistula. End of vein to side of artery.

the brachial artery (see Fig. 7.14). Alternatively the basilic vein, which normally runs deep between the muscles on the medial aspect of the upper arm, can be brought to the surface and anastomosed onto the side of the brachial artery (see Fig. 7.15). To do this operation the surgeon must make an incision all the way from the axilla down to the elbow.

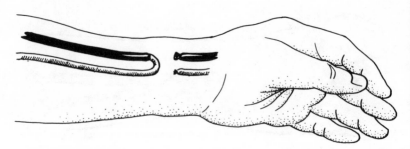

Fig. 7.12. End-to-end AV fistula. The vessels are joined in a smooth curve. The artery comes round to meet the vein.

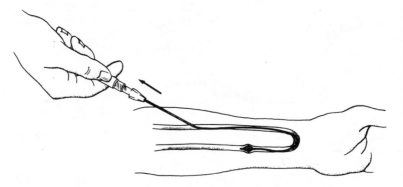

Fig. 7.13. Percutaneous declotting of an end-to-end AV fistula with a size 3 Fogarty catheter.

When the operation is complete the incision is closed behind the vein which will be anterior to it but just under the skin.

Fistulas can also be made in the leg. Attempts to make a fistula at the level of the ankle, using the posterior tibial artery and the long saphenous vein, have rarely been successful; but proximal fistulas in the thigh, using the long saphenous vein brought round in a loop and placed on the femoral artery, have worked well for some patients (see Fig. 7.16). We have not been very keen on this type of fistula, nor have we had much success with it. The medial aspect of the thigh is an awkward place to insert needles for dialysis and, when painful hematomas develop here, they interfere with walking.

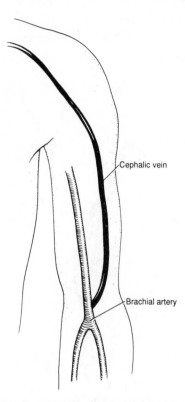

Fig. 7.14. Upper arm cephalic vein fistula.

Fistula substitutes

The patient's own veins should always be used for fistula construction if at all possible, but for a patient who is lacking any useful veins there are some fairly successful prosthetic substitutes. The two commonest substitutes are bovine carotid artery (processed in such a way as to make it acceptable for grafting into humans) and a purely synthetic material called polytetrafluorethylene (PTFE). This latter material is a kind of teflon cloth fashioned into a tube about 5 mm in internal diameter, and sold widely under the trade names Goretex and Impra. Most comparative studies of bovine carotid artery and synthetic PTFE have shown the latter's superiority in terms of the success of the fistula and its long-term survival.

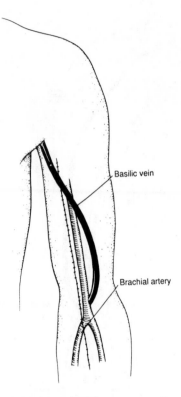

Fig. 7.15. Upper arm basilic vein fistula. The basilic vein has been lifted out of its normal position and placed under the skin, anterior to the incision on the medial aspect of the arm.

These graft substitutes can be used in two ways. Firstly, they can be used simply as a connecting tube or conduit to conduct blood from an artery to the vein which will serve as the site of needle puncture for dialysis. Secondly, the graft can act as the vein substitute and can itself be repeatedly punctured by the fistula needles. Neither bovine carotid artery nor PTFE stands up to being punctured repeatedly by needles nearly as well as one's own veins, so, if it is possible to find a length of vein to receive the needles, it always pays to do so.

Another disadvantage of bovine carotid artery is that in some patients it seems to undergo a chronic rejection reaction, probably due to the fact that it contains tissue from an animal of a different species. Both these substitute materials are placed in subcutaneous tunnels and anastomosed to the patient's own blood vessels. Two commonly used prosthetic fistulas

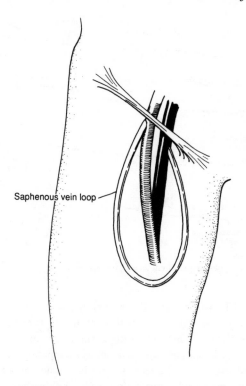

Fig. 7.16. Saphenous vein loop on the medial aspect of the upper thigh.

are shown in Fig. 7.17. The straight graft from the radial artery to the antecubital vein is very nice to use, but has a higher failure rate than the loop graft from the brachial artery travelling down the forearm and back to the antecubital vein.

Some special points about the use of PTFE should be mentioned.

1 In contrast to the operation for construction of a standard radial artery fistula at the wrist, which can be done under local anesthetic, insertion of PTFE grafts requires a general anesthetic or a brachial plexus nerve block. If the anesthetist has difficulty with the nerve block he will want to administer a general anesthetic anyway, so it is fair to assume that all these patients should be kept in a fasting state before surgery unless you are otherwise instructed.

2 When anastomosing PTFE to native vessels there tends to be a lot of oozing of blood from the prosthetic material through the stitch holes. This however is only temporary and soon stops.

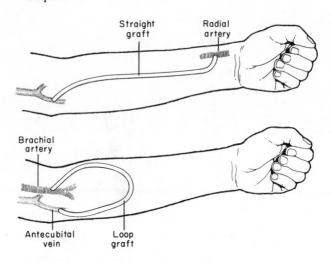

Straight graft   Radial artery

Brachial artery

Antecubital vein   Loop graft

Fig. 7.17. Two types of prosthetic arteriovenous fistula.

3 When PTFE is first inserted it is slightly porous and for the first few days a lot of plasma water escapes through the walls of the graft into the surrounding tissues. This can cause alarming edema of the arm at the site of the PTFE insertion but it is always temporary and will subside within about two weeks. Patients should be warned about it before the operation and reassured about it afterwards. Within about two weeks the whole of the inside of the graft material becomes lined with a layer of cells identical to vascular endothelium. At that point it becomes watertight and the surrounding edema fluid is reabsorbed and disappears.

4 Holes made in PTFE with fistula needles do not close as well as holes made in natural veins after the needles are removed. There is a tendency for false aneurysms to develop. A special section on the technique of needling fistulas appears on p.261.

5 Infections in or around a prosthetic graft are much more serious than those that occur in relation to natural arteries and veins. If prosthetic graft infections are treated very early and effectively they can usually be cleared up but, once they advance to the point of pus formation and a discharging sinus, it is virtually impossible to eradicate them. The only way to get rid of the infection is to get rid of the foreign body, in other words the whole graft or as much of it as possible has to be surgically excised. This is a difficult operation because the graft is usually very securely stuck under the skin.

6 PTFE grafts tend to stay patent for long periods provided that they

have a high blood flow. A high blood flow entering the arterial side of the graft is fine but a high flow emerging from the venous end seems, in a proportion of patients, to damage the intima of the patient's own vein. This chronic intimal damage leads to a build up of thrombus on the vein wall with a consequent narrowing of the vein at this point. The venous narrowing will be detected during dialysis as a high venous pressure which gradually gets higher as the weeks go by. It can be demonstrated radiologically by means of injected contrast medium. At this point it is probably wise to ask the vascular surgeon to revise the venous anastomosis because if this is not done the fistula will eventually clot up completely. In fact when a fistula does clot spontaneously during an interval between two dialyses there is nearly always a structural cause for it. It is easy to declot a fistula surgically but if the narrowed vessel is not dealt with it will quickly clot again.

7 Occasionally a forearm loop fistula will take so much blood away from the brachial artery that not enough blood will flow on towards the hand—this is called a steal. It will lead to ischemic symptoms in the hand. The hand will feel colder than the normal hand and there may be pain in the hand both during dialysis and when the hand is exercised. This is a form of intermittent claudication and may lead to the necessity to narrow the fistula so that it takes less blood or possibly the fistula may need to be closed completely.

8 One other rare but important complication of AV fistulas is high output cardiac failure. The flow through a fistula from the artery to the vein goes straight back to the right side of the heart and in effect whatever is the volume of this blood flow it is added to the total cardiac output. If the normal resting cardiac output is 5 litres/minute and the flow through a fistula is 700 ml/minute, the resting cardiac output is likely to rise to about 5.7 litres/minute and this is likely to be well tolerated by a healthy heart. If, however, a patient has a PTFE loop fistula with a flow of 1.5 litres/minute and we were to construct a new fistula 'as a spare' because the first one is giving trouble, and the new fistula is in a proximal upper arm or upper thigh position and also has a flow of 1.5 litres/minute, it is quite likely that the resting cardiac output would rise to 8 litres/minute and this will put the patient into heart failure—so-called high output cardiac failure. This is why it is not really feasible to make two fistulas for a patient just in case one fails. It is very rare for one fistula, even if it has a high blood flow, to cause heart failure (though we have seen this), but it is relatively common to induce heart failure if you make two. When high output cardiac failure occurs from this cause, it is nearly always predominantly left ventricular failure with

pulmonary congestion. It leads to breathlessness both at rest and on exertion and often a chronic troublesome cough. If cardiac failure occurs from this cause one has no alternative but to ligate or dismantle one of the fistulas.

Whichever type of fistula is constructed for long-term hemodialysis we should always attempt to have it ready well before it is needed. Fistulas all take time to heal up and mature. If one knows that a patient is going to need a fistula, arrangements should, if possible, be made to do the operation weeks or months before dialysis is required. If the need for dialysis cannot be foreseen or a patient arrives in hospital with hitherto undiagnosed end-stage renal failure, one cannot construct a fistula and use it immediately.

Some temporary method for vascular access must be used until the fistula is ready. Fistulas made using natural veins can usually be used within two weeks if the veins are good. Prosthetic vein fistulas such as PTFE grafts usually take 3−4 weeks before they can be used. The decision when to start using a fistula is usually made jointly by the medical and nursing staff who examine the patient at each dialysis.

One other important point relates to the timing of fistula operations. Fistulas have a tendency to clot during the first 24 hours after major surgery in other areas (e.g. abdominal surgery). Therefore if a patient needs a fistula but also needs major surgery, it is sensible to do the major surgery first. Once the patient is stable after major surgery it is fine to go ahead with the fistula construction.

The Bentley Dia-tap and the Renal Systems Hemasite

In those patients for whom construction and maintenance of an AV fistula has proved extremely difficult or impossible, there is available a very cleverly conceived alternative. This device, manufactured in a slightly different way by two different companies, consists essentially of an in-line T junction, in which the horizontal part of the T is incorporated into the stream of fast flowing blood of an upper arm fistula. The vertical limb of the T protrudes through the skin and in the intervals between dialysis is blocked off. In order to carry out a dialysis a special two-pronged probe is lowered into the device as shown in Fig. 7.18. One probe draws blood out of the vessel from the upstream side while the other probe delivers blood downstream in the opposite direction.

Connections and disconnections for dialysis are entirely painless and predictable because the nurse only has to manipulate the prosthesis. Liberal amounts of iodine-containing antiseptic are used and the prosthesis is protected in the intervals between dialysis by a cap or hood to

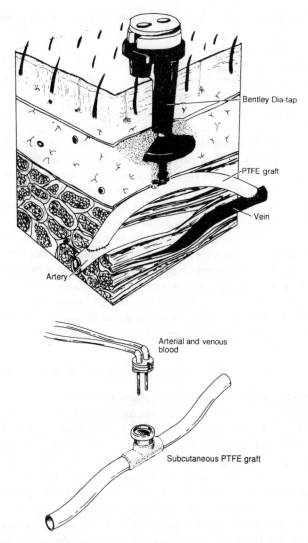

Fig. 7.18. a) The Bentley Dia-tap, taken from an illustration by courtesy of Bentley Laboratories.
b) The Renal Systems Hemasite.

keep the area clean. The device is much appreciated by patients who have been through endless ordeals of painful needling of unsuccessful fistulas. When the device is working well, it is a joy to use. The underlying weakness, however, is the same as that of a shunt. A foreign body is protruding from the skin and this may at any time give rise to infection.

Clotting may also occur though usually much less frequently than with shunts.

The device can either be implanted into an upper arm vein such as the basilic vein, having first anastomosed the basilic vein to the brachial artery, or the device mounted on a length of PTFE graft can be implanted under the skin of the upper arm. The lower end of the PTFE graft is anastomosed to the brachial artery and the upper end to the basilic vein. In either case the only part of the device visible on the outside is the little polished plate emerging through the skin into which the connections are made for dialysis. Neither of these devices is recommended for use in the forearm and the main reason seems to be that they need a very high blood flow to maintain patency. An additional reason is the difficulty of stabilizing the position in the forearm. It seems better if it is anchored to a deep vein which does not move much.

There is no doubt that the devices have functioned well in a number of patients for long periods without clotting or infection. We believe that, despite their very high cost, they have a role to play in a limited number of patients with very special vascular access problems.

Excellent detailed instructional material is available from the manufacturers to show the surgeon how the device should be implanted, and also for the nurses showing how it should be used for dialysis.

Temporary vascular access and central venous catheters

Ideally every patient requiring long-term hemodialysis for end-stage renal failure should be provided with an arteriovenous fistula before it is needed and this will continue to function throughout the period during which hemodialysis is needed. Even when the patient receives a successful renal transplant we do not usually tie off the fistula but leave it intact as an insurance policy in case the transplant ever fails. Actually, fistulas often close spontaneously after a successful transplant. This probably has something to do with the return to completely normal blood coagulation and hematocrit. Unfortunately, the ideal fistula is not always possible and there are many occasions when an alternative means of temporary vascular access will be required. These situations can be cited as follows.

1 In acute renal failure one is not always able to use a shunt. With the present trends in acute renal failure the patients are tending to be older and more arteriopathic with numerous complications. The arteries or veins or both may be unusable or the patient's blood pressure may be too low to provide a good flow through the shunt.

2 Patients may arrive in hospital in end-stage renal failure and there has not been time to create an arteriovenous fistula in advance.

3 Established AV fistulas may clot or fail unexpectedly.

4 Patients receiving regular long-term peritoneal dialysis, usually CAPD, may develop peritonitis requiring temporary removal of the peritoneal catheter and a short period of 2−3 weeks on hemodialysis. Alternatively, peritoneal dialysis patients may need elective or emergency abdominal surgery, requiring a temporary switch to hemodialysis.

5 Transplant patients may at any time require dialysis if the kidney fails to function adequately for whatever reason. The previously used fistula may have clotted.

6 Access to the circulation may be required at short notice to provide hemodialysis or hemoperfusion for the treatment of poisoning. Usually only one or, at most, two treatments are required. Obviously it does not make sense to put in a shunt, thus destroying two blood vessels, for the sake of one or two dialysis treatments.

7 Plasmapheresis, sometimes called plasma exchange, is becoming increasingly widely used as a treatment for a number of kidney diseases as well as for other conditions. In this procedure large volumes of blood are removed from the body, the plasma is separated from the red cells and the red cells are returned to the circulation. The treatment is usually carried out every day for several days at a time. Shunts are often still used for this procedure but in our opinion this is rarely justified because of the waste of blood vessels.

For all of these acute situations we now have well tried and convenient solutions in the form of central venous catheters. The femoral catheter has been available as a vascular access method ever since the early 1960s. It is only since the late 1970s that the subclavian catheter has become widley accepted as a temporary vascular access device. It has been largely responsible for making the silastic-teflon shunt obsolete in the management of end-stage renal failure. The use of both these devices was made possible by an ingenious method known as the Seldinger technique. In the intervals between dialyses the connections of the catheters can be capped off by means of Luer-Lock injection caps through which heparin can be injected to maintain patency.

The femoral catheter

This device, which is basically a wide bore plastic tube with a tapered end and a number of side holes, was largely popularized by Dr Stanley Shaldon in the earliest days of hemodialysis for end-stage renal failure. It is often called the Shaldon femoral catheter. Its advantage is that it can be inserted into any patient at a moment's notice and with a minimum of risk. It does not matter that the patient is critically ill, profoundly hypotensive, or in gross pulmonary edema. Even the presence of a bleeding tendency is not a contra-indication to its use as long as some care is used during the insertion. The only contra-indication to its use is the presence of recent operations in the groins to repair the femoral arteries or perhaps the presence of infected burns in these areas.

The big disadvantage of the femoral catheter is that it cannot, for obvious reasons, easily be left in place from one dialysis to the next, especially in an ambulant patient who wants to go home or back to work. The main role of a femoral catheter is to provide access for one or, at most, two dialyses in an ill patient who is confined to bed. Repeated separate punctures of the femoral vein at every dialysis for insertion of a catheter is unacceptable to most patients and their staff; and this practice has been made unnecessary by the development of the subclavian catheter technique. The procedure for femoral catheter insertion is as follows.

Since the femoral vein runs in the groin just medial to the femoral artery (which can easily be located by palpating the pulse), the assistant, who may be the hemodialysis nurse, shaves the area as far as the midline. It makes no difference which side is used for the insertion except that a right handed operator will usually find it easier to work on the right femoral vein of the patient. The bed should be raised to a height convenient for the operator so that no stooping is needed (see Fig. 7.19). (This applies to all technical dialysis-related procedures carried out in the patient's bed.)

The operator will wear a mask, sterile gown and gloves and will clean the area with iodine, povidone iodine or some other skin sterilizing agent. The area is draped with sterile towels. Local anesthetic is infiltrated into the skin as far as the femoral vein. A small opening in the skin is made with a scalpel blade. The next step is for the operator to pass the Seldinger needle into the femoral vein. This is any gauge 16 needle (about 2 inches long) which has a plastic cuff. There are many different makes which are suitable to serve this purpose and the medical staff will usually state their preference. Once the needle is in the vein and dark venous blood can be withdrawn into a syringe, the needle is removed while the plastic cuff is advanced into the vein. Now the Seldinger guide wire is advanced through the cuff into the vein. It should pass easily right up into the inferior vena cava without any obstruction. The guide wire has a soft, floppy tip at one end and this is the part of the wire which enters first. The rest of the wire is relatively stiff. The guide wire you

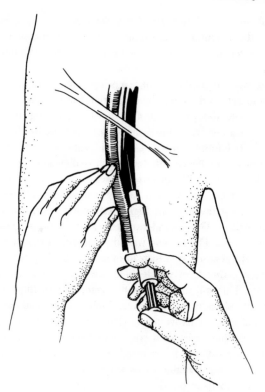

Fig. 7.19. Insertion of femoral catheter. The Seldinger-type needle is first inserted into the femoral vein while the left hand palpates the artery.

need is 70 cm in length and the gauge is 0.038 inches. Once the wire is in place, the plastic cuff is withdrawn over the wire. The femoral catheter is passed in over the wire, through the skin and up into the vein. The wire is then withdrawn. The operator confirms that a free flow of dark venous blood can be aspirated through the catheter and then the catheter is flushed with heparinized saline. It is then held in place with a dressing which serves to keep the skin exit site clean and also prevents the catheter from slipping out. The dressing we use for femoral catheters is the same one which we developed for subclavian catheters. This has come to be known as the double Op-Site dressing (Op-Site is the dressing manufactured by Smith and Nephew) and it will be described fully in the section on subclavian catheters. A number of other similar dressings are now available. They are all transparent, adhesive, sterile and apparently a good barrier to the entrance of micro-organisms.

Central venous catheters for dialysis can be used to withdraw blood to take it to the machine, to return blood from the machine, or to do both alternately by means of a device called a single-needle machine, of which more later.

If the catheter is used only for removing blood from the central large vein, we must return the blood by a different route, perhaps a vein in the arm. The trouble about using an arm vein for returning the blood is the danger of damage to arm veins if this is done repeatedly. Another option is to place two femoral catheters into the same femoral vein, one just above the other. The lower catheter (which is allowed to protrude farther from the skin than the higher one) is used to remove blood for dialysis while the higher catheter is used to return it. Alternately one can use a 20 cm catheter for the first one higher up, and a 15 cm catheter for the second one below. The second catheter can then be inserted fully and not left protruding. The trouble with this method is that we are making two holes in the femoral vein instead of one. A third option is to insert a double-lumen catheter, of which there are now several types available, into the vein. This will make a slightly bigger hole in the vein but there will be two blood pathways. However, double-lumen catheters are fairly expensive and most of us would be reluctant to insert one for only one dialysis. For all these reasons it is clear that one should, if possible, use the same femoral catheter for removal and return of the blood and to do this we should have available to us single-needle machines or devices. These are described on p.241.

If the operator decides to place two single-lumen catheters in the same vein, the second one should be placed below and after the first. This way there should be no danger of hitting the first catheter when inserting the Seldinger needle for the second. Because of this potential danger some operators do not insert either catheter until both guide wires are in place.

Heparinizing femoral and subclavian catheters

Femoral catheters for dialysis are usually used only once and then removed, whereas subclavian catheters are usually left in place and used repeatedly for an average of about three weeks. If a femoral catheter is used for dialysis immediately after insertion, and removed after dialysis, it will not need to be heparinized. However, if a catheter, either femoral or subclavian, is inserted, and dialysis is delayed for more than an hour or so, or if it is left in place after dialysis to be used again one or two or three days later, then something must be done to prevent it from becoming blocked by blood clot.

For a long time it was our practice when heparinizing a catheter to fill the deadspace of the catheter with a heparin solution equal in volume to the internal volume of the catheter. The deadspace of a single-lumen subclavian catheter (we use the same catheter for insertion into the femoral vein) is almost exactly 1 ml. Our practice, which we advocated to others, was to fill the deadspace of the catheter with 5000 units heparin in a total volume of 1 ml. This was injected with a fine needle through the injection cap of the catheter, immediately after insertion if dialysis was to be delayed or after dialysis if the catheter was to be left in place. We always assumed that the heparin stayed largely within the confines of the catheter and did not cause systemic anticoagulation by becoming dissipated through the side holes. However, our studies during the winter of 1984 showed that this technique does cause marked prolongation of the activated partial thromboplastin time both at 5 minutes and 1 hour after the injection. This might be dangerous if a patient is going for major surgery such as a kidney transplant or a bilateral nephrectomy immediately after dialysis.

We therefore changed our method and used pure heparin (5000 units in 0.5 ml) undiluted with any sterile saline. This method caused no significant systemic anticoagulation in any patient, presumably because the small volume of heparin stays initially in the proximal part of the catheter, diffusing only slowly into the distal section. Furthermore we found that with this method there is no increase in episodes of catheter clotting. This rather laborious explanation is given to explain why we now advocate heparin 5000 units in 0.5 ml (0.5 ml of a 10 000 unit/ml heparin) for all single-lumen catheters which have a 1 ml deadspace.

The subclavian catheter for temporary vascular access

When a patient needs regular hemodialysis for end-stage renal failure, but does not have a functioning AV fistula, a subclavian catheter or cannula is now accepted as the best method for temporary access to the circulation. A subclavian catheter, like the femoral catheter, is inserted by the Seldinger technique over a guide wire. It is introduced by a subclavicular route to the subclavian vein and it emerges from the skin through a subcutaneous tunnel. Fig. 7.20 shows the anatomy of the subclavian veins and superior vena cava. The catheter can be inserted equally easily from either side. The vein is entered by penetrating the chest wall in the angle below the clavicle and above the first rib. Unlike the femoral catheter the subclavian catheter can be left in position for as long as necessary because, in this position on the anterior chest wall, it can be anchored safely and conveniently. It does not interfere with dressing or

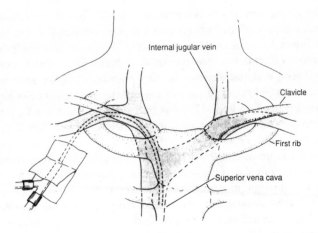

Fig. 7.20. Showing the position of the subclavian veins behind the clavicles. The catheter can be inserted equally easily from either side.

any normal activities and is concealed by a shirt or blouse. The patient can go home and back to work after dialysis. The only restriction is on swimming and having a shower. But the patient can sit in a bath to wash. The femoral catheter, being close to the perineum is at risk from infection. Being in the angle of the groin it interferes with walking. The subclavian catheter is in a clean site where it does not interfere with movements of the arms.

The disadvantages of the subclavian catheter compared with the femoral catheter are as follows.

1 The patient must be lying flat during the insertion in order to avoid air embolus. A patient in severe pulmonary edema cannot lie flat. For this reason it is our belief that subclavian cannulation for hemodialysis should never be attempted in a patient who has overt pulmonary edema.

2 Very occasionally, even with an experienced operator, there is a danger of a pneumothorax. It is therefore a calculated risk to attempt subclavian cannulation if the patient has a diseased or damaged lung on the opposite side of the chest.

3 Subclavian cannulation is a calculated risk in a patient on a ventilator because of the danger of pneumothorax in such a patient. This is why we always use femoral cannulation for patients receiving dialysis for severe poisoning. These patients are nearly always on ventilators. Furthermore a patient in this clinical situation is always supine, is not going anywhere, and will only need at most one or two dialyses. A femoral catheter is not, therefore, a disadvantage.

4 If one inadvertently punctures the femoral artery while attempting femoral vein cannulation one can apply pressure to stop the bleeding. If, on the other hand, one punctures the subclavian artery by mistake, one has to hope that the bleeding will stop spontaneously because it is not accessible to digital pressure. For this reason we make it a rule never to heparinize the patient for hemodialysis immediately after an accidental subclavian artery puncture. We always postpone hemodialysis for 24 hours. One patient had a near fatal hemothorax when we ignored this rule.

5 Safe cannulation of the subclavian vein requires more skill and experience than cannulation of the femoral vein. Therefore, if dialysis is needed urgently for an ill patient in the middle of the night, the inexperienced resident should not attempt subclavian cannulation. This is a technique for experts and those who have been very carefully instructed and supervised. The first dialysis can always be done through a femoral catheter. The subclavian catheter can then be inserted by an expert when the patient is more stable, usually the next day.

In practice we now use subclavian cannulation for nearly all temporary vascular access problems with two exceptions.

- Patients who are in respiratory distress and cannot lie flat. The usual cause for this is pulmonary edema.
- Patients receiving dialysis or hemoperfusion for poisoning, and receiving only one treatment for whatever reason.

Subclavian catheter insertion

Insertion of a subclavian catheter is now a very frequent procedure performed by the medical staff associated with a hemodialysis unit. Among a large group of patients in a busy center there will always at any one time be some who do not have a functioning fistula. In skilled hands the insertion takes about 20 minutes and dialysis can be started very soon afterwards. The insertion can be done wherever the patient is able to lie flat on an operating table, or stretcher, or on a bed which can be raised to an appropriate height. The procedure should be painless apart from the initial discomfort of local anesthetic. We find that most patients do not need premedication with a tranquilizer, but there is no objection to this being given to someone who is frightened or anxious.

The equipment required is most conveniently made available in two packs: 1, a sterile tray of surgical instruments including bowls for skin cleaning solutions and heparinized saline, and towels or paper drapes; 2, a pack containing all the other sterile disposable components one needs for the procedure.

Comprehensive packs or sterile trays are also available commercially which provide the operator with everything needed for the procedure. The nurse can save time and avoid aggravation by making sure that all the equipment is ready before the procedure starts.

One can also save time by asking which side the catheter is going to be inserted, checking the patient's chest wall, and shaving hair from the subclavicular region of hairy chested men.

The patient should lie completely flat without a pillow and with the face turned to the opposite side. An absorbent pad should be placed under the neck and shoulder to save the sheets from being soiled with iodine and blood. The operator first cleans the skin. We use aqueous tincture of iodine followed by alcohol, but many US centers feel strongly that povidone iodine should be applied and allowed to dry on the skin. These points tend to be dictated by hospital policy and I know of no evidence to show that either method is microbiologically superior. Our method undoubtedly provides quicker sterilization of the skin for a doctor who is in a hurry. It is also esthetically more pleasant for the patient. Who wants dried povidone iodine left on the skin of the chest wall? The area is then draped with sterile towels and local anesthetic is infiltrated into the insertion site and the subcutaneous tunnel.

Why have a subcutaneous skin tunnel?

Many centers have questioned the necessity for a subcutaneous tunnel. In our view there are three reasons why catheters should always be tunnelled for subclavian insertion. Firstly, the tunnel provides a longer physical barrier to the entrance of infection. At the time of going to press we have seen reports of two prospective controlled trials which show that a subcutaneous tunnel reduces the infection rate. Secondly, if the catheter is tunnelled it emerges from a flat area on the chest wall below the clavicle and this makes it easier to apply the dressing securely. It is also more comfortable for the patient. The third and most important reason relates to the consequences of the catheter slipping out or being pulled out by mistake. If a catheter slips out and there is no skin tunnel, the patient is left with an organized track leading directly to a central vein. The patient will bleed through this opening if he is lying flat or may suffer a fatal air embolus if upright. If, on the other hand, there is a tunnel under the skin about 5 cm in length, it will tend to close as soon as the catheter is removed. One of our patients had a bad dream and pulled out his catheter during the night while sleeping in bed at home. The skin tunnel soon closed and bleeding was minimal. This argument becomes even more compelling when one is using a double-lumen catheter with a larger outside dimension. If there is no tunnel there will be a wide gaping hole leading directly to the vein from the skin opening under the clavicle.

The tunnel can be made in two ways. Either one can make a 1—2 cm skin opening under the clavicle and tunnel outwards and downwards from this with a hemostat (this method we recommend) or alternatively the operator can use a longer Seldinger-type needle (more than 8 cm) and start tunnelling from the position at which he would like the catheter to emerge. The advantage of this is that the guide wire goes straight through the tunnel into the vein. The disadvantage is that it is harder to direct the needle accurately into the vein from a position so far out. These are really technical matters, only of concern to the operator, but nurses should be aware of the implications of not making a tunnel. The other point is that if there is no tunnel the standard 20 cm catheter will enter further into the superior vena cava and the tip will end up inside the right atrium. If your medical staff are adamant that tunnels are unnecessary they will need a supply of shorter catheters. Actually catheters should be supplied in a variety of different lengths to suit different patients.

Once the cannula is in place it is flushed with heparinized saline and capped. If dialysis is not going to be performed immediately it should also be heparinized, see page 220. The small incision at the insertion site is closed with one stitch. The application of the dressing is important. The best method we know is the 'double Op-Site' technique (see Fig. 7.21). This requires a little manual dexterity. Every hemodialysis nurse will become very good at it because changing the dressing once a week or more often if necessary is usually the nurse's job. First, the skin around the cannula exit site should be clean and dry. At the time of a new insertion a small square of gauze is placed over the incision. One dressing is placed under the silastic section of the catheter and reflected back, adhesive side up. A second dressing is placed above and over the catheter, the lower half adhering to the upturned adhesive surface of the first dressing. The catheter will then be held between two layers of sterile, transparent, adhesive dressing. It will be very secure and needs no sutures to hold it in place. The skin site can be observed continually for signs of infection. Our routine is to change the dressing once a week and more often if necessary. Some patients sweat more than others and this may cause the dressing to come loose earlier than usual. Oozing of blood under the dressing is an additional reason for a new dressing. If there is any sign of infection at the time of a dressing change, a culture should be taken from the skin site before the skin is cleaned and a new dressing

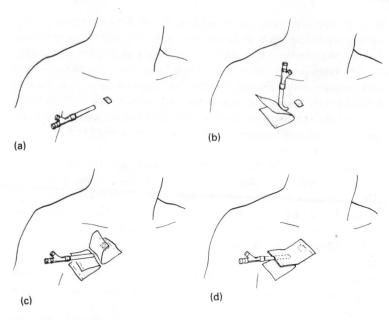

(a)

(b)

(c)

(d)

Fig. 7.21. a) The catheter in place with a small gauge square covering the incision. b) The first Op-Site dressing under the catheter. c) The second Op-Site dressing brought down onto the first. d) The catheter is held firmly as it emerges between two layers of sterile Op-Site. The exit site is protected against the entrance of organisms.

applied. The attention of the medical staff should be drawn to any exit site infection. The options are to leave it alone and observe it, treat with an antibiotic, or remove the catheter after dialysis.

The last job to be done after each new subclavian insertion is to arrange a chest X-ray to make sure the catheter is in a satisfactory position. It is the job of the doctor who inserted the catheter to look at the X-ray to satisfy himself that all is well. However, before the patient goes for an X-ray the nurse should place safety tapes on the connections and apply clamps to the silastic extensions. The use of Luer-Lock caps and safety tapes, as well as clamps on the tubing of the catheter, may seem excessively cautious but we have heard of at least one patient bleeding to death at home because the connection of his subclavian catheter came apart during the night.

Changing subclavian catheters

Once a subclavian catheter is inserted it is left in place and used at each dialysis for as long as necessary whether this period turns out to be three days or five months. Catheters are constructed in such a way that they will be durable and they should not wear out or break. In the early days we used to change them routinely once a week with the idea of reducing the infection rate; but then we did a controlled trial of changing versus no changing and found that the infection rate was identical in the two groups. Since then we have done no routine changing to reduce infection. However, some subclavian catheters become blocked by blood clot and under these cicumstances the best way of getting dialysis started quickly is to do a cannula change.

This procedure requires most of the same preparation as a new insertion. The patient must lie flat. After simple handwashing the nurse removes the Op-Site dressing. It is easy to peel it off the skin but it is usually necessary to cut it off the silastic tubing with scissors, taking care not to cut the silastic tubing itself. The doctor carrying out the change will clean the skin in the usual way and thoroughly soak the catheter at the same time with an iodine-containing solution. The area is draped with sterile towels. The silastic portion is clamped with a hemostat and the silastic is cut through between the clamp and the rigid Y piece.

Now, a new guide wire is passed down the catheter through the open cut end of the silastic. Once the guide wire is in and protruding beyond the distal end of the catheter, the catheter is removed. It is sensible to cut off the terminal 5 cm or so of the catheter with sterile scissors and send this for culture. If there is a positive growth of organisms it may serve as a guide to which antibiotic to use in the event that the patient develops a clinical infection. Now a new catheter can be advanced over the guide wire. Once it is fully in position with the silastic flush with the skin, the guide wire can be removed. The catheter is flushed and capped and the dressing is applied in the usual way.

We do not usually carry out a chest X-ray after a catheter change because we assume that the guide wire followed the old catheter and that the new catheter was led into the correct position by the guide wire.

Removing a subclavian catheter

A subclavian catheter should be removed as soon as we are sure that it is no longer needed. If one is waiting for a fistula to mature, it is wise to use the fistula once or twice. Sometimes we carry out a dialysis using the subclavian catheter to remove blood via the 'arterial' line to the machine and we put one needle in the fistula for the venous return. At the next dialysis we may put both needles in the fistula in order to be confident that the fistula is working well. Then, after the dialysis the subclavian catheter is removed. Catheter removal is a hemodialysis nurse's procedure.

After simple hand washing and putting on a mask, the Op-Site dressing is removed. The patient must then lie flat. Sterile gloves are put on and a small gauze pad is made by folding a four-by-four gauze square. Simply press gently over the skin exit site with your gauze pad while the catheter is steadily withdrawn. There will be no pain, no bleeding and no dramatics. The hole in the vein can only bleed through the skin tunnel and it takes very little pressure to close the tunnel. Pressure can be kept on for 2–3 minutes by the patient who can then be sent home with a small dry dressing over the skin opening. The patient can replace this later with a band-aid and will be relieved to start having showers again. Actually we have just started using shower 'capes' to cover the anterior chest wall to keep it dry while the patient takes a shower. We do not think that this practice will cause infection.

Care of subclavian catheters in the intervals between dialysis

In the intervals between one dialysis and the next a subclavian catheter requires no attention. It is heparinized, as described on p.220, and it should remain capped, taped and clamped. If, however, the patient is ill in hospital and requires intravenous infusions it may be more appropriate to use the catheter than to damage peripheral veins with peripheral infusions.

It is quite legitimate to use the subclavian catheter for an iv infusion as long as one remembers two things. Firstly, the iv infusion set must have a Luer-Lock connection and it should be taped. The usually snug fit iv infusion set may become accidentally disconnected and if this happens the patient may bleed to death or suffer a fatal air embolus, depending on his position (supine or upright) at the time. Secondly, one should recognize that every disconnection and reconnection with a catheter carries a risk of contamination and the possibility of bloodstream infection. Therefore, these procedures should be kept to a minimum and they must be carried out by a careful aseptic or antiseptic technique. This is described in the section on initiating and terminating a dialysis.

Subclavian catheter complications

The advantages of subclavian cannulation for temporary vascular access need no emphasis. The convenience to patients and staff and the avoidance of damage to blood vessels, which were such a feature of silastic teflon shunts, are now recognized worldwide. The only argument that can be raised against the use of subclavian catheters is the potential for serious complications. Fortunately, serious complications are largely preventable. Disconnections and air embolus have been discussed already.

1 Infection

All central venous blood lines have the potential for causing bloodstream infection, and subclavian catheters are no exception. Organisms may enter from the skin exit site, from contamination during connections and disconnections, or they may be carried in the bloodstream and settle on any blood clot which is attaching to the catheter. The patient will develop a fever with diurnal temperature swings and become vaguely unwell. If there is no other obvious cause for the fever, the catheter should be suspected and two blood cultures should be taken at least five minutes apart, either from the blood lines if the patient is on dialysis, or from a distant vein if the patient is off dialysis. Blood for culture should not be drawn through the cap of the cannula because organisms found here may just be local contaminants. A positive blood culture—usually available within 24 hours—will confirm the diagnosis. The correct treatment is to remove the catheter. Most authorities would also advocate administering an appropriate antibiotic. Others would always use antibiotics if they find *Staphylococcus aureus* but would withhold antibiotics with *Staph. epidermidis*. They would argue that removing the catheter in this case is enough to get rid of the infection. In any event a new subclavian catheter can be inserted on the opposite side one or two days later in time for the next dialysis.

Infection is by far the commonest complication of subclavian cannulation but not by any means the most serious. We have never seen one which failed to clear up. Our policy has been to use an appropriate antibiotic in every case of proven bloodstream infection. If on the other hand the infection is confined to the skin exit site, simple removal of the catheter will always clear up the infection. The incidence of infections can be kept low by careful attention to good hygiene.

2 Trauma

As has been implied already, trauma can be largely avoided by making sure that only skilled or carefully supervised doctors are authorized to insert catheters. Very occasionally there will be a *traumatic pneumothorax*. As long as it is recognized no serious harm will come to the patient. It should be treated by insertion of a chest tube drain until the lung is fully re-expanded. Inadvertent *subclavian artery puncture* will not usually cause problems as long as the patient does not receive heparin. In practice this means postponing hemodialysis for 24 hours. If hemodialysis is necessary immediately to save life it must be done without heparin and with very careful observation of the patient for signs of bleeding into the chest. See p.249 for heparin-free dialysis.

Perforation of the wall of the superior vena cava has occurred in a number of patients, not usually during the time of insertion of the catheter but after one or two uneventful dialyses have already taken place. Sometimes this was clearly due to a catheter being pushed back in when it had slipped out to some degree. The unprotected and semi-rigid catheter tip then went through the vein wall. This is not noticed unless the patient is on dialysis at the time or until dialysis is started later. Then when blood is being returned through the catheter during the venous return phase it is pumped into the hemithorax, into the lung itself causing massive hemoptysis, into the pericardium causing cardiac tamponade, or into the mediastinum causing severe pain and an effect similar to pericardial effusion and tamponade. Any of these situations can prove rapidly fatal if they are not detected. The moral is that a subclavian catheter should *never* be pushed back in (no matter how tempting it is to do so) if it is seen to be slipping out. The medical staff should be called and a guide wire can be passed down the catheter. The catheter can then be returned safely to its correct position or even better the catheter, which may be slightly contaminated by slipping out, is removed completely and replaced by a new one.

More worrying than these cases of perforations caused by catheters being pushed back in are those which appear to have happened spontaneously. We have wondered whether the tip of the catheter can erode its way through the vein wall as it repeatedly stiffens and relaxes under the influence of alternating positive and negative pressure of the single-needle machine.

We ourselves have seen two deaths from subclavian cannulation in our nine year experience of this technique. A catheter was placed deep into the heart of a young female of small stature and it found its way through the wall of the right atrium. Apparently patients hardly ever survive this injury. It was clearly much too far in. The correct position for the tip is at or above the entrance to the right atrium. Another catheter with its tip in the cavity of the right atrium caused the build-up of a ball thrombus which ultimately became big enough to block the tricuspid valve. The patient died at home.

We feel strongly that all subclavian catheters in future should be made 'idiot proof' by having floppy tips which are incapable of perforating anything even if they are incorrectly used. Also, catheters should be available in a range of different lengths to suit small and large patients.

Finally, if a patient with a subclavian catheter complains of chest pain or some other unexplained symptoms such as hypotension shortly after the start of dialysis it is essential to rule out some catheter-related injury as the cause. The dialysis should be stopped and the medical staff should be called at once to investigate.

3 Thrombosis

A well recognized complication of subclavian cannulation is *thrombosis of the subclavian vein*. This may show itself as edema and congestion of the arm and may appear only after the catheter has been removed. Any hemodialysis nurse who notices edema of the arm in a patient with a subclavian catheter should immediately draw it to the attention of the medical staff. It can be demonstrated radiologically by means of a subclavian venogram and, if diagnosed early, it responds well to heparin as does a deep vein thrombosis in the leg. However, because there are excellent collateral venous channels in the upper arm, the condition may be quite silent and may only come to light weeks or months later when dilated superficial veins are seen on the upper arm and chest wall. At this stage the thrombus is organized and will not dissipate with anticoagulants. Fortunately this condition seldom causes any serious disability even if there is an AV fistula in the same arm increasing the blood flow. In such cases the fistula arm may remain swollen and uncomfortable. If the patient has a successful transplant and the fistula clots spontaneously or is deliberately ligated the edema will usually subside completely.

One other type of thrombotic phenomenon that has been observed, other than the simple blocking of the catheter by clot, is a bunch of clot clinging to the outside of the catheter in the superior vena cava. This condition can be suspected if the catheter is giving a poor flow and changing it makes very little difference. It also can be demonstrated radiologically by a venogram and is seen as a large space-filling defect in the superior vena cava around the catheter. Clearly in this type of case there is a danger of pulmonary embolus from clot which becomes dislodged. It is perhaps surprising that we have never seen a proven case of pulmonary embolus from a subclavian catheter. This probably means that the natural fibrinolytic processes in the lungs can cope with numerous small clots and cannot be taken as evidence that pulmonary emboli never occur. If a large amount of clot is demonstrated in the superior vena cava we would recommend that the patient should be started on full heparin treatment and the catheter should be removed 24 hours later.

Double-lumen central venous catheters

The obvious and compelling advantage of a double-lumen central venous catheter is that, having two independent blood pathways, it can be used with a standard extracorporeal blood circuit and there is no need for a single-needle machine. There is also no need to damage arm veins in a search for a venous return. There is, at present, a quite proper sense of caution about unduly enthusiastic acceptance of double-lumen catheters because, being larger, they make a bigger hole in the vein wall. They have been criticized by those who say that it is not justified to dispense with the inconvenience of single-needle machines if double-lumen catheters are more dangerous. Actually there is no reason why they should be more dangerous provided that they are well designed and manufactured and also properly used. At present there are two main types. Firstly, there is the concentric or coaxial configuration of a tube within a tube; and secondly, there is the double-D configuration in which two pathways run side by side divided by a central septum. Both types suffer from the problem that one or both pathways may become blocked by blood clot. In the case of a coaxial catheter the inner tube can be removed to allow declotting. With a double-D configuration it is harder to declot the catheter mechanically. Furthermore, with this latter type the side holes obviously cannot be circumferential and they may therefore end up lying against the vein wall, thus blocking the flow.

At the time of writing double-lumen catheters are still being developed and perfected but they show a great deal of promise. In our opinion the most important advice we can give about them relates to their safety aspect. If a double-lumen subclavian catheter is used it is more important than ever to use a subcutaneous tunnel. If a large bore catheter, emerging from the chest wall just below the clavicle, were to slip out or be pulled out accidentally, there would be a wide open, well organized hole leading directly into the subclavian vein. This would allow massive air embolus or massive bleeding, depending on the patient's position at the time. If, however, there were a 5 cm subcutaneous tunnel, this would tend to close spontaneously or could be closed immediately by a little subclavicular pressure.

One of the most useful aspects of double-lumen catheters in our hands has been the ability to carry out continuous slow ultrafiltration for patients with acute renal failure in the intensive care unit. This topic is discussed on p.278. Double-lumen catheters are also very convenient when used in the femoral vein when one or, at most, two treatments are required for hemodialysis or hemoperfusion in the management of severe self-poisoning.

The extracorporeal circuit and its monitoring

When a nurse first joins a hemodialysis unit and looks closely at a dialysis in progress she tends to be disconcerted by the maze of blood tubing and the numerous dials and switches. A good teacher will point out that the essential part of the process is quite simple.

The dialyser

She will point first to the dialyser, easily recognizable by its shape, which is provided with two blood lines, one for the entry of blood from the patient and the other for the exit of purified blood which will return to the patient. The dialyser is also provided with two (larger bore) dialysate lines, one for bringing pure dialysate to the dialyser and the other for carrying away the spent dialysate which has picked up impurities from the patient's blood. This will be carried away down the drain. This is why modern kidney machiens are called 'single-pass systems'. The dialysate goes through the dialyser once only and is discarded. This allows the blood coming from the patient's body to be dialysed against fresh dialysate continuously throughout the whole duration of the treatment. The blood flow rate through the dialyser should generally be at least 200 ml per minute and the rate of flow of dialysate approximately 500 ml per minute. Identify the dials which display the flow rates.

Arterial and venous blood lines

Next the teacher will direct attention to the patient's arm. A needle near the wrist is drawing blood from the dilated vein of the AV fistula. This is called the 'arterial' needle and the tube attached to it carries a red mark symbolic of arterial blood. Higher up the arm is another needle attached to a blood tube with a blue mark. This is the venous line returning blood from the dialyser to the patient. The uremic blood entering the arterial line is extracted from the fistula near to the artery and is in effect coming straight from the heart. The purified blood coming from the dialyser returns to the vein upstream from the arterial outflow and is swept on by the fast flow in the fistula up into the great veins to the right side of the heart where it rapidly becomes mixed with the general circulation.

Blood pump

It can be seen that the arterial line leads to a peristaltic blood pump. This is a pump with rollers which compress the tubing and in effect massage the blood along in one direction. The part of the arterial line in the blood pump is rubbery expanded tubing called the blood pump segment, designed to return to its former shape as soon as the roller has gone over it. You will see that there is a knob to turn to make the blood pump go faster or slower. Blood flow is variable from extremely slow (a steady drip) to as high as 400 ml/minute. The blood pump can be adjusted to whatever speed is required. This blood pump is the power unit drawing blood from the patient through the dialyser and back into the patient.

Sterility

All the components of the extracorporeal circuit must be sterile on the inside so that blood during the purification process does not become microbiologically contaminated. The inside of the blood circuit must also be chemically clean so that the blood does not become chemically contaminated.

Anticoagulation

When blood comes in contact with an artificial surface it tends to clot. In order to prevent this happening during dialysis we administer a continuous infusion of heparin to keep the blood anticoagulated. This heparin infusion line (a very small diameter tubing) will be found entering through a T-junction in the arterial line between the blood pump and the dialyser. It is usually administered from a 20 or 30 ml syringe whose plunger is being steadily pushed home by a syringe pump. The amount of heparin delivered can be controlled by the concentration of the heparin solution in the syringe as well as by the syringe pump speed. The syringe pump speed is manually adjustable but constant at a given setting. It is the nurse's job to control the heparin administration according to the patient's needs. This will have been decided by prior discussion with the medical staff.

Heparin infusions have sometimes been administered upstream of the blood pump, between the arterial needle and the blood pump. This is undesirable because the blood tubing has a negative pressure at this point and a break in the heparin infusion circuit could lead to the entry of air. The heparin infusion should always enter beyond the blood pump into a segment of the blood circuit which has a positive pressure. However, this also means that the heparin infusion pump must be capable of pumping against a high positive pressure without any change in infusion speed. We now have blood which is being pumped, anticoagulated and purified. What else has to be controlled and monitored?

Temperature

The blood going though the dialyser has to be kept at body temperature. This is controlled by the dialysate temperature. Remember that the dialysate is completely surrounding the blood compartment of the dialyser. If the dialysate is too cold it will cool the blood. If it is too hot it will heat the blood and hemolyse the red blood cells. Dialysate rising above 42°C will do this. So the dialysate is thermostatically regulated at a temperature of 37−38°C. The dialysate temperature should be constantly visible on a dial.

Pressure

There are three main reasons for monitoring pressure in the extra-corporeal circuit. The first is that the relative pressures in the blood compartment and in the dialysate compartment determine the total hydro-static pressure gradient across the dialysis membrane (the transmembrane pressure) and hence the amount of water lost from the blood into the dialysate during the period of the dialysis. The second reason is related to patient safety.

Blood leak detector

The blood compartment pressure must always be higher than the dialysate pressure. In this way if a leak should develop in the membrane it will be detected as a trace of blood in the dialysate. Every dialysis machine has a blood leak detector for this purpose. If the pressures were reversed and a leak were to develop in the membrane, non-sterile dialysis fluid could enter the blood compartment and cause septicemia. We once saw this happen in the early days when we were using a primitive dialysis system. The patient fortunately survived.

The third reason for measuring pressure is in order to be kept informed of what is happening on the arterial and venous sides of the dialysis circuit.

Venous pressure

Beyond the dialyser, in the venous line returning to the patient, is a blood chamber with an airspace above it. Leading from the top of this chamber is a pressure monitoring line running to a venous pressure dial on the machine. The pressure in this chamber (continuously displayed on the venous pressure dial) reflects the positive pressure in the blood compartment of the dialyser. It is determined by the blood flow rate through the dialyser and the restriction to flow offered by the venous fistula needle. Most dialysis circuits also have a fine mesh filter at the bottom of the venous pressure chamber the purpose of which is to trap solid particles to prevent them from returning to the patient. When clotting occurs in any part of the dialysis circuit, it usually starts in the filter. Clotting in the filter would also cause the venous pressure to rise. However, if there is no clotting (easily seen by the presence of fibrin on the walls of the chamber), in the venous filter, a high venous pressure means obstruction at the level of the fistula needle or beyond. An obvious exception would be kinking of the blood tubing itself or a clamp left on the blood line by mistake. Obstruction beyond the level of the fistula needle is most commonly due to narrowing of the vein at the outflow end of the fistula but it could also be due to the needle being dislodged from the vein so that the venous blood is being pumped into the interstitial tissues. On the other hand a sudden fall in the venous pressure could be caused by the fistula needle coming right out of the patient or by a complete disconnection of the fistula needle from the venous blood line. On the venous pressure dial there are upper and lower limits which can be set. If these limits are exceeded, a venous pressure alarm will sound and the appropriate light will draw attention to the problem. When the alarm goes off, the blood pump is also switched off automatically and the dialysis can only be restarted by the nurse or somebody identifying the problem.

The whole dialysis system is based on monitoring of this type which draws one's attenion to faults which develop during dialysis. If this were not so it would be necessary for someone to be watching all aspects of the dialysis all the time and one full-time nurse would be needed for each patient. Nowadays we take all this sophisticated monitoring for granted but we should remember that in the early pioneering days of hemodialysis patients bled to death when blood lines became accidentally disconnected. Blood would be pumped onto the floor at the rate of 200 ml/minute or a litre in five minutes. If the nurse's back was turned nobody noticed because there were no pressure alarms. Much as we would like to see dialysis machines simplified, we accept the necessity for monitoring because we cannot afford the manpower to watch the machines all the time. Nurses must be free to attend to other patients while dialysis is in progress. Patients who dialyse themselves at home must be able to go to sleep, secure in the knowledge that the machine will wake them if something goes wrong.

Arterial pressure

Examination of the arterial line between the arterial fistula needle and the blood pump will reveal another blood chamber with air above it and a pressure monitor line leading to an arterial pressure dial. The pressure in this part of the circuit will be negative rather than positive because blood is being rapidly carried away by the blood pump. In general the faster the blood flow the greater the negative pressure but a restriction of flow through the fistula needle will also increase the negative pressure. This may be due to bad positioning of the fistula needle or possibly just a poor fistula with a low flow through it. A more serious reason would be sudden death or cardiovascular collapse of the patient, which also leads to poor or absent flow in the fistula. The least serious cause would be a kink in the blood tubing.

It can be seen that all arterial and venous pressure alarms must be investigated at once, if for no other reason than to get the dialysis started again. Many patients, even if they do not carry out their own dialysis completely unassisted, are capable of responding appropriately to an arterial or venous pressure alarm. They have been trained to look for and identify the problem and correct the cause. They can then get their own dialysis going again, so saving a nurse from having to intervene.

Subclavian and femoral catheters do not cause an alarm in the event of circulatory arrest.

When a patient is being dialysed through a shunt or through needles in an AV fistula, sudden circulatory arrest or sudden severe fall in blood pressure will cause abrupt loss of flow in the shunt or fistula and this will lead to an arterial negative pressure alarm. This in turn will draw the nurse's attention to the patient's predicament. If, however, the patient is being dialysed through a central venous catheter, either subclavian or femoral, the catheter is lying in a central venous pool of blood. Even if blood flow ceases in the central venous system due to a cardiac arrest, the catheter will continue to supply blood to the extracorporeal circulation. There will be no development of arterial negative pressure. This problem was brought dramatically to our attention in the following way. A patient, whose kidney transplant had recently failed, was being dialysed in the main hemodialysis unit with a subclavian catheter for temporary vascular access. Shortly after the start of the dialysis he expressed a desire to go to sleep. He curled up on his side and pulled his sheet over his head to shut out the light and the noise. Half an hour later his nurse went to carry out routine monitoring of his vital signs. She pulled his sheet back to uncover his arm and found him dead. We had unknowingly been dialysing a corpse and no alarm had sounded. Attempts at resuscitation were not surprisingly unsuccessful since he could have had his cardiac arrest any time up to half an hour before. The central venous catheter had not killed the patient but it had failed to draw attention to his cardiac arrest. The moral of this horrifying story is that patients being dialysed through central venous catheters must never be allowed to have their heads covered during dialysis. Their vital functions should be constantly visible and, as an extra precaution in an unstable patient, it may be felt wise to attach a portable cardiac monitor. Someone should be able to observe this constantly.

The air embolus monitor

We all know that it is dangerous for air to enter the veins and this tragic accident has killed patients in the early days of dialysis. It must never be allowed to happen. One of the main ways of protecting the patient from the possibility of air embolus is the air embolus monitor. This will be seen as a solid sensor mounted on the venous pressure chamber opposite the column of blood. If the level in the chamber drops due to the entry of air, the sensor will detect an airspace instead of a solid column of blood. A good air detector will also detect foam. If the level of blood falls below the air detector sensor, an alarm will be triggered. This alarm will simultaneously clamp the blood line below the venous chamber, stop the blood pump, and set off a visible and audible alarm. This device, which is an essential part of every extracorporeal circuit, should reliably prevent any air which may have entered the extracorporeal circuit from reaching the venous line which is returning the blood to the patient. It goes without saying that the air detector should be in place and switched on throughout the whole period of the dialysis. The emergency treatment of air embolus is described on p.287. A number of physical principles have been used to try to make the perfect air detector. The perfect air detector should detect foam but should not be activated by saline. Furthermore it should not be so sensitive that it is frequently triggered by tiny bubbles causing false alarms. If this happens the patient may be tempted to turn it off just in order to get some peace. Once it is turned off it cannot perform its proper function. A number of patients owe their lives to the proper functioning of an air detector.

The most reliable type depends on the use of ultrasonic sound waves which are better transmitted by liquid than by air. The device is particularly efficient because it detects foam as well as streams of bubbles.

The older air detectors which depended on a beam of light being picked up by a light-sensitive photocell were unreliable because foam usually obscured the light source and so did layers of fibrin on the inside of the bubble trap. Air could thus pass through without the alarm being activated.

Pressure monitor lines must be isolated. Pressure in the bubble traps is monitored by means of a small-bore air-filled line leading from the airspace of the bubble trap to a meter in the machine. If blood were to fill and displace this airspace it could run right up the pressure line into the machine. If the same thing happened with a different patient's blood at a subsequent dialysis the first patient's blood could contaminate the second. In this way blood-borne diseases such as hepatitis B could be spread from one patient to another. It is for this reason that you will see disc-shaped separators designed to interrupt the flow of blood to the meter in the machine. These separators, which are disposed of together with the blood lines at the end of dialysis, can transmit air pressure but will obstruct blood flow.

The dialysate negative pressure. The early coil dialysers which were used for many years depended for the removal of water on development of positive pressure within the blood compartment. This we achieved by pumping blood into the dialyser and restricting the outflow pathway (the venous blood line) with an adjustable clamp. Hence they were called positive pressure dialysers. Modern dialysers are all contained in a rigid box called the dialysate compartment. Hydrostatic pressure for fluid removal is generated by exerting a negative pressure on this dialysate compartment. This is done by actively drawing the dialysate out through the dialysate outflow line, while restricting the lumen of the inflow pathway. This dialysate negative pressure is displayed continuously and is adjustable up to a maximum of about 500 mmHg. There will also be a positive pressure in the blood compartment, continuously monitored as already mentioned. The two pressures added together constitute the total transmembrane pressure and this in turn dictates the amount of fluid removed. We will see later how to remove a given amount of fluid accurately during the course of a dialysis.

De-aeration or de-gassing of dialysate. The product water used to make dialysate usually contains a considerable amount of dissolved air, especially during winter, because more air dissolves in cold water. When the dialysate is warmed to body temperature the air comes out as small bubbles. This is a nuisance for several reasons.

• Air gets into the dialysate compartment of the dialyser and prevents contact of dialysis fluid with the membrane, effectively reducing the dialysing surface.

• Air interferes with the ability to generate negative pressure in the dialysate compartment because it is expandable.

• Air can cross the membrane into the blood compartment and block the fibers of a hollow fiber dialyser.

• An air−blood interface encourages clot formation and this may lead to the development of micro-emboli which may be carried to the lungs and interfere with gas exchange.

• A large amount of air or foam will find its way to the venous bubble trap and lower the blood level where it will have to be removed regularly. If it is not detected it will activate the air detector or cause an air embolus to the patient.

For all these reasons the dialysate has to be de-aerated and in practice the best way to do this is to heat it to body temperature and subject it to a strong negative pressure. The air which is released must then be vented. Only after this has been done can the dialysate be allowed to run into the dialyser. Modern dialysis machines have very efficient de-aeration systems.

Disinfection of the dialysate pathway

Dialysate for hemodialysis does not have to be sterile. Bacteria in the dialysate cannot cross the intact dialysing membrane into the blood. If there is a hole in the membrane, blood will leak out into the dialysate and be picked up at once by the blood leak detector. Non-sterile dialysate will not pass into the bloodstream because the pressure across the membrane is, and always must be, in the opposite direction. Nevertheless, heavy bacterial growth in the dialysate can be harmful and must be prevented. Dialysate at body temperature is an excellent culture medium, so a method must be developed for disinfecting the dialysate flow pathway regularly. In a busy dialysis unit, with two or three shifts of patients following in quick succession, the disinfection is normally done once every 24 hours at the end of the working day. Bacteria also have a tendency to grow in the deadspaces of de-ionizers and this can contribute to the contamination.

Sterilization can be done by sending heated water at about 95°C through the dialysate pathway or by using disinfectants such as formaldehyde or sodium hypochlorite. Heating is generally less popular because the hot water may lead to caramelization of the glucose in the residual dialysate and this will then stick to vital parts of the fluid pathway. Formaldehyde is an extremely efficient disinfectant but is unpleasant because of the fumes which are liberated and these may affect nurses and other personnel working in the area. There are also, in many countries, by-laws which restrict the amount of formaldehyde which one is allowed to discharge into the drains and sewers. Sodium hypochlorite is widely used and effective and is currently the most popular agent for the purpose but it does have the disadvantage of being corrosive to certain metals with which it comes in contact. Glutaraldehyde is now being used to good effect and has the double advantage of being effective as well as esthetically and socially acceptable. It seems to be relatively non-toxic. Whatever method is used to disinfect the dialysate pathway there must be a foolproof system for cooling it down if it has been heated (hot dialysate can hemolyse the blood and kill the patient) and for removing the sanitizing agent after the disinfection is complete. This is normally done by flushing the whole system with dialysate at normal body temperature for a stipulated period of time before dialysis is allowed to start.

Single-needle systems

The majority of dialyses for end-stage renal failure in the last 20 or more years have been performed by using either a silastic-teflon shunt (which has an arterial outflow and a venous return) or by inserting two needles in an AV fistula, one for arterial outflow and one for venous return. In either case one blood pump is adequate to draw the blood out of the patient and propel it through the dialyser and back into the patient. However, from an early stage it was realized that there would be a great advantage in being able to carry out dialysis by using only a single conduit or blood pathway. For example, it would be very useful to be able to perform dialysis through a single catheter in a large vein or through a single needle in a fistula. No patient would wish to have two catheters inserted in central veins if one would do. Also, it is usually fairly easy to put one needle in a fistula but it may be difficult to insert two. And perhaps fistulas would last longer if they received only half the number of needle punctures.

In 1972, Dr Klaus Kopp in Germany showed that it was also possible to draw blood through a single blood pathway, propel it through the dialyser, and then return it through the same single pathway back to the patient. This meant having an alternating flow in opposite directions through the single pathway. The principle is demonstrated in Fig. 7.22.

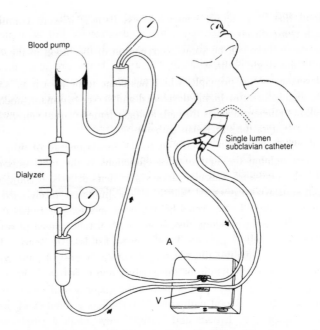

Fig. 7.22. Diagram of the Vital Assist single-needle device. The clamp on the Vital Assist box alternately clamps the arterial and venous lines.

During the 'arterial' phase of the cycle blood is drawn out of the patient by the blood pump while the clamp V occludes the distal end of the venous return line. Blood is filling the system but it cannot escape at the other end. Since blood is not compressible the extra volume is accommodated by compression of the airspaces at the top of the arterial and venous bubble traps, and also to a minor extent by distension of the dialyser. Although the old coil dialysers were fairly distensible the modern hollow fiber dialysers are not, so the extra volume is really dependent on the bubble traps. During the second phase (venous return) of the cycle, the clamp V is released and clamp A is simultaneously applied to the arterial outflow line. This allows the dialysed blood to rush back into the patient down the single pathway and the dialysis circuit is partially emptied by expansion of the compressed air in the bubble traps. Once this extra blood has returned to the patient the venous clamp closes, the arterial clamp opens and the cycle is repeated. The blood is pumped continuously and the clamps operate alternately. This ingenious principle allows the dialysis circuit to be supplied with blood from a single pathway. The main limitations of the method are:

- Blood flow is generally somewhat less than if it were continuous through two pathways.
- Inevitably there will be some recirculation of the blood in the deadspace of the single pathway.

Nevertheless this principle, which has come to be known as 'single-needle dialysis', is now highly developed and serves two main functions:

- It allows efficient dialysis through a single-lumen central vein catheter such as a femoral or subclavian catheter.
- It allows us to use one needle in an AV fistula instead of two.

In our opinion the first of these functions is the most important. Nearly all temporary vascular access for hemodialysis is now done through subclavian catheters. Silastic-teflon shunts are rarely used now for patients with end-stage renal failure, even on a temporary basis. The advantages of using only one needle in an AV fistula instead of two are fairly controversial. If patients have a good fistula it is nearly always possible to insert two needles. If this is not easily possible, the patient probably needs a new fistula or the existing one needs to be improved. Although this is only our opinion, in fact the majority of dialyses are still performed with two blood pathways. Nevertheless a number of dialysis units, particularly in Britain and Europe, now adopt a single-needle system routinely for all their dialyses. Whether one agrees with this policy or not, it is hard to avoid the necessity for single-needle systems for some dialyses in some patients. Therefore, one needs a minimum understanding of and familiarity with them. We now have experience of three different single-needle systems and between them they illustrate most of the currently available technology.

The first single-needle system to be widely used (it is also very simple and cheap) was the Vital Assist (Renal Systems, Inc.). This has the advantage of not requiring special blood tubing sets and consists essentially of a clamping device set in a box. The blood lines coming from the patient are set in the top of the box and are clamped alternately. The cycle time can be varied within limits but the triggering of the clamps is activated by the pressure in the venous bubble trap. Because blood is not compressible, one depends on the small amount of air in the top of the arterial and venous bubble traps to provide the filling volume of the extracorporeal circuit while the venous clamp is on. This filling volume or 'stroke volume' can be calculated by dividing the blood flow rate through the pump by the cycling frequency. If the blood flow rate is 300 ml per minute and the clamps are activated 30 times per minute the stroke volume should be 10 ml. We know that with each cycle the blood in the deadspace of the catheter will be pumped around again or 'recirculated'. There will also be some recirculation of venous blood back into the arterial line in the split second between the opening of the venous clamp and the closing of the arterial clamp.

We have found that we can achieve a fairly efficient dialysis if the blood flow rate is 300 ml per minute or more and the pressure drop on the dial is at least 30 mmHg. This will give a stroke volume of at least 10 ml. Then, if 2 ml of blood in each cycle recirculates there will be 20% recirculation and one will still have an adequate dialysis. However, if the blood flow through the subclavian catheter is at all sluggish due to partial thrombus obstruction, or the flow through the fistula needle is inadequate due to poor flow through the fistula, it is well-nigh impossible to obtain a good dialysis. We depended on Vital Assist machines for a number of years and in general we obtained satisfactory results in spite of the inherent difficulties and the unavoidable degree of recirculation; but, when the Vital Assist is used without proper skill and knowledge, recirculation may be almost complete. The other disadvantage of the Vital Assist machine is that the necessity of generating high venous pressures to accommodate the stroke volume causes an unavoidable high ultra-filtration pressure and consequently a substantial obligatory fluid loss. This may have to be accepted and compensated for by increased infusion of normal saline into the extracorporeal circulation. Excessive turbulence in the venous drip chamber caused by the large rise and fall in pressure causes much foaming and consequently clotting at this site. Also, a rise in the blood level could block the venous pressure monitor line. To some extent these difficulties can be obviated by having a larger venous drip chamber and hence room for greater expansion in the extracorporeal circuit.

The second system we tested and used for a number of years was the pressure-pressure cycled double pump system developed by Bellco (see Fig. 7.23). This was a great step forward because the presence of two large expansion chambers allows a stroke volume of at least 40 ml. This means that the small volume of recirculated blood is a very small percentage of the total. The blood pumps, which are occlusive, also act as blood line clamps while they are stopped. Experience taught us that the Bellco system, properly used, provides a good dialysis every time. Recirculation has been demonstrably low, as shown by many independent studies in different centers and because of the presence of expansion chambers, high venous pressures, and therefore high ultrafiltration, can be avoided.

The disadvantages of the Bellco system which became apparent to us were as follows.

Firstly, the venous blood pump was downstream from the air detector.

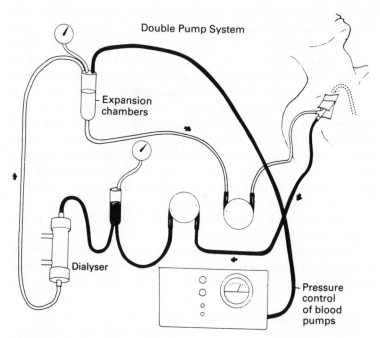

Fig. 7.23. The Bellco single-needle system. Note that there are two blood pumps and two expansion chambers, but no air embolus monitor downstream of the venous blood pump.

This allows the possibility that air could enter the circuit beyond the air detector and before the blood pump, thus leading to an air embolus. This accident happened in one of our patients but fortunately it was detected before it reached the patient. Secondly, because there is no arterial and venous pressure monitoring between the blood pumps and the subclavian catheter or the fistula needle, one remains unaware of large pressure fluctuations due to partial catheter obstruction or a partly blocked needle. The development of high positive pressure during the venous return phase could cause the blood line to blow apart. The third disadvantage of the Bellco system is that it is an extra bulky and expensive piece of hardware which has to be accommodated at the patient's bedside. Also the special blood tubing sets with their expansion chambers are more expensive than conventional blood tubing sets.

The third single-needle system of which we now have experience is the Cobe double-pump system (see Fig. 7.24). Modelled on the Bellco system, it has been further refined and improved. Like the Bellco system there are arterial and venous expansion chambers, and the arterial and venous blood pumps are triggered by preset pressures. However, in addition there are arterial and venous bubble traps between the blood pumps and the patient which allow pressure monitoring at these points, and the air detector is correctly positioned beyond the venous blood pump to ensure reliable prevention of air embolus. In addition there are blood line clamps close to the patient, and synchronized with the blood pumps, which effectively restrict recirculation. Now that we can effectively monitor these pressures we are realizing that we must accept high positive and negative pressures (up to 300 mmHg) in order to obtain good blood flow and stroke volume.

Finally the double pump module is integrated with the whole machine so that the system is very compact.

Although the Cobe double pump single-needle system is the best of those we have tested, we know that a number of other manufacturers have similar systems incorporated into their machines.

Control of anticoagulation

If blood is taken out of the body and allowed to sit in any container, no matter how smooth or inert or sterile it is, it will clot. If it is circulated fast through a smooth plastic tube such as the silastic of a shunt, it may stay fluid without clotting for long periods. The modern hemodialysis circuit has areas of relatively slower flow, such as the dialyser itself (a hollow fiber dialyser has a much greater cross-sectional area than the blood tubing), areas of relative stagnation such as the bubble traps of a conventional dialysis circuit, and the expansion chambers of a single-needle system. If no anticoagulant is used, clotting will start very quickly in the fibers of the dialyser and in the bubble traps and expansion chambers. From the earliest days of hemodialysis it was found that anticoagulants were needed to keep the system from clotting. The earliest pioneers such as Abel, Rowntree and Turner in the US and Dr George Haas in Germany used hirudin, the natural anticoagulant of leeches. They had to grind up the heads of hundreds of leeches to obtain enough hirudin to carry out dialysis. Hirudin was unreliable and too toxic for clinical use. Dialysis did not become successful until heparin became available as an anticoagulant during World War II.

Heparin has remained the standard anticoagulant for hemodialysis ever since, and is likely to remain so even though hemodialysis has been performed successfully with an antiplatelet agent called prostacyclin.

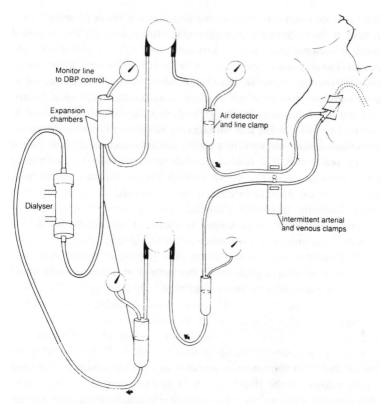

Fig. 7.24. The Cobe double blood pump single-needle system.

Prostacyclin is extremely expensive, very unstable, and causes hypotension on the basis of vasodilation. Its only advantage over heparin is that it does not seem to precipitate bleeding.

The one major disadvantage of heparin is that it may precipitate bleeding from a potential bleeding site such as a recent wound which has stopped bleeding, and it may greatly aggravate and increase any bleeding which is already occurring. We should all develop a healthy respect for the dangers of heparin and in general we should never use more heparin than is strictly necessary.

When carrying out a dialysis, heparin is usually administered as a bolus intravenous injection to prime the system and then as a continuous intravenous infusion into the arterial line beyond the blood pump and before the dialyser. If the patient has no special risk of bleeding we give enough heparin to be sure to prevent clotting. If there is a special risk of bleeding we use the minimum dose of heparin throughout the dialysis.

The gold standard for assessing the anticoagulant effect of heparin on a patient is the activated partial thromboplastin time (APTT). A normal result is about 30 seconds (normal range 27−33). To obtain full anti-coagulation this figure should be twice to two and a half times normal (60−80 seconds). However, this test involves sending a blood sample to a hematology laboratory and the test requires the skills of a trained hematology technician. In the early days of hemodialysis we used to assess the effect of heparin by taking a blood sample from the extra-corporeal circuit, putting it in a clean glass tube and seeing how long it would take to clot. The tube was usually surrounded by a water bath at body temperature and one had to keep tipping the tube at frequent intervals to see whether clotting occurred. Normal blood usually clots within 3 minutes or so by this method. It was generally believed that the clotting time should be prolonged to about 20 minutes during hemo-dialysis. This method is unsatisfactory because it takes too long to get a result. One should have a method giving a quick result which allows one to act on it immediately. Secondly the method of watching while blood clots in a glass tube takes too much of a nurse's time. There is a tendency to forget about it and miss the point at which clotting occurs.

Equipment is now available for use in the hemodialysis unit which depends on measuring the activated clotting time (ACT-Hemachron). The result is available within a few minutes and can be acted on immediately. For routine anticoagulation in a patient who is not bleeding we try to maintain the Hemachron ACT in a range of 220−250 seconds. When we are trying to restrict heparin to a minimum we aim for a range of 180−210. Sensitivity to heparin varies from one patient to another but in the same patient tends to remain stable. A new patient starting on dialysis should have a series of ACTs done, perhaps at hourly intervals during the first 3−4 dialyses, and these should be compared with the predialysis ACT. Heparin should be given in whatever amount is required to maintain the ACT at about 2−2½ times normal. After this it might be sensible to repeat the ACT about once a month. In this way the individual patient's heparin requirements become known and routine heparin orders can be written. Less heparin may be needed when using more biocom-patible membranes such as cellulose acetate and polyacrylonitrile (PAN). An ACT of 1½−2 times normal may then be adequate. It is not uncom-mon to use 3000−4000 units of heparin in a 3−4 hour dialysis and only 1000−1500 units during minimal heparinization. Some of us remember in the old days using as much as 10 000−15 000 units during a dialysis. Heparin requirements are usually somewhat greater during single-needle dialysis, probably due to the lower overall blood flow and the stop/start motion and increased turbulence which leads to foaming and the formation of clots.

An alternative approach to minimizing heparin, in cases in which bleeding is a danger, is so-called regional heparinization. In this technique heparin is infused continuously into the arterial blood line and protamine, the antidote of heparin, is infused continuously into the venous line close to the patient. If the right doses and infusion rates are used the dialyser compartment and venous bubble trap will be kept anticoagulated but the protamine will at least partially counteract the heparin in the patient's own circulation.

It should be possible by this method to keep the patient's blood clotting time close to normal while the extracorporeal circuit remains sufficiently anticoagulated to prevent clotting. Regional heparinization is a lot of work to supervise and has largely gone out of fashion because the results seem to be no better than minimal heparinization. In fact with regional heparin one usually ends up using a greater total amount of heparin (to overcome the protamine).

Heparin-free dialysis

The danger of bleeding from heparin, especially if the patient already has a bleeding problem, makes the idea of carrying out dialysis without heparin particularly appealing. Prostacyclin has already been mentioned but at the time of writing it does not seem to be widely applicable. It is still a very expensive research tool.

From our vantage point it seems to us that there are three practical approaches to heparin-free dialysis.

1 A more biocompatible membrane. It is more or less agreed that some dialysis membranes are less likely to provoke blood clotting than others. Of the membranes we have tested the most promising seems to be cellulose acetate. For example, the hollow fiber dialysers from Cordis-Dow, the CDAK 4000 and the 3500, have been used repeatedly by a number of different centers with great success with either little or no heparin. The same thing would not be possible using a membrane of cuprophane or regenerated cellulose.

2 Regular saline flushing. The rationale of this approach is that it takes time for platelets and fibrin to be deposited on foreign surfaces. The build-up occurs gradually and progressively. If, after half an hour of dialysis, you flush the whole system with a bolus of 100−200 ml of normal saline, you will wash most of the platelets and fibrin off the membrane. If this is done regularly every half hour or so the build-up will be inadequate for the system to clot. Although the concept seems ridiculously simple it seems to work.

3 A fast blood flow rate. It has been shown in studies by Fuji in Japan, using a scanning electron microscope, that when blood flows over a dialysis membrane for a standard period of time at a normal blood flow rate of 200 ml per minute, a certain number of platelets will stick to the membrane. If the same experiment is repeated using a blood flow rate of 400 ml per minute there will be hardly any platelets on the membrane at the end of the test period. It seems that a fast enough rate of blood flow over the membrane effectively prevents platelet adherence.

We have tested this concept during three hours of hemodialysis in a number of patients and have shown that we can use a fast flow rate to prevent clotting during completely heparin-free treatment.

We did this in a manner sugested to us by Fuji. The fast flow through the dialyser was achieved by introducing a shunt or by-pass in the extracorporeal circuit from the venous line beyond the venous bubble trap to the arterial line proximal to the blood pump as shown in Fig. 7.25.

The blood pump speed can then be increased from the normal 200 ml per minute in a standard dialysis to 400 ml per minute. We now have 400 ml per minute going through the dialyser, of which 200 ml per minute is directly from the patient and 200 ml is coming through the by-pass line and is recirculating. We wondered what effect this would have on the clearances of toxic solute such as creatinine and urea. On the one hand a fast flow rate should increase the efficiency of dialysis while on the other hand a 50% recirculation would be expected to reduce efficiency, since the gradient across the dialysis membrane would be less. We therefore measured the clearances during standard dialysis and during recirculation dialysis at 400 ml per minute. It turned out that clearances of small molecular weight substances were 15% less during recirculation dialysis than during normal dialysis. This is probably a small price to pay for the privilege of dialysing a patient without heparin.

The one place where clotting still seems to occur to some extent is in the venous bubble trap. This is probably due to a combination of stagnation and turbulence. We are now working with a re-designed bubble trap which causes less turbulence and, because of its slimmer shape, less stagnation. At the time of writing the method has still not been perfected to the point where it can be recommended for wide clinical use, but it

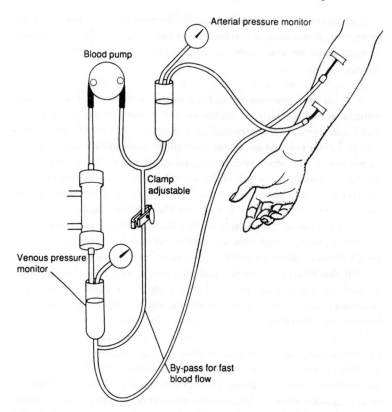

Fig. 7.25. Circuit diagram of shunt used for fast-flow, heparin-free dialysis.

seems clear that some of these principles or a combination of them will be exploited successfully to provide heparin-free dialysis whenever it is required in the future.

Hemodialysis for end-stage renal failure

Logistics and organization

At the hub of all hemodialysis is the hospital-based unit, containing usually 10–20 patient stations, and sometimes more. Most large centers also have a home dialysis program and frequently also a self-care program. The guiding principle is that every patient should be as self-sufficient and independent as possible, each according to his or her own ability.

Training patients for home dialysis is carried out in one or more special training rooms in which the patient and partner can receive concentrated instruction from the same nurse assigned to them for every dialysis.

Patients without partners who are trained to do unassisted self-care dialysis in a center outside normal working hours or in a satellite facility are trained in a similar way, usually by one assigned nurse in a concentrated one-to-one manner during each dialysis.

Ideally there should always be space in the in-center hospital program for patients whose other forms of treatment have run into trouble. Such patients may need temporary short-term help on hemodialysis or more long-term help until a way can be found to make them independent again, either by means of a second kidney transplant or by going back onto some form of home dialysis. The worrying thing is the gradually increasing number of patients who have tried all other forms of treatment repeatedly and have repeatedly had to come back to in-center hemodialysis because there is no other alternative. It is only by a policy of very active renal transplantation and home dialysis for everyone who can possibly do it that we will continue to be able to provide treatment for everyone who needs it.

New patients starting on hemodialysis will start in the center program but preferably even before they reach end-stage renal failure we should be making plans to move them out of the center. If very early renal transplantation can be anticipated, either from a living related donor or from a cadaver donor (in this country patients with blood group A never have to wait long for a kidney), there is no point in instituting self-care training. But, if the wait for a kidney transplant is likely to be a long one, plans should be made for home hemodialysis, self-care hemodialysis or CAPD.

Strategy for new patients

Any patient starting on hemodialysis for the first time is an unknown quantity and should be treated rather in the same way as the patient with acute renal failure being dialysed for the first time. The care and skill required will depend on how much initial preparation has been done and how uremic the patient has become. There is a tendency nowadays to start dialysis earlier, before patients become too ill, because in this way it will take less time to rehabilitate them. To some extent we will be guided by blood levels of urea and creatinine, and also the creatinine clearance, but clinical indicators are even more important. Symptoms such as loss of appetite, nausea, loss of energy, and pruritus should not be ignored. If these symptoms persist in spite of a protein-restricted diet, dialysis should not be delayed. Uremic complications such as polyneuritis make dialysis more urgent and, if the patient develops a pericardial friction rub as a sign of pericarditis, dialysis must be started at once. We should not even delay for 24 hours. The same applies to neurological manifestations such as asterixis. See p.277.

If end-stage renal failure has been anticipated there should be evidence of a negative hepatitis B antigen test in the chart. The patient should also have an AV fistula constructed and this should by now be mature enough to use.

During the first dialysis the patient should be watched carefully, just like a case of acute renal failure. We should look out for dialysis disequilibrium and take steps to prevent seizures. The first dialysis should be kept short for this reason and if necessary the patient can be dialysed again the next day.

Once the patient is beginning to feel better we can arrange a regular dialysis schedule which, for the vast majority of patients, will be 3−5 hours of dialysis three times a week. Once dialysis is started the patient's own renal function and urine output usually decline abruptly, probably mainly because of the loss of the osmotic diuretic effect of the high blood urea. The patient will then have to restrict fluids in order to avoid becoming fluid overloaded in the intervals between dialysis. A fortunate minority, usually only five to ten per cent of those placed on regular hemodialysis, will continue to exhibit a useful degree of residual renal function. This phenomenon most often occurs in patients with polycystic kidney disease and tubular and interstitial disorders, and occasionally in diabetics. They are fortunate in that only one or two dialyses are needed each week to supplement their residual renal function, and because of their good urine output they frequently do not need much salt or water restriction.

Diet and fluids

Most patients on hemodialysis, no matter how well they are dialysed, will require diet and fluid restrictions. In this our patients will be helped enormously if we are lucky enough to have the services of a dedicated dietitian. Most large centers have at least one dietitian specializing in the problems of kidney disease and renal failure. Dietary protein which up till now has been restricted to 0.4−0.6 g/kg of body weight per day can now be liberalized to 1 g/kg. Patients with severe chronic renal failure, not yet requiring dialysis, rarely become hyperkalemic. They seem to be able to excrete their potassium load provided they still have a good urine volume. However, once these patients start dialysis, urine output drops and with it potassium loss. If these patients do not now restrict potassium intake there will be a danger of hyperkalemia in the intervals between dialysis. Dietary potassium restriction will now therefore be necessary. Patients must be warned about high potassium foods and will have to continue to be careful as long as regular hemodialysis continues. If a dialysis is missed for any reason in a patient who has been receiving dialysis regularly, there is a danger of fatal hyperkalemia. If there is a deliberate intention to miss a dialysis for some legitimate reason, such as going on a trip, the patient can be protected from hyperkalemia by oral ingestion of an exchange resin such as Kayexalate. This can be taken in a dose of 15 g mixed with water three times a day, starting after the last dialysis. The serum potassium can usually be reliably kept down for a week by this means.

Phosphate restriction, which is now practiced by everyone with chronic renal failure, because hyperphosphatemia is generally acknowledged to be a nephrotoxic influence, must be continued in patients on dialysis but for a different reason. Hyperphosphatemia in patients on regular dialysis stimulates the parathyroids into a state of overactivity, thus predisposing to osteitis fibrosa. More importantly it leads to the deposition of calcium and phosphate in the tissues. This soft tissue calcification, which may cause pruritus and red itchy eyes due to calcium deposition in the skin and under the sclera, also occurs in the walls of blood vessels, in the joints, causing an acutely inflamed joint (rather like gout), and in the conducting system of the heart. One of our patients many years ago (before the importance of keeping down the plasma phosphate was fully appreciated) developed such severe soft tissue calcification in the heart that he developed complete heart block which would not even respond to a cardiac pacemaker. At autopsy his whole heart resembled a large rock. This is the most compelling argument in favor of plasma phosphate control in dialysis patients.

Just as a high plasma phosphate must be prevented we should also avoid letting it go too low. This may happen if a very ill dialysis patient is in an intensive care unit for a long time on total parenteral nutrition which contains no phosphate. Prolonged hypophosphatemia can cause rapid development of osteomalacia—calcium and phosphate are rapidly mobilized from the skeleton. It can also have very adverse effects on neurological function, mainly obtundation and coma, a form of metabolic encephalopathy. Always consider the possibility of hypophosphatemia in a patient on prolonged parenteral feeding.

Sodium restriction is necessary in all hemodialysis patients unless they happen to be excreting large amounts of sodium, which is extremely unusual. Most are oliguric and often virtually anuric. Any sodium taken in the diet will therefore stay in the body. Extra salt intake, by making patients thirsty, will lead to extra fluid intake. Salt and water will expand the extracellular fluid volume, leading to peripheral edema, hypertension, heart failure and pulmonary edema. Peripheral fluid retention in the form of ankle edema is not so serious but once edema starts forming in the lungs this is a sign of a failing heart, especially the left ventricle. As one would expect, left ventricular failure revealing itself as breathlessness due to pulmonary congestion and edema is much more common in older patients with ischemic heart disease and hypertension. Failure to comply with sodium and water restriction will consequently have more devastating effects in this group of patients. Although the vast majority of hemodialysis patients must restrict salt and water, even here one finds exceptions and each patient must be considered as a separate problem. We had one patient in end-stage renal failure after attempted suicide from ethylene glycol ingestion who, even after being on dialysis for months, was losing so much salt and water in his urine that he needed large numbers of salt tablets to stop him from being hypotensive from volume depletion!

Dietary supplements

Dialysis removes undesirable substances from the blood but unfortunately it does not have the discrimination to conserve some substances which are desirable. Hence water soluble vitamins such as ascorbic acid and the B complex are dialysed out. If the patient's diet is not supplemented with these they may become deficient. Thus, it is necessary for patients to take a preparation containing the vitamins B complex and C. The necessity for vitamin C was vividly demonstrated to us when one of our patients developed florid scurvy with a massive ecchymosis on his thigh. He admitted when pressed that he had not taken his vitamins for two years. Vitamin A should not be included in this; it has been shown that vitamin A, which is fat soluble, is actually contra-indicated in hemodialysis patients because it tends to raise the plasma triglycerides, which are usually already too high.

It used to be common practice to give folic acid (which is also water soluble) as a supplement to hemodialysis patients. However, there are now at least three good studies which show that this is not necessary, at least in patients who are eating normally.

Vitamin D is necessary in nearly all dialysis patients. This is dealt with separately under dialysis bone disease.

Oral iron is known to be as effective as parenteral iron in helping the anemia of patients on hemodialysis. One ferrous sulphate tablet (300 mg) per day is appropriate for most patients to replace their iron losses but it may be not enough for some patients and too much for others. Therapy is best guided by serum ferritin levels (see anemia, p.304).

Dialysing stable patients with end-stage renal failure

When you first started to dialyse patients on your own you will begin with stable patients who have been dialysed many times before. The patient, on seeing a new nurse, will probably be as nervous as you are. It will give you both confidence if you have taken the trouble to find out a little about the patient from the patient's medical and nursing record and also preferably from one of the senior nurses or at least from someone who knows his or her idiosyncrasies. You should be aware of any special problems such as a tendency to react adversely to first use dialysers, to develop leg cramps or become hypotensive or hypertensive on dialysis, and any special points about the fistula. You should also be aware of what medications the patient is receiving and whether there are any routine orders for drugs or infusions to be given during or at the end of dialysis. If the patient is to receive a blood transfusion during dialysis you should find out whether the blood is ready in the blood bank or whether the samples for crossmatching have to be taken before dialysis begins.

Most long-term, regular hemodialysis patients have routine blood tests before and after dialysis once a month. Between these times no blood work is done unless it is specially ordered by the medical staff. An exception is blood to carry out clotting tests to determine heparin requirements. In many patients, the heparin dose is established and unchanging so that no clotting tests are required.

Introduce yourself to the patient and reassure the patient by demonstrating some of your knowledge about his or her case. Carry out the predialysis observations of weight, blood pressure (lying and standing), pulse and temperature and record these on the dialysis chart. The weight compared with the patient's ideal dry weight will tell you how much fluid has to be removed during dialysis.

Well trained and disciplined patients who comply with diet and fluid restrictions gain no more than 1 kg in the short intervals between dialysis during the week, and no more than 2 kg during the long gap at the weekend. This makes it easy to remove enough water during the course of dialysis to return the patient to his ideal weight without inducing any hypotension. If, on the other hand, the patient has gained 4–5 kg in weight (most often during the weekend) the patient will be fluid overloaded, perhaps to the point of heart failure, at the beginning of dialysis and may also be hypertensive. Dialysis is likely to be unstable and uncomfortable for the patient because of the large amount of ultrafiltration required and the consequent hemodynamic disturbance. Some patients arrive for dialysis so fluid overloaded as to be in overt pulmonary edema. They may have to be propped up in order to breathe and may even need oxygen. Your medical staff may wish to examine the patient prior to starting dialysis and they may want an arterial blood sample for blood gas analysis.

If the patient has a raised temperature the medical staff should also be informed so that they can look for the cause. The search will probably include taking blood cultures from the blood lines, two separate samples at a five minute intervals, once the patient is on dialysis. The patient should settle down on the bed or chair in whatever position is most comfortable. You should raise the bed to the level at which you can work most comfortably on the patient's fistula.

Now turn your attention to the machine. If your dialysis unit practices dialyser re-use, you must check that the dialyser is labelled with the patient's name. Even a dialyser being used for the first time should have the patient's name on it in some clearly recognizable way which will not become detached.

The extracorporeal circuit now has to be primed with sterile saline and dialysate must be run through the dialysis compartment. Check that you have the right dialysis concentrate and that the concentrate feedline is in the container. If the dialyser is still filled with formaldehyde as a sterilizing agent for re-use this has to be removed by passing dialysate through it for a required number of minutes and a litre of sterile saline must be flushed through the blood compartment. When this is done you must test the saline emerging from the venous blood line to make sure all the formaldehyde has been removed. The best and most sensitive test for this purpose is Schiff's reagent which reliably detects one part per million.

Many dialysis machines deliver a dialysate with a predetermined fixed sodium concentration, anything from 135–140 mmol/litre, depending on what your medical staff believes to be most appropriate. Some modern machines can vary the dialysate sodium concentration and you have the privilege of dialling in the sodium concentration you want. Check that you have what you want and that the conductivity is correct.

Calculating the fluid removal

We do not all have the luxury of modern equipment which automatically removes the correct amount of fluid once you have calculated how much needs to be removed per hour. The total volume to be removed can be calculated as follows:

Excessive weight to be removed = 1.5 kg	=	1500 ml
Volume of saline used for priming the extracorporeal circuit	=	300 ml
Normal saline used for rinsing the blood back into the patient after dialysis	=	400 ml
Intake during dialysis including oral and intravenous	=	500 ml
TOTAL		2700 ml

With some equipment you simply dial in the number of hours the dialysis is to run, e.g. 4 hours and the figure 2700. The machine does the rest, regardless of which dialyser you are using. With another machine you may have to divide the figure 2700 by 4 to obtain an hourly rate (675 ml per hour) and again the machine does the rest. For older negative pressure machines you must know the ultrafiltration factor of the dialyser. If the dialyser allows the passage of 5 ml water per hour for every mmHg of trans-membrane pressure, then the ultrafiltration factor (UF) is 5. To determine the trans-membrane pressure (TMP) required to remove 2700 ml of fluid in 4 hours, the calculation is as follows. First divide the total volume to be removed by four. This gives the volume to be removed per hour (i.e. 675 ml). The hourly volume should then be divided by the UF. (675 divided by 5 = 135 mmHg.) Bear in mind that the TMP is the sum of the positive pressure in the blood compartment (the venous pressure) and the negative pressure in the dialysate compartment. These added together give you the TMP. In practice what one does first of all is to set the blood pump at the best speed one can reasonably obtain without developing an unduly high arterial negative pressure or venous positive pressure. In general a positive venous pressure up to 150 mmHg is quite acceptable. To get a really good dialysis one should have a blood flow over 200 ml/minute—and higher if possible. So once you have the blood pump turned up to the desired speed, read the venous pressure (usually about 100 mmHg) and add whatever negative pressure you need to reach the desired TMP.

If, during the course of the dialysis, the patient's blood pressure starts to drop too low, a decrease in the TMP for 5−10 minutes will often allow it to stabilize. If this is not enough to bring it up you may have to infuse a bolus of saline from the saline bag. An alternative is to infuse 10–15 g of mannitol. This, by raising plasma osmotic pressure, will draw water into the blood compartment from the interstitial tissue. It thus allows you to raise blood pressure without greatly increasing body water.

Some dialysis units have very accurate weighing beds (or chairs) so that you can observe the patient's weight loss continuously to the nearest 10 grams. To accomplish the same result another way some machines show you in a volumetric cylinder exactly how much fluid you have removed.

French technology developed by Rhone-Poulenc in Lyon has developed an ingenious method for controlling exactly the amount of water removed by ultrafiltration during dialysis. The principle is that the dialysate in contact with the membrane of the dialyser is always kept isolated from the dialysate inflow from the proportioning machine as well as from the dialysate outflow going to the drain. The machine has an enclosed inner circuit circulating dialysate through the dialyser. At regular short intervals the dialysate in this circuit is replenished with fresh dialysate while the dialysate lines to the dialyser itself are momentarily clamped off. This means that the only fluid removed from the extracorporeal circuit is that which is pumped out by a separate ultrafiltrate pump from the inner circuit of the dialysate and measured volumetrically. The method is illustrated diagrammatically in Fig. 7.26. Outstanding advantages of this method are:

• Fluid removal during dialysis does not depend on any complicated calculation of ultrafiltration factors but is completely and accurately controllable and under direct vision.

• The machine can operate just as easily with dialysers having a very high ultrafiltration factor or with more conventional dialysers having lesser degrees of permeability.

If you have neither of these refinements but wish to assess how you are getting on, it is quite legitimate to ask the patient to step out of bed onto a scale. This tactic is naturally only applicable to healthy patients who will not faint when they stand up!

All these methods are designed to help you to bring the patient down to his or her ideal weight by the end of dialysis. However, an experienced dialysis nurse will learn to review the patient's ideal weight continually. If, in order to bring the patient down to his supposed ideal weight, you find that you are inducing leg cramps during dialysis and postural hypotension at the end of dialysis, the patient has probably gained dry weight and you are only reaching the 'ideal weight' by reducing body water. The ideal weight should therefore be adjusted upwards by half to one kilogram.

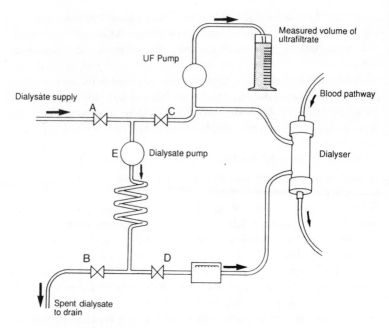

Fig. 7.26. The Rhone-Poulenc method for control of fluid removal. During dialysis both the dialysate clamps A & B are closed to isolate the dialyser from the dialysate supply. Clamps A & B open to allow fresh dialysate into the coil when clamps C & D close. In this way we know that the measured volume of ultrafiltrate can only have come from the patient via the dialyser. It is physically impossible for it to have come from the dialysate supply.

This can be done immediately by an infusion of normal saline before the blood lines are completely disconnected or the patient should be told to drink a little extra and the adjustment can be made at the next dialysis.

If, on the other hand, a patient arriving for dialysis is ostensibly at his ideal weight but you observe that he has puffy eyes, swollen ankles, distended neck veins and is manifestly breathless (perhaps with hypertension as well) then you know that the patient has lost dry weight and gained water. The ideal weight needs to be adjusted downwards. If the patient is distressed by pulmonary edema and it is necessary to remove fluid urgently, the patient can literally be bled into the extracorporeal circuit by allowing the saline from the venous blood line to be drained out before the venous line is connected to the patient. This will reduce the patient's blood volume by about 300 ml and produce almost immediate relief of the pulmonary congestion.

In practice we are always on the alert for changes in body water which are often quite slight and subtle. The medical staff must approve a decision to change the ideal weight, but we find that the more experienced a hemodialysis nurse becomes, the more she will make these suggestions herself as a result of assessing the patient. We teach our nurses how to examine for the presence of edema and a raised jugular venous pressure and some of them become very expert. Also, as a result of dialysing the same patient many times the nurses get to know them very well. They become very good at deciding whether patients need more or less water in their bodies.

Cannulating the AV fistula for dialysis

The most important manual skill of a hemodialysis nurse is the ability to place needles in a fistula. It is a skill which comes from watching someone and then doing it yourself and having plenty of practice. The patient's arm should be resting comfortably on a waterproof sheet or pad and a sphygmomanometer cuff should be placed on the upper arm. Pumping the cuff up to diastolic pressure will distend the vein to make it easier to cannulate. Fistula needles are all basically similar, having a stainless steel, thin-walled, wide-bore needle with an open bevelled end sharpened to a point. The other end of the needle is attached to a flexible plastic tube and at the junction of the needle and the tube there is a pair of flexible plastic wings used to tape the fistula in place on the patient's arm. The gauge of the needles varies from 14 (large) to 17 (small), the most common being 15 and 16. Fig. 7.27 shows the various component parts.

The placing of needles should be done as a sterile procedure, and in our opinion this should include skin preparation with an antiseptic, draping with sterile towels, the wearing by patient and nurse of a mask and sterile surgical gloves for the nurse. Some centers do not wear a mask or gloves but simply use a 'no touch' technique. We are not aware of any controlled trial to test the necessity for a sterile technique to prevent infections at fistula skin sites. We only know that in our program such infections are exceedingly rare. Nearly all centers have a sterile disposable tray for starting dialysis which includes disposable drapes, gauze squares and skin antiseptic containers.

The use of local anesthetic in the skin prior to inserting fistula needles is variable from center to center and patient to patient. Initial infiltration of the skin with local anesthetic should make cannulation itself painless, but it means giving two pricks instead of one, and some people say that the anesthetic makes it harder to judge where the point of your needle is. Often this issue is decided by the patient's personal preference.

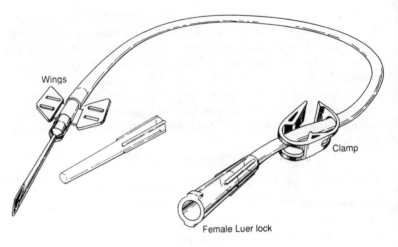

Fig. 7.27. The component parts of a fistula needle.

The next decision is whether the fistula needle should be primed with heparinized saline prior to insertion or whether it should be left dry. The advantage of heparinized saline is that it discourages clotting in the end of the needle. Next you should decide whether you wish to insert the needle with the bevel facing upwards or downwards. See Fig. 7.28.

It may seem more natural to insert the needle bevel up. The problem with this is that fistula needles tend to have a coring effect—cutting a piece of tissue out of the skin and out of the vein as they enter. It can easily be appreciated that this is more likely to happen with the bevel up method. If you insert the needle bevel down, the heel of the needle will probably slide through the gap made by the point. There will be a slit in the skin and in the vein but no core of tissue will be physically removed. This becomes crucially important when putting needles in prosthetic grafts such as bovine carotid artery and PTFE. These materials are more easily damaged by faulty needle techniques. If you cut a core out of a PTFE graft there will be a circular hole in the wall which may become a false aneurysm (called 'false' because the wall of the aneurysm is really formed by the overlying skin) (see Fig. 7.29). This will have to be repaired surgically.

When you insert the needles for dialysis, one will be close to the arteriovenous anastomosis and this will be used for the outflow via the arterial tubing set to the kidney machine. The other will be further away,

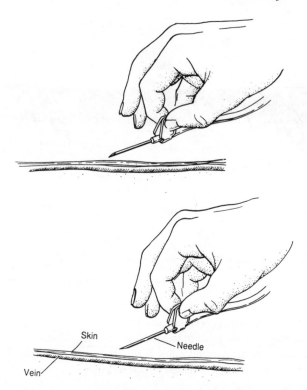

Fig. 7.28. Insertion of a fistula needle. a) Bevel up tends to be associated with coring. b) Bevel down causes less vein wall damage.

downstream from the anastomosis, bringing back purified blood which will return to the heart. It might seem logical to place the arterial needle so that its open end is pointing towards the AV anastomosis while the venous needle will be pointing up the arm in the direction of flow of blood. In practice we have found that it is better to have both needles pointing in the direction of the blood flow. In this way, when the needles are removed at the end of dialysis, the blood flow tends to close the hole in the wall by pushing back the flap created in the vein wall (see Fig. 7.30). The blood flow through the needle during dialysis seems to be equally good whichever way the arterial needle is pointing.

Another helpful point of technique is to try, if you can, to go through the skin and tunnel under it a short distance before dipping down again into the vein. This helps to prevent you from pushing straight through both walls of the vein and out the other side. It also helps you to stop the

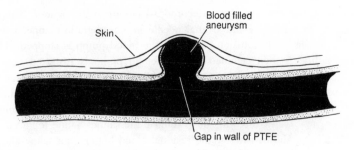

Fig. 7.29. False aneurysm caused by needle damage to a PTFE graft.

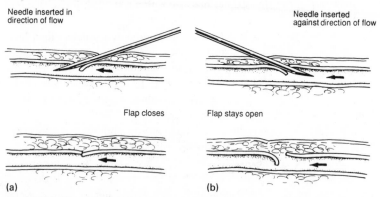

Fig. 7.30. a) Fistula needle inserted in direction of flow. b) Needle inserted against the direction of flow.

bleeding at the end of dialysis when the needle is removed, because the skin puncture will not immediately overlie the vein puncture.

Finally, be sure to go through a clean area of skin each time. Some dialysis units advocate going through the same needle track at each dialysis because they say it reduces trauma to the vein. If you decide to follow this practice be sure to remove any scab from the skin first. If you go through a scale or crust, it could be concealing a bead of pus which would then be inoculated into the bloodstream. We have seen at least one case of staphylococcal septicemia clearly related to this cause.

Taking the patient off dialysis

When the patient has had the required number of hours on dialysis and the appropriate amount of fluid has been removed, the next step is to return all the blood in the extracorporeal circuit to the patient. This is done by first flushing the arterial needle in a retrograde manner using saline in the saline infusion bag while the blood pump is stopped. The arterial line is then clamped and the blood pump is restarted slowly. Saline from the saline bag is pumped through the dialyser and back to the patient. After about 400 ml of saline have gone through, the lines will be only faintly pink and very little blood is left in the circuit. Some centers now follow this with air to remove the saline. Saline followed by air has been shown to clear the residual blood better than saline alone. However, the difference in residual blood is not substantial and the danger of the air rinse method is the danger of accidental air embolus. Furthermore, air in the dialyser makes it difficult to flush for subsequent re-use.

After the wash-back is complete, the arterial and venous blood lines are disconnected from the fistula needles. The blood lines together with the dialyser and the whole extracorporeal circuit are removed from the machine, placed in a container of some kind to avoid blood spillage, and taken away. In most centers the dialyser will be re-used, and the blood lines will be discarded in waterproof bags.

The patient's observations will be repeated and recorded—weight, temperature, pulse and blood pressure lying and standing.

Removal of the fistula needles is normally done with non-sterile gloves, the purpose of which is simply to protect your hands. Pressure is maintained on the needle puncture sites with pads of folded gauze dressings until the bleeding has stopped. If possible steady pressure should be applied without occluding the flow through the fistula itself. If fistula clamps are used, as in some units, one should check to make sure that the bruit is audible after the clamp is removed. A band-aid is placed over the needle puncture and kept on for a few hours after the patient goes home.

Assessing the adequacy of dialysis

In any patient on long-term dialysis there is a responsibility to assess regularly the adequacy of treatment. Freedom from uremic complications such as pericarditis, insomnia and pruritus is a good start, but one would also like to see evidence of positive good health. Until recently we have relied on experienced clinical judgment backed up by a regular (usually monthly) profile of biochemical estimations carried out before and after dialysis.

In the 1970s Doctors Sargent and Gotch pioneered the concept of what has become widely known as 'urea kinetic modelling'. This is an attempt to quantify mathematically the dynamics of uremia control in the hemodialysed patient. Although there are undoubtedly numerous uremic toxins, some better known and studied than others, they chose to study urea as a marker of protein catabolism and the thoroughness of its removal by dialysis. Urea estimations are readily available in all hospital laboratories and have traditionally been used in assessing all patients with renal failure.

The modelling concept assumes that urea equilibrates well throughout the body under dialysis conditions so that it can be considered to be in one compartment or 'single pool'. Using the mass balance equation,

Accumulation = input − output

or stated another way,

(Change in content) = (generation) − (removal)

it is possible to derive further equations mathematically which enable one to estimate urea generation rate (G) and from this the protein catabolic rate (PCR). It is now possible to compute these values, using appropriate software in a microcomputer, provided that the results of certain basic measurements are known. These include blood urea values (pre- and post-dialysis for one mid-week dialysis and pre-dialysis for the next), intra- and inter-dialytic time periods for the same cycle, weight gain and urine volume over the interdialytic period, and blood and dialysate flow rates. From these parameters residual renal clearance and dialysis clearance can be calculated, and in turn the urea generation rate and the protein catabolic rate.

The benefits attributed to the modelling concept include the following.
1 Ability to assess objectively the adequacy of dialysis. Using these calculations, Sargent and Gotch claim very convincingly that they can predict, without even knowing the patient, whether dialysis is inadequate, adequate or excessive. This is not only important for the individual patient but also cost-effective. In some cases we may be able to cut down dialysis time without sacrificing patient well-being.
2 The ability to assess and monitor protein nutrition. The stated goal in protein nutrition is to maintian dietary protein intake (DPI) between 0.8 and 1.4 g/kg/24 hours and to ensure that intake is adequate for zero or positive protein balance. In the stable dialysis patient DPI = PCR. If these values are significantly different we can deduce that the patient's intake is either inadequate or excessive. The calculation will thus help to identify patients who are in need of dietary counselling.

3 Ability to detect technical aberrations during dialysis. This is done by comparing the estimated dialyser performance with the expected performance using previously tested and known dialyser performance data. If the performance is lower than it should be we have an obligation to search for potentially correctable factors such as excessive recirculation in a fistula, inadequate blood flow rates due to inaccurate blood pump calibration, or abnormal clotting in the dialyser.

From being an interesting research concept in the 1970s, urea kinetic modelling is being used increasingly in many dialysis centers for routine clinical monitoring. The concept of kinetics has also extended to related procedures such as heparin delivery, plasmapheresis, and hemoperfusion in cases of poisoning.

Dialyser re-use

Modern negative pressure dialysers are beautifully manufactured commercial products intended to be used for one dialysis and then thrown away. The companies which make them and sell them would naturally like us to do this and they state specifically that they take no responsibility for the product if it is re-used. However, dialysis costs have always been a source of concern to all health care organizations; and the cost of a new dialyser is a large part of the cost of a dialysis. Many centers have, for this reason, been re-using dialysers for many years, but as health care budgets are being more tightly controlled all over the world the necessity to re-use dialysers becomes more compelling. Re-use should not in our opinion be the responsibility of the hemodialysis nurse. This is a misuse of her time. Her skills are better employed in the care of patients. Special personnel, most appropriately under the supervision of the chief technologist, will do the re-use. In our center the re-use is performed by technical assistants who, when not performing re-use, assist the nurses in the dialysis unit and assist the technologists with preventive maintenance on the machines. Only a fraction of the money saved by re-use is necessary to pay the salaries of these technical assistants.

Objections to dialyser re-use have come from some patients' organizations who wish to protect their members from inferior treatment; and from medical and administrative staff in hospitals who do not want to be exposed to the danger of litigation arising from an accident due to faulty re-use.

With regard to the first objection, it has been shown repeatedly that centers that re-use dialysers have lower rates of mortality and morbidity than centers that use new dialysers every time. The reasons for this are not entirely clear but we do know that reactions to the dialysis membrane, complement activation leading to white cell sequestration in the lungs, are common in new cuprophane dialyers but hardly ever occur in re-used dialysers.

We ourselves in this center, and many other groups, have shown that dialysers re-used many times function just as well as new ones in terms of their ability to clear small and middle sized molecules from the blood and to remove water by ultrafiltration.

Some centers still use formaldehyde as a sterilizing agent during re-use and we know from our previous experience with formaldehyde in non-disposable Kiil dialysers that repeated exposure of a patient's blood to small amounts of formaldehyde can lead eventually to the formation of a red cell antibody called anti-N. Anti-N antibody formation was very common in the days of Kiil dialysers but is rather uncommon in modern dialysis units which practice re-use of disposable hollow fiber dialysers. This is probably because formaldehyde can be removed from hollow fiber dialysers so completely. In our center only 6% of patients' on dialyers regularly re-used with formaldehyde develop anti-N antibody and this antibody does not cause the patients any problems anyway. We can therefore, with complete honesty, reassure patients that re-use is in their best interests.

On the point of possible accidents resulting from re-use, let us consider the worst that can happen. But before we do this let us describe briefly how re-use is done. It should be stated here that hollow fiber dialysers are more suitable for re-use than multilayered flat-plate dialysers. The exact re-use method will differ from one center to another, manual or automated, and a number of good automated re-use machines now exist but the basic principles are the same.

1 Each dialyser, when first taken out of its packet, should be labelled indelibly with the patient's name and reserved thereafter for that patient only. Then, when any dialysis is started, it should be the responsibility of the nurse carrying out the dialysis to check the identity of the dialyser. Dialysing a patient with another patient's dialyser does not have the same serious implications as an incompatible blood transfusion. The objections are more esthetic than medical, rather like using another person's tooth-brush, but a strict code of practice should ensure that everyone gets his own.

2 When a dialysis is over and the blood has been returned to the patient with a saline rinse, the dialyser and blood lines should be placed in a container to prevent any dripping on the floor. The complete circuit is then taken to the re-use room where the lines are discarded and the dialyser is submitted to the re-use process.

An air rinse following the saline rinse is somewhat more efficient than the saline rinse alone in reducing the amount of blood left in the dialyser, but filling the dialyser with air interferes with the subsequent flushing process, so most programs which employ re-use have given up using an air rinse.

3 The next step depends on whether there is someone available to start the re-use process immediately. If there is no one available straight away, the dialyser should be capped (blood ports and dialysate ports) and it should be put in a refrigerator at 4°C. This is to prevent any growth of bacteria in the blood compartment which might occur if the dialyser is left lying around at room temperature. Subsequent sterilization with antiseptic would of course kill any bacteria which grow in the dialyser but dead bacterial protein left in the blood compartment after the sterilization could cause a pyrogenic reaction. Refrigerating the dialyser when no one is available to deal with it (e.g. at the end of an evening dialysis shift) will avoid the necessity of discarding it and wasting it.

4 The essence of the re-use process is flushing the dialyser, the dialysate compartment and the blood compartment with very pure water. The water does not really need to be chemically pure since very little of the water will be left in the dialyser at the end. Purity in this context means freedom from micro-organisms and pyrogens and freedom from particulate matter.

We learned this lesson the hard way. We had no trouble with our re-use method until some extensive building alterations were started in the hospital. We then encountered one or two pyrogenic reactions in patients on re-used dialysers. We realized that pyrogens in the old hospital plumbing system were being dislodged from the pipes and were entering the dialysers in the water we were using for flushing them. This problem was immediately solved by introducing an ultrafilter into the line to prevent the entrance of pyrogens. Not only did this prevent pyrogenic reactions but it also greatly improved the efficiency of the re-use technique because we were no longer blocking up the fibers of the dialysers with fine particulates.

5 What criteria should one use to decide whether a dialyser is clean enough? Most of us teach our re-use personnel to look at a dialyser and assess the number of blocked fibers which will look like a red or black thread going down the center. This 'eyeball' check has proved to be just as reliable as more scientific measurements which depend on 'residual fiber volume'.

6 Once the dialyser is clean it is primed with formaldehyde 3% solution, both compartments are capped and it is left on the rack at room temperature until it is needed for the next dialysis.

7 The process of removing the formaldehyde before the next dialysis is described on p.257 under instructions for starting dialysis.

8 At least three other antiseptics have been used successfully for dialyser re-use, glutaraldehyde, agents that liberate chlorine, and peracetic acid mixed with hydrogen peroxide. The latter is being used increasingly widely. Although we do not have experience of long-term use of these agents for this purpose, it is likely that they will displace formaldehyde. Formaldehyde is undesirable because of the fumes it causes, and a number of cities now have by-laws restricting the amount of formaldehyde which one is allowed to discharge into the drains. Each time a dialyser is used a mark should be placed on it by the re-use technician indicating whether this is the third or fourth use, etc. The re-use personnel have a duty to keep a record of the number of times each dialyser is used and usually there will be guidelines about the maximum number of uses which are permitted. In our unit we have a record which tells us exactly how many times each dialyser has been used for each patient, going right back to the inception of the program in 1977.

9 Dialysers, it is generally agreed by everyone, should not be re-used in patients who are carriers of hepatitis B. We have also stopped dialyser re-use for a period of 165 days when we found a case of hepatitis B positivity among our patients, because this meant that the rest of the patients were in quarantine. Re-use is an unacceptable extra risk if the patient's blood may be carrying hepatitis B.

If the above principles are adhered to there should be no harm coming to any patient as a result of re-use. There may inevitably be the rare instance of someone being dialysed with someone else's dialyser— undesirable but not serious. A pyrogenic reaction is a possible consequnce of failing to refrigerate a dialyser while it is waiting for processing but this should never happen. If it is left out at room temperature for anything more than a few minutes after dialysis it should be discarded. Theoretically if dialysers are repeatedly flushed under high pressure there might be an increase in fiber rupture and subsequent blood leakage at the next dialysis. All our dialysers are pressure tested before they are filled with the sterilant. Blood leaks are so rare as to be insignificant. The worst that could happen is that a dialyser is flushed but inadvertently not filled with sterilant. It might then harbor live bacteria which could induce septicemia in the patient. In an eight year period of dialyser re-use we have not seen a single episode of bloodstream infection attributable to this cause.

In our opinion dialyser re-use is here to stay and must inevitably be adopted by all centers until or unless someone comes up with a better idea.

The details of our manual method for re-use are described in Appendix 3 on p.413.

Hemodialysis for acute renal failure

What sort of patient will it be?

Most people believe that peritoneal dialysis is the treatment of first choice for uncomplicated acute renal failure. But there are a number of conditions which make peritoneal dialysis unwise or impossible. Conditions which come to mind are recent abdominal surgery, intra-abdominal infection, multiple previous operations or intra-abdominal events that have resulted in the presence of many adhesions, retroperitoneal hematoma or any condition that leads to such a high catabolic rate that peritoneal dialysis will be inadequate. An example of this would be multiple trauma leading to massive tissue breakdown. Any superimposed infection will increase the catabolic rate still further.

If many of the simple or uncomplicated cases of acute renal failure are dealt with by peritoneal dialysis, it follows that those which need hemodialysis will usually be complicated and demanding. The dialysis will often require considerable thought and planning on the part of the medical and nursing staff. Often the patient will be in an intensive care unit or on some other ward in the hospital, so a nurse must be sent out with a machine and will normally carry out the hemodialysis single-handed.

The vascular access

First the medical staff will have to decide which type of vascular access they wish to provide. If this is a shunt, someone has to be found who has the skill to put it in. That individual has to decide which limb to use and the nursing staff will usually provide the necessary equipment. The operation takes about an hour and can be done, if necessary, at the bedside. More often these days a subclavian catheter is inserted. If it is a single-lumen catheter, we will usually use a single-needle system rather than puncturing an arm vein for the venous return, but the practice varies very much from one center to another. If the patient is too ill to lie flat for subclavian insertion the first one or two dialyses should be conducted through a femoral catheter. Once the patient's condition has stabilized a subclavian catheter can be inserted.

In our opinion it is likely that a double-lumen subclavian catheter will be the most commonly used device in the future. It has the advantage of simplicity of insertion as well as providing two blood pathways without recirculation. It should also be applicable to almost every patient regardless of the state of the peripheral blood vessels.

Is the patient hepatitis B negative?

The nursing staff will want to be reassured that the patient has a negative hepatitis B antigen test. If none has been done and dialysis is needed urgently we will have to go ahead without it and assume that the patient might be positive. This means taking extra precautions, and a machine that cannot and will not be used for any other patient until the result of the patient's test is known. This is why we try to brainwash all the junior hospital medical staff to request hepatitis B testing as soon as possible on all patients who might conceivably need dialysis. Then, with a bit of luck, a result will be available before the first dialysis is needed.

What equipment will be needed?

The equipment used will naturally depend on what is available. Some centers still use batch systems for treating acute renal failure. The Travenol RSP (recirculating single pass) was a very good concept and continues to be used very effectively. The disadvantage is the need to trundle a heavy tank full of dialysate along the corridors and in and out of elevators. Of course one could wait to fill the tank with tap water when one reaches the ward (as we used to do in the old days) but it is generally agreed that this is no longer justified. Dialysate must be constituted from pure water even in acute renal failure.

Our own system now consists of taking a single patient proportioning machine with its own portable reverse osmosis unit mounted on the same set of wheels. The disposable plastic tubing sets (arterial and venous blood lines), dialyser, saline bag and heparin infusion are usually all set up in the main unit before the nurse leaves to carry out the dialysis. She will also take with her a cart on which to transport all the other items such as sterile trays, drugs, dialysis record keeping equipment, doctor's orders, etc.

We usually send one nurse and one nursing aide out together to start the dialysis (it takes two to move all the equipment). The assistant can come back to the main unit once the dialysis is started.

The dialysis orders

Whereas most dialyses for end-stage renal failure can be started by the nurses without doctor's orders because the method is routine and understood by everyone, a dialysis for acute renal failure must be individually planned and preferably discussed thoroughly by the doctor and the nurse who will be doing it. The head nurse of the unit will usually also have some suggestions to make. The chances are that she will be far more experienced than either of the other two. The only person more experienced than her is the medical director or consultant in charge who may or may not be supervising the dialysis personally. Nurses should make a point of insisting on proper discussion of the dialysis plan. Medical residents tend to feel threatened by nurses who ask too many questions but this need not be done aggressively and many lives have been saved by nurses who asked the right questions and obtained clear and well thought out instructions. The first obvious yet frequently neglected question, which to an inexperienced resident may sound impertinent but which on reflection is very sensible, is why is the dialysis being done—or stated differently—what aims are we hoping to achieve? Is the dialysis being done mainly for uremia (the blood urea is very high) or for fluid removal (the patient has life-threatening pulmonary edema), for hyperkalemia, for metabolic acidosis or for a combination of any of these? The aims will dictate the strategy.

The composition of the dialysate will depend on the patient. The sodium concentration for acute dialysis is usually $130-135$ mmol/l on the assumption that most patients are in positive sodium balance and will need sodium removal. Most patients are hyperkalemic but by no means all of them are. If the serum potassium is high the dialysate potassium will be low—often as low as 1 mmol/l; but if the potassium is low, perhaps as a result of gastro-intestinal losses in diarrhea, a low dialysate potassium will lower the serum potassium still further, causing muscular weakness and dangerous cardiac arrhythmias. Therefore the doctor will decide on the potassium level only after knowing the patient's serum level. Whether to dialyse using acetate or bicarbonate will depend to some extent on local policy but there is an increasing tendency to use bicarbonate in acute renal failure since it is more physiological and generally better tolerated. Acetate can cause troublesome hypotension, and in the first dialysis for acute renal failure you never know quite how acetate is going to affect the patient. There is more predictable correction of the metabolic acidosis with bicarbonate and patients will be hemodynamically more stable. A good general rule is 'if in doubt use bicarbonate'.

Very occasionally we may wish to change or modify other components of the dialysate such as the calcium in a case of hypercalcemia or even magnesium but usually these do not need to be considered. Most centers now use physiological concentrations of glucose in dialysate but there may occasionally be an argument for increasing the glucose concentration to avoid lowering the plasma osmotic pressure too fast. See dialysis disequilibrium, p.276.

Orders should also be obtained from the medical staff as to what blood tests should be drawn pre- and post-dialysis. If blood sampling is done on any patient with renal failure, it makes sense to do it at the beginning or end of dialysis when we have to obtain access to the circulation anyway. Venepunctures for blood tests in the intervals between dialysis should be largely avoided in order to conserve the veins and avoid unnecessary disconnection or invasion of subclavian catheters. In this way infections from subclavian catheters will be reduced.

Fluid removal

The next thing you need to know from the medical staff is how much the patient's weight needs to be lowered by removal of water. In cases of gross pulmonary edema and heart failure you may wish to remove as much as 3−4 kg during the dialysis. If fluid removal is the first priority you may wish to spend the first hour doing pure ultrafiltration and if so the medical staff should write a specific order for this.

Water can be removed during dialysis by hydrostatic means, simply by increasing the trans-membrane pressure. As you dialyse the patient you will also be removing water from the blood compartment of the dialyser and this is actually depleting the water of the intravascular compartment of the patient. But during dialysis you are also rapidly removing toxic solutes and this is rapidly reducing the osmotic pressure of the blood. The more efficient the dialysis, the greater is the reduction in plasma osmotic pressure. It will take time for equilibration to occur between the plasma and the interstitial fluid, so at first the plasma osmotic pressure will be lower than the osmotic pressure of the interstitial water. This means that water will move out of the plasma (the area of low osmotic pressure) into the interstitial space (the area of high osmotic pressure). If water is moving simultaneously from the plasma to the dialysate and from the plasma to the interstitial space, blood volume will fall rapidly. This rapid reduction in blood volume will usually cause a dramatic fall in blood pressure, even to the point where the patient may become unconscious from underperfusion of the brain. This will have to be corrected immediately by infusion of normal saline into the extra-corporeal circuit, which of course defeats the object of the exercise because the patient is still overhydrated with net excess of salt and water in the body.

How can one remove water in cases of overhydration without inducing hypotension? The best way is to carry out pure ultrafiltration without dialysis. This is done by maintaining a strong negative pressure in the dialysate compartment while at the same time stopping the inflow of dialysate. The blood flow through the dialyser is maintained at the same rate, and water and low molecular weight solutes will filter through into the dialysate compartment and down the drain. Sodium is removed with the water in isotonic concentrations but the plasma osmotic pressure is not lowered. This means that as fast as water is removed from the plasma into the dialysate more water will enter the blood compartment from the interstitial space. This acquisition of water from the interstitial space will maintain the blood volume and prevent a fall in blood pressure. Whether or not this theory is completely accurate or represents a slight oversim-plification, the method certainly seems to work in practice. By doing pure ultrafiltration for the first hour of dialysis it is possible to remove 3–4 kg of water without any significant hypotension. Once the excess water has been removed and the pulmonary edema has been corrected, it is possible to proceed with dialysis. The only penalty one pays for the benefits of this strategy is loss of dialysing time, and this is not serious. If blood pressure falls during dialysis there are other things you can do. The most obvious and easy thing to do is to raise the plasma osmotic pressure and thereby draw water into the intravascular space from the interstitial space. The time-honored way to do this is by infusion of a small volume of mannitol in high concentration. Mannitol is a relatively harmless and inert sugar— usually supplied as a 10% sterile solution (in plastic bags or 50 ml glass ampoules). In due course it is metabolized but in the short term it is beneficial because it is osmotically active. The other thing you can do to help to maintain blood pressure is to give an infusion of albumin. Salt-poor human albumin is hideously expensive (rather like infusing pure gold into the patient) but if the patient has a low albumin level it may be necessary. It has been shown that pulmonary edema is aggravated by a low plasma albumin level and can be improved by raising the albumin level. This is because colloids stay within the intravascular space and exert 'colloid osmotic pressure' to draw water from the pulmonary inter-stitial space into the pulmonary capillaries. They will similarly reduce peripheral edema but this is not so threatening to the patient as pulmonary edema. Remember throughout all this that water depletion of the intra-vascular space is not the only cause of hypotension during dialysis. Acetate is a vasodilator and causes a reduction in peripheral resistance. Acetate is particularly likely to cause hypotension in those patients with cardiac conditions who are unable to mount an appropriate increase in cardiac output in response to a fall in peripheral resistance. However, if blood pressure falls and you are not using acetate, you have to think of other causes. Remember that heparin may provoke bleeding and this is especially likely to occur if the patient already has a potential bleeding source such as a peptic ulcer or recent abdominal surgery.

Apart from the composition of the dialysate and the amount of water that has to be removed, you need to know how long the patient has to be dialysed and what about the anticoagulation?

Generally, it is rather unwise to dialyse the patient for too long at the first dialysis if uremia is very severe. This is because of a condition known as dialysis disequilibrium.

Dialysis disequilibrium

It is necessary to remember that when we are dialysing a patient we are only dialysing the plasma. The capillary walls are a semipermeable mem-brane between the plasma and the interstitial fluid, so in due course the interstitial fluid equilibrates with the plasma. Then, through the cell walls, the products of uremia in the intracellular water pass into the interstitial water. However, during dialysis changes in the intracellular fluid lag behind changes in the extracellular fluid. At least for a while intracellular osmotic pressure remains higher than extracellular osmotic pressure. This difference in intracellular and extracellular osmotic pres-sure will be greater if the initial uremia is very severe, if the dialysis is very efficient and if the dialysis is prolonged. The longer the dialysis continues the greater the difference will become. It is believed that the relatively high intracellular osmotic pressure draws water into the cells and brings about cell swelling. This does not matter in most parts of the body but it does matter in the brain. Increased brain cell swelling leads to drowsiness, mental confusion, twitching and eventually major seizures. This sequence of events is known as dialysis disequilibrium. Drowsiness and mental confusion are not serious as long as the mechanism is understood and the patient is looked after, but major seizures can sud-denly convert a patient who is seriously ill into one who is critically ill.

Seizures may cause cerebral hypoxia, vomiting and inhalation of vomit into the lungs and possibly respiratory and cardiac arrest.

Hence the danger of dialysis disequilibrium and the need to prevent it. Always consider the possibility of dialysis disequilibrium in a patient being dialysed for the first time especially if the blood urea is very high. The more efficient the dialysis and the longer it is continued the greater the danger of disequilibrium. Also some individuals have a lower threshold for epilepsy than others. Generally infants and young children are especially prone to seizures and also very old people, or anyone with previous brain damage. How should dialysis disequilibrium be prevented and how can a patient be protected? Here are a few suggestions based on what we know about the condition.

1 When dialysing a very uremic patient for the first time it is wise not to be too efficient or go on for too long. It makes sense to reduce the blood flow rate through the dialyser (or use a lower surface area dialyser) and reduce the dialysis time. One can also reduce the dialysate flow rate. There are no hard and fast rules about this and each center will work out its own guidelines. The dialysate flow rate can also be reduced from 500 ml/minute to 300 ml/minute.

2 Look out for signs of drowsiness, mental confusion and any twitching such as myoclonic jerking. Asterixis is also a helpful sign to observe repeatedly. To test for asterixis ask the patient to hold his arms out straight in front, palms towards the floor. Then ask him to tip his hands up, palms facing forwards and maintain that position. If the patient cannot maintain this position but instead the hands keep dropping down towards the horizontal, the patient has asterixis. This is a non-specific sign of metabolic encephalopathy, also seen in severe liver disease and sometimes called 'liver flap', but in the clinical setting of acute renal failure it is a helpful indication of the severity of the uremia or the degree of dialysis disequilibrium. If, during the course of the first dialysis when the uremia is being corrected, the asterixis is getting worse, it is probably safe to assume that dialysis disequilibrium is developing.

3 Mannitol, which is so useful in preventing hypotension during fluid removal, also helps to prevent dialysis disequilibrium if given repeatedly or continuously into the blood pathway. It helps to maintain plasma osmotic pressure, but its use has to be restricted in order to avoid giving too much. Your medical staff should tell you how much you can give. A high dialysate glucose level will accomplish the same purpose but it does so by making the patient hyperglycemic and the extent to which this happens is rather unpredictable, depending on the patient's own endogenous insulin response. For this reason we tend not to use a high dialysate glucose level even in acute renal failure.

4 Anticonvulsants such as phenytoin sodium and phenobarbitone are very helpful in this clinical setting, especially if given prophylactically before fits occur. It will do no harm to suggest these to the medical staff so that they can at least be considered.

5 Patients are best kept in a fasting state until the first dialysis is over, because of the danger of vomiting and inhalation. In patients receiving peritoneal dialysis for acute renal failure it may be wise to pass a nasogastric tube to empty the stomach before dialysis is even started. This is because peritoneal dialysis compresses the intra-abdominal contents and may provoke vomiting for purely mechanical reasons. Vomiting may also occur during the first hemodialysis so if in doubt it may be safer to empty the stomach before you start.

6 The patient should certainly have one-to-one nursing at the first dialysis and frequent observation of all vital signs.

Slow continuous ultrafiltration in the management of acute renal failure

When acute renal failure is treated by hemodialysis, the frequency of dialysis sessions is dictated by such factors as the rate of rise of blood urea and serum potassium and the necessity to remove fluid. Even if a patient is highly catabolic with a rapid rise in plasma urea and potassium levels, these can usually be controlled by daily dialysis. However, there is a group of patients with oliguric acute renal failure in whom, for various reasons, the gastro-intestinal tract cannot be used for feeding. These patients are usually being nursed in an intensive care unit and have intra-abdominal problems, often the complications of abdominal surgery. They may have numerous other complications including respiratory failure leading to the need for artificial ventilation. Such patients will lose weight very rapidly if they are not nourished, and in this clinical setting the only way to provide nutrition is by the intravenous route. Adequate parenteral nutrition cannot usually be contained in a volume much less than three litres in 24 hours. This means that even if dialysis is being done daily the patient will come to dialysis in a positive fluid balance of at least three litres and may be verging on, if not in, actual pulmonary edema.

During a three to four hour dialysis all this extra water has to be removed. This may be hard to do in an ill patient who has less than normal cardiac function. Rapid fluid removal carried out simultaneously with efficient dialysis will tend to cause troublesome hypotension. To some extent this problem can be alleviated by performing ultrafiltration first to remove water and then hemodialysis for the uremia. The rationale for this so-called sequential ultrafiltration and hemodialysis has already been discussed on p.275. However, there is another way to tackle this problem which has gradually been gaining favor in the last few years. This approach is based on the idea that removing fluid continuously and steadily over 24 hours is likely to be better tolerated by the patient than having it removed rapidly during a three hour dialysis. The method employed is slow continuous ultrafiltration (SCUF).

In practice, what happens is that a simplified extracorporeal circulation is allowed to run through a highly permeable filtration device. The filtrate, which is an ultrafiltrate of plasma, containing mainly water as well as sodium in isotonic concentrations, is removed at a controlled rate. Several different filters have been used for this purpose as well as several different ways of obtaining access to the circulation.

The two most widely used methods are those popularized by Dr Paganini in Cleveland and the late Dr Kramer in Germany. In Dr Paganini's method illustrated in Fig. 7.31, a silastic-teflon shunt is connected by a very short extracorporeal circuit to a hollow fiber filter (Amicon Diafilter 20). The patient's own arterial and venous pressure difference is enough to perfuse the circuit without a blood pump. The volume of filtrate is regulated by a simple adjustable screw clamp on the filtrate outflow line. An hourly volume of 100−200 ml will provide a 24 hour volume of 2.4−4.8 litres. To achieve this the patient must have a good shunt and an adequate arterial pressure. To prevent clotting in the filter it is necessary to infuse heparin continuously into the arterial line through an infusion pump. Anything from 5000−20 000 units of heparin may be needed in each 24 hour period. The supreme advantage of the method is that optimal hydration can be maintained throughout the 24 hours. Hence it should be possible to avoid iatrogenic pulmonary edema as well as the necessity to remove fluid during dialysis. Avoidance of pulmonary edema will improve blood gas exchange and will often allow discontinuation of artifical ventilation at an earlier stage than would otherwise be possible. The only disadvantage of the technique is the need for continuous instead of intermittent heparin. This may not be serious if the patient has no source of bleeding but it may be disastrous and impossible to continue in the face of bleeding gastric erosions or a bleeding peptic ulcer. What we need now is a method for carrying out SCUF day after day with no heparin at all.

Two other important points have to be remembered. Firstly, SCUF is not a substitute for hemodialysis. Although it removes sodium and water very efficiently it does not rid the patient of very much potassium (since potassium is present in the filtrate in small concentrations) or

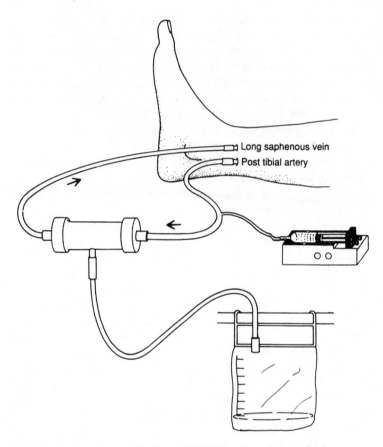

Fig. 7.31. Slow continuous ultrafiltration (SCUF) using a shunt in the leg.

other uremic solutes. Dialysis will still be needed for uremia and hyper-kalemia with about the same frequency as before and these must be monitored just as closely as before. Dialysis will not, however, be needed for fluid overload. Secondly, it must be remembered that sodium is being removed by SCUF in physiological concentrations (close to 140 mmol/l) and therefore any replacement solution, including the intravenous feeding, must contain sodium in physiological concentrations (140 mmol/l).

In the management of oliguric acute renal failure we are so used to restricting sodium intake that we may be inclined to forget that we need a high sodium replacement fluid during the performance of SCUF.

The second well-known method of vascular access during the performance of SCUF is the technique popularized by Dr Kramer. This

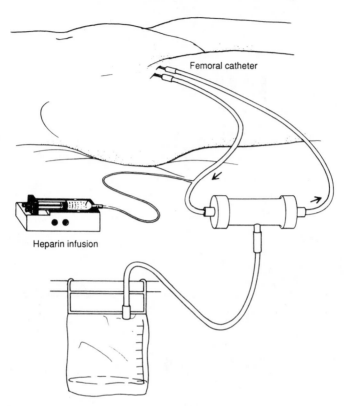

Fig. 7.32. SCUF using femoral catheters, Kramer's method.

involves introducing wide bore catheters into the femoral artery and
femoral vein as shown in Fig. 7.32. Again one relies on the patient's own
blood pressure to perfuse the circuit. Apart from the vascular access
method, the technique is in all respects the same.

If it is not possible to use a shunt or femoral artery and vein
catheters, as for example in a patient who has had bilateral femoral artery
surgery, we have adopted a third method for the performance of SCUF,
illustrated in Fig. 7.33. This method employs a double-lumen subclavian
catheter to draw blood from and return it to the central venous system.
Because there is no head of pressure to propel the blood we have to use
a blood pump. As soon as one does this one creates a negative presure
proximal to the blood pump and therefore a potential danger of air
embolus.

Therefore, we will need an air detector as on a dialysis machine. We

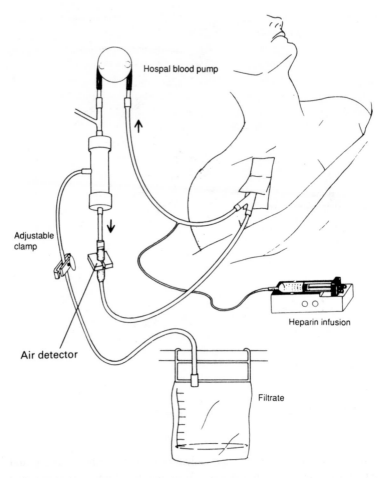

Fig. 7.33. SCUF using a blood pump and a double-lumen subclavian catheter.

will also need a method for monitoring the venous pressure as a means for early detection of obstruction on the venous side of the circuit. Having done this we have created a system which is beginning to look suspiciously like a kidney machine. It is not traditionally the job of ICU nurses to perform hemodialysis; and yet it is not feasible for the hemo-dialysis nurse to stay with the SCUF equipment 24 hours a day. The whole purpose is to devise a system which is very simple and requires very little attention for long periods of time. A number of groups in different parts of the world are solving the problem in their own way.

Furthermore, intensive care nurses are showing themselves to be equal to the task of monitoring the SCUF.

In our unit the nephrologist or renal fellow provides the vascular access and the hemodialysis nurse sets up the equipment and gets it going. Once it is running smoothly it is left to the ICU nurse to monitor it and adjust the filtration rate as well as the heparin infusion rate. We have found that intensive care nurses are so highly trained and used to looking after gadgets that they have not objected to being in charge of this simplified extracorporeal circuit. The advantage of having fingertip control of fluid removal from minute to minute and hour to hour outweighs any disadvantage of having an extra piece of equipment to look after. Our hemodialysis nurses come to check on the progress of the SCUF routine twice a day, whether or not the patient is due for a hemodialysis. One filtration device can be used in the interval between one dialysis and the next and it is even possible to re-use the filtration device (in the same way as one would re-use a dialyser) when the hemodialysis is over and it is time to initiate the SCUF once more.

There is no doubt that the use of SCUF makes the care of these patients a great deal easier. The reason that the clinical outcome is so often disappointing and that so many of these patients die in spite of receiving optimal care for their renal failure is that this group of patients tends to have a high incidence of lethal complications such as widespread intra-abdominal sepsis.

Hemofiltration

Some years ago a number of different nephrologists, notable among them Dr Lee Henderson, conceived the idea that blood purification could be achieved by filtration rather than by osmotic diffusion. If a filtration device could be used, rather similar to that described above with a high permeability for water and solutes, undesirable soluble metabolites could be removed by filtration. In order to achieve adequate blood purification it would be necessary to remove fairly large volumes of filtrate. (We should remember that in the first step towards the production of urine the kidneys produce a large volume of glomerular filtrate—about 180 litres a day). The second important step in urine production is selective reabsorption of a large part of the water and essential solutes. If we purify the blood by filtration outside the body, we also have to return to the body an almost equivalent volume of water and essential solutes. In fact this can and has been done—more extensively in Europe than in North America—and the process has come to be called hemofiltration.

In practice one can achieve blood purification equivalent to that which can be obtained by hemodialysis by doing 3−4 hours of hemofiltration three times a week. During each treatment, in which a high blood flow rate of about 300 ml/minute is desirable, a filtrate is produced of about 20−25 litres, and a physiologically composed replacement solution of similar volume is infused into the bloodstream. If the intention is to remove fluid during the treatment it is a simple matter to re-infuse somewhat less than the volume being removed. No dialysate is used. Instead of about 120 litres of non-sterile dialysate we need about 23 litres of sterile replacement solution of a quality fit for intravenous infusion.

The sterile physiological replacement solution can be infused proximal to the filtration device (pre-dilution) as shown in Fig. 7.34 or distal to the infusion device (post-dilution) as shown in Fig. 7.35. The post-dilution method is generally more popular. The volumes of filtrate being removed and of replacement solution being returned are so large that it is important not to let them get out of step. If one did get too far ahead or too far behind it would be easy to cause pulmonary edema from fluid overload or hypovolemic shock from fluid removal. Hence the equipment must have a failsafe method for keeping the patient in balance. In practice this is usually done by a system of balancing the weight of fluid removed against the weight of fluid returned. The method has been very successfully applied in patients with end-stage renal failure for long periods of time. What are the advantages and disadvantages of the method as compared with conventional hemodialysis?

The first advantage is that no dialysate is required. Instead one only needs a supply of sterile intravenous replacement solution. Actually this is more expensive and difficult to achieve than the supply of dialysate. For reasons of expense a number of units are actually preparing their own replacement solution rather than buying it commercially. One way to do this is to pass a non-sterile solution such as a dialysate through a bacterial filter. The production of the sterile replacement solution is a science in itself and considerable work is still being done on it. At present it remains a difficulty which is inhibiting the more widespread adoption of this method of treatment.

The other main advantages of the method, claimed by those who advocate hemofiltration in preference to hemodialysis, are as follows:
1 Hemofiltration is well tolerated hemodynamically. Patients tend not to have episodes of hypotension during treatment.
2 Hemofiltration produces better control of hypertension. Patients on long-term hemodialysis with refractory hypertension have had their blood

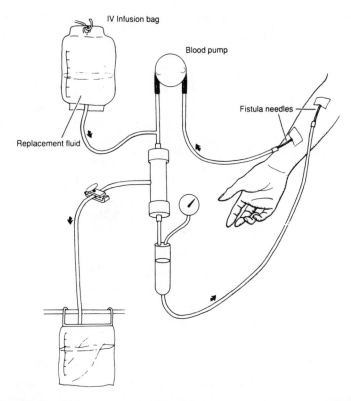

Fig. 7.34. Pre-dilution hemofiltration. The replacement fluid enters the circuit before the dialyser.

pressure well controlled by hemofiltration. The explanation for this is not entirely clear but it may have something to do with the fact that hemofiltration removes (because of the more highly permeable membranes) a series of larger molecules in the middle molecular weight range (500–3000) which may be important in uremia and its complications. 3 Probably for the same reasons it is believed that hemofiltration is more effective than hemodialysis in treating uremic polyneuritis which is thought to be caused mainly by retention of uremic substances of middle molecular size.

It seems too early to predict what will be the ultimate place of long-term hemofiltration in the management of end-stage renal failure. A lot might depend on improved technology for producing the sterile intravenous replacement solution more reliably and more cheaply.

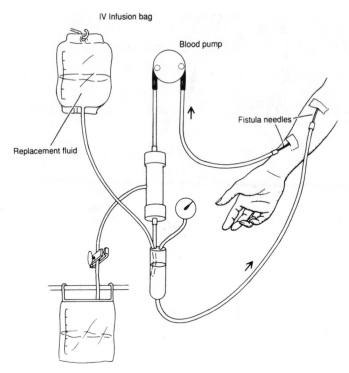

Fig. 7.35. Post-dilution hemofiltration. The replacement fluid enters the circuit after the dialyser.

Continuous hemofiltration in the management of acute renal failure

This method is a logical extension of what has already been developed. If a patient is being treated for acute renal failure with slow continuous ultrafiltration (SCUF) we still have to carry out a conventional dialysis every one or two days. SCUF is not a substitute for hemodialysis since it does not correct uremia or hyperkalemia. It merely prevents overloading by salt and water. It would be an attractive idea if we are already doing SCUF to step up the volumes of filtrate to a litre per hour (24 litres a day) and replace volume for volume with sterile intravenous replacement solution. This process would not only prevent fluctuations in hydration, it would also maintain continuous blood purification by continuous and effective removal of uremic substances. It would be a close approximation to what is achieved by normal kidneys, though of course the level of blood purification would not be as good.

Many people believe that this continuous, low-efficiency hemofiltration is the best and most physiological way to treat a complicated case of oliguric acute renal failure and that in future we will all have the skill, experience and appropriate equipment to do it whenever it seems indicated. The basic disadvantage of the need for continuous heparin applies equally to this method as it does in the case of SCUF. The aim should be to devise a method for carrying out both these treatments without heparin.

Hemodiafiltration

Hemodiafiltration is one further variant which combines the principles of dialysis by diffusion with filtration which is convective transport of solute. Essentially what is done is to carry out hemodialysis using a standard dialysate with a high permeability filter such as is used for hemofiltration. The transmembrane pressure is adjusted to provide removal of solute and water by filtration and the replacement solution is infused to replace whatever volume is required. Advocates of this technique claim that it has the advantages of both hemodialysis and hemofiltration. Because it is so highly efficient and is also extremely well tolerated by the patient, treatment times can be cut down with no loss of patient well-being. The method is still in a relatively early stage of development and we may hear a lot more about it in the future. A limitation to this process of progress-ively shortening the dialysis time by providing ever more efficient blood purification may be imposed by the time it takes for other fluid compart-ments of the body to equilibrate with the blood. To take an absurd example, there would be no point in lowering blood urea and creatinine to normal all in the space of one hour, because as soon as treatment is discontinued the levels would rebound back up as uremic substances continued to diffuse out of the cells and from the interstitial fluid into the plasma. The search for faster and faster methods of treating patients is probably governed by a law of diminishing returns.

Acute emergencies on dialysis

Air embolus

Air entering the venous circulation inadvertently in any appreciable amount goes straight to the right side of the heart. The heart is not designed to pump air and so for a while the air is just churned up and there is little forward progress of blood to the lungs. The patient will complain of chest pain and collapse with hypotension. Before long the air—blood mixture of froth is pumped into the lungs and starts to return to the left side of the heart. Patients seldom die in this initial phase of cardiovascular collapse. The danger is that air or froth will enter the carotid vessels and be pumped into the brain where it will block blood flow and cause death of brain tissue. Air elsewhere in the body causes only temporary loss of perfusion.

Emergency intervention if carried out quickly enough will usually save the patient's life. If air is spotted moving along the venous blood line, clamp the line immediately and turn off the blood pump. No emergency demands greater speed than this. Next, place the patient head down—head lower than the chest. This is one reason why beds which tilt head downwards are essential in hemodialysis units. The purpose of the head down position is to encourage air and froth which is entering the aorta to by-pass the blood vessels going to the head. Then give the patient 100% oxygen to breath and call for medical help. The medical staff may wish to infuse low molecular weight dextran intravenously to improve capillary perfusion of the brain. They may wish to place the patient in a compression chamber to administer hyperbaric oxygen (the device used for emergency treatment of decompression sickness) if one is available. Even if the patient is virtually comatose and desperately ill some remarkable recoveries have been seen after this disaster.

The most important steps taken to prevent air embolism have been the banning of bottles with air intake lines for infusion of saline in dialysis patients and the provision on all kidney machines of reliable air embolism monitors. Most of the fatal episodes of air embolism which occurred in the early days were the result of air entering through the air intake of an empty bottle of saline used for infusion. It is worth remembering that the same thing could happen through using a bottle of albumin for infusion during dialysis. When plastic bags empty they suck flat and do not allow entry of air.

The other thing to remember is that the only fatal cases of air embolus that have occurred in recent years were the result of deliberate or accidental deactivation of the air embolism monitor. The air embolism monitor will only function if it is switched on. To leave it switched off is to risk the patient's life.

Acute massive hemolysis

Hemolysis of a substantial amount of the patient's blood during hemodialysis is so rare that most dialysis nurses have never seen it happen. Such classical causes as copper poisoning from copper pipes are so well known that no dialysis unit ever allows any copper to be incorporated in any part of the plumbing. In the old days when batch systems were used routinely for hemodialysis, patients were occasionally dialysed against pure water because someone forgot to put any concentrate in the tank. Blood emerging from the venous side of the dialyser was totally tanslucent and the colour of claret wine because there were no surviving red cells. Overheating of the dialysate has caused deaths from hemolysis within recent memory and we ourselves had some episodes of massive hemolysis during the winter of 1983, the cause of which has not yet been fully resolved. The hemolysis was associated with methemoglobin which makes the blood turn an almost brownish black color and the patients looked as though they were cyanosed. Diagnosis depends on having one's suspicions aroused. If a patient becomes ill and the blood in the venous line looks peculiar at all, take a sample and spin it down in a centrifuge. If the supernatant plasma is pink or brown instead of the usual pale yellow, you know that hemolysis has occurred. The main danger to the patient is the hyperkalemia caused by massive liberation of potassium from the destroyed red cells. Emergency treatment consists of exchange transfusion to replace the destroyed red cells and then emergency dialysis to deal with the hyperkalemia. If the condition is not suspected and the patient is allowed home there is a danger of hyperkalemia causing cardiac arrest at home before the next dialysis.

If you are ever in the situation of discovering a case of hemolysis in a patient on hemodialysis, stop the dialysis immediately and call the medical staff. It is also important to throw nothing away. All the components of the extracorporeal circuit including the dialyser, the blood lines, the heparin and saline infusions must be kept for examination and analysis. You will also need samples of the blood and dialysate.

Chest pain in a patient on dialysis

This symptom must always be taken seriously and is always a reason to call a doctor unless the patient is a known angina sufferer who is simply having another familiar attack. Attacks of angina may be precipitated by the sudden development of arrhythmia on dialysis so always check the rhythm of the pulse. In a patient receiving dialysis via a subclavian catheter, always suspect the possibility that the chest pain is caused by the catheter. Fatal cardiac tamponade can occur if the catheter inserted from the right side enters the pericardial cavity. A hemothorax may also occur. Most of these traumatic complications should not lead to death of the patient if the cause is accurately identified in time to take appropriate action. Chest pain within the first few minutes of dialysis may also be due to the first use phenomenon already discussed on p.180 under the section on dialysis membranes. However, if you are in any doubt ask a doctor to see the patient.

An acute myocardial infarction occurring on dialysis is a reason to discontinue the dialysis and move the patient to a coronary care unit for observation until the condition has stabilized.

Cardiac arrest on dialysis

Most in-center dialysis units, being part of a busy, modern hospital, will have cardiac resuscitation teams at their disposal which can be called in an emergency. Not infrequently there may be only one nurse in the unit observing a number of different patients. If she sees a patient collapse and she diagnoses cardiac arrest, she does not have time to carry out cardiopulmonary resuscitation and phone for the arrest team at the same time. For this reason all modern dialysis units in hospital centers should have a clearly visible cardiac arrest button on the wall or at the nursing station which can be pushed in an emergency. This will immediately indicate to the central telephone exchange that a cardiac arrest has occurred in the hemodialysis unit. It is the telephone operator's responsibility to summon the arrest team while the nurse can get on with the business of resuscitating the patient. If you diagnose an arrest your actions in order of priority should be as follows.

1 A hard thump on the center of the sternum will occasionally restart the heart.

2 If not, and if you are alone, get the patient flat at once and summon the cardiac arrest team.

3 Put in an airway and start cardiopulmonary resuscitation (CPR).

4 As soon as any help arrives ask for a board to place behind the patient's chest and that the bed should be lowered to the most advantageous position for you to do external cardiac massage.

5 Once the arrest team takes over the CPR you will be free to take the patient off dialysis. Retransfuse the patient through the arterial line and after the blood has been returned to the patient leave the venous cannula intact for intravenous infusion purposes.

In all well run, modern hospitals courses in CPR are made available to all clinical personnel, medical and nursing, on a regular basis. Revision courses for hemodialysis nurses at regular intervals, probably once a year, should be obligatory.

Major seizures on dialysis

Major seizures in patients on dialysis can occur for a number of reasons. However, your first responsibility is to make sure that the patient is safe. First make sure that the patient's involuntary movements have not dislodged the fistula needles. If a needle has been pulled right out or dislodged into a subcutaneous interstitial site, you have to stop the blood loss or the development of a large perivascular hematoma. Turn off the blood pump, clamp the lines, and exert pressure over a bleeding site.

Next make sure that the patient has a clear airway. Meanwhile someone should be calling the medical staff, who should come immediately and give an order for an intravenous anticonvulsant. Diazepam is safe and reliable for this purpose.

By far the commonest cause of major fits on dialysis is acute hypotension due to volume depletion. This is turn causes cerebral hypoxia. Most patients do not have seizures in response to acute hypotension—only those patients with what we call a low threshold for epilepsy. The nurses in any hemodialysis unit soon get to know which patients do have a low epilepsy threshold and they become accordingly very vigilant to make sure that such patients are carefully watched to prevent serious hypotension.

If a major seizure in a patient on dialysis does not have an obvious explanation, one has to start thinking about possible causes. Is this a very uremic patient manifesting dialysis disequilibrium? Is this an elderly arteriopathic patient who has suffered a stroke? Could it be a fault in composition of the dialysate? We know that both high sodium concentrations and low sodium concentrations can cause cerebral disorders. If there is any doubt it is essential to obtain an independent conductivity measurement of the dialysate and probably a chemical analysis also. Obtain a sample of venous blood and centrifuge it to make sure there is no hemolysis.

The explanation for the seizure must be found and corrected.

8

Chronic Medical Problems in Dialysis Patients

Robert Uldall

The problem of hepatitis

There are two commonly recognized forms of viral hepatitis. Infectious hepatitis, now called hepatitis A, is a comparatively mild illness, occurring sporadically or epidemically in the community. It is spread by the fecal-oral route, has a relatively short incubation period of 3–6 weeks and seldom leads to death or chronic liver disease. There is no easy diagnostic test and no specific therapy but spontaneous recovery nearly always occurs. Serum hepatitis, or hepatitis B, is an illness which may be asymptomatic and subclinical, may be associated with a chronic carrier state, may be associated with disabling morbidity, may lead on to chronic aggressive hepatitis, or may be fulminating in onset and rapidly fatal. It is a disease mainly associated with hospitals, and often acquired in hospitals, and it has a long incubation period varying from 1 to 6 months, with an outside limit of 165 days. It is spread by blood or blood products and usually by the parenteral route. Anyone who has anything to do with other people's blood is at risk from catching the disease. The classical mode of transmission is by receiving a blood transfusion from an infected patient or a carrier, but various other possible avenues exist. The following list is by no means comprehensive but gives an idea of the widespread nature of the danger.

• Patients in hemodialysis units are having their blood removed from their circulation regularly in large amounts and for long periods as part

292

of their treatment. These patients may be in poor general health and therefore probably have reduced resistance to infection. They also have blood transfusions though not as often as in the early days of dialysis. An infected blood transfusion is a large inoculum. Five hundred ml of blood is capable of transmitting a very large dose of virus. As little as a tiny drop of blood on a contaminated needle has been known to transmit infections.

• Patients undergoing cardiac surgery receive very large multiple blood transfusions.

• Drug addicts who inject themselves with drugs intravenously tend to share needles and have poor standards of hygiene.

• Commercial tattooing is dangerous because of the same lack of attention to sterility.

• Sexual promiscuity, particularly that which is associated with anal intercourse, is dangerous because of incidental blood inoculation. Hence the high incidence of hepatitis in male homosexuals.

• Promiscuity and drug addiction tend to go together and this makes the danger greater.

• Patients coming from underdeveloped countries, especially from Asia, have a high incidence of hepatitis B carrier state.

• Hospital workers most at risk are those who repeatedly handle blood. The two most vulnerable are the staff of hemodialysis units and the technical staff in chemical pathology laboratories.

• Staff who work in peritoneal dialysis units are at somewhat less of a risk but peritoneal dialysis effluent has been shown to be infective so that the precautions applied to hemodialysis units should also be applied wherever peritoneal dialysis is performed.

• Hepatitis B can almost certainly be, and probably has been, transmitted by transplantation of a cadaver kidney. Fortunately since Blumberg in 1964 discovered the Australia antigen, now known more correctly as hepatitis B surface antigen, or HBsAg for short, we now have a very reliable identifiable marker for hepatitis B which can be demonstrated in the blood of any person who is actively infected or is an asymptomatic carrier.

The third form of hepatitis with which we have to concern ourselves, and which has acquired real importance, in hemodialysis patients especially, is, for lack of a better name, called non-A non-B. This is usually a mild and often subclinical disease, the mode of transmission of which is the same as that of hepatitis B. As yet there is no distinctive serological marker by which it can be recognized, so diagnosis is by exclusion.

Testing for hepatitis B antigen

There are really only three methods which need to be considered here.

1 Cross-over electrophoresis

This is a rapid screening test which can be carried out in about 90 minutes with simple unsophisticated equipment. Staff have to be trained to do it but it is not an expensive test to run. It will only be expensive if a clinical department demands a 24 hour emergency service which could necessitate calling in a technician. This method might be appropriate for a small hospital doing a limited number of tests, particularly if a service is not available from a large central laboratory. It is not as sensitive as the other methods but will nevertheless pick up 90–95% of all positives. There are no false positives.

2 Radioimmunoassay

This is 10 000 times more sensitive than cross-over electrophoresis. It is the standard method now used by all large laboratories and all blood transfusion services but it is only economical if fairly large numbers of samples are tested. The result can be available in 4–5 hours but it is not a good test for checking one blood sample in the middle of the night. Laboratories may run a batch of samples once or twice a week. If an isolated result is required urgently (i.e. the same day) it probably pays to run all the other waiting samples at the same time, since the cost of the technician's time is the same for one test as it is for fifty. HB antibody status is also obtained by radioimmunoassay. There is now a reliable method for the detection of HBsAg by radioimmunoassay from a drop of dried blood on a filter paper. The potential usefulness of this technique has not yet been fully explored.

3 Immuno-electron microscopy

This is the most sensitive and at the present time the most definite and reliable of all the methods for detecting HBsAg. However, it is extremmly difficult and time consuming and can really only be used as a research tool. It is the only method which can reliably detect hepatitis A and it is likely to be the most useful technique for delineating the entity of non-A, non-B hepatitis. On occasion one may have a patient who is strongly suspected of having hepatitis B in whom the diagnosis cannot be proved by radioimmunoassay. This may be because all the antigen is being mopped up by antibody. In such a case immuno-electron microscopy might be expected to give an answer.

The prevention of hepatitis B in the renal unit depends on the following:

1 Hepatitis B vaccination. Now for the first time we have a hepatitis B vaccine both in Europe and North America. It is given intramuscularly in three separate doses at the start, one month later and six months later. It seems to produce active immunity in 95% or more of healthy recipients without renal failure. They become and remain antibody positive. They will probabaly have lifelong protective immunity to hepatitis B. This is good news for all health care workers including nursing, technical and medical staff who work in dialysis units. The vaccination is expensive but most people believe that it will save money in the long run because we can stop doing routine HBsAg testing in anybody who becomes antibody positive. Unfortunately the vaccine is not so routinely successful in inducing immunity in patients who are already on hemodialysis. One large study of the North American vaccine showed that only 50% of patients became antibody positve and the incidence of hepatitis B in this group was no lower than in those who failed to respond. However, results in Europe have been more encouraging. The Pasteur Institue vaccine reduced the incidence of hepatitis B infection in antibody positive patients by 53% and the Dutch vacine by 78%. It is still not clear what impact will be made on the hepatitis problem by recent introduction of vaccines. It is likely that they will provide considerable protection for staff. In view of the relative failure of patients on hemodialysis to respond to the vaccine, it has been suggested that a program of active vaccination should be carried out on all patients with early renal impairment who are expected to end up on dialysis eventually. Perhaps in this way we will ultimately succeed in achieving active immunity against hepatitis B in the majority of the dialysis population. However, in the meantime we have to continue a program of prevention based on constant vigilance.

2 All possible steps must be taken to prevent the entry of hepatitis B virus into the renal unit by appropriate screening tests for HBsAg.

3 One must assume that at any time any patient receiving treatment for renal failure may be incubating the disease and is therefore potentially infective. The logical consequence of this assumption is that all blood or anything which may be contaminated with blood must be regarded as potentially dangerous and possibly lethal.

All the precautions which are now widely adopted and almost universally accepted both in North America and Europe follow from these three basic principles. It is also important to be aware of the fact that hepatitis B virus can exist for long periods outside the body and it is not killed by phenol or alcohol-containing disinfectants. The virus is killed as far as we know by hypochlorite, formaldehyde and glutaraldehyde. It is also killed by heat sterilization and autoclaving. The live virus can enter open cuts or abrasions on hands. It can probably pass through intact mucous membranes; it can be ingested and cause infection by the oral route (though this must be uncommon). There is even evidence of one well documented outbreak in which infection occurred by aerosol contamination. Several patients in a confined area contracted the disease when a bottle containing infected blood shattered on the floor.

The hepatitis B virus has been shown to pass through the intact semipermeable membrane of a dialyser, from the dialysate into the blood compartment or in the opposite direction. Nevertheless the usual route of infection is by parenteral injection such as pricking oneself with an infected needle. Outbreaks have been caused in pathology staff receptionists who were inadvertently cutting their hands on the sharp edges of pathology requisitions which were contaminated with blood spilled on the outside of their containers.

Having discussed what is known about hepatitis B vaccination, prevention will be considered under two headings:

1 Prevention of entry of virus to the renal unit.
2 Blood precautions in the renal unit.

At the outset the younger generation in various hospital disciplines may be tempted to ask why all these precautions are necessary. The disease is not very conspicuous these days. Why all the fuss? Only a few years ago outbreaks of hepatitis were common and often serious. Patients as well as medical and nursing staff in various parts of the world died of it. Hepatitis B, like cholera or poliomyelitis, will only remain unobtrusive as long as we remain eternally vigilant. It is worth noting that in Britain the rising incidence of hepatitis B in dialysis patients was halted only after the institution of a comprehensive nationwide prevention program. The incidence of hepatitis in patients fell from nearly 5% in 1970 to 1.4% in 1972 and among staff from 1.3% in 1970 to 0.4% in 1972.

The main features of this prevention program were published in a classic document in 1972, the report of the Advisory Group under the chairmanship of Lord Rosenheim. The recommendations of the Rosenheim report have received wide publicity in all centers and in all countries which take the hepatitis B problem seriously. Every renal unit should have copies of this report and should draft its own code of practice based on the prevailing local conditions.

Prevention of entry of infection into the renal unit

The keystone of prevention is the hepatitis B surface antigen test, still sometimes called the Australia antigen test.

Infection may enter in one of two ways. A patient receiving treatment may receive infected blood or blood products. Several different blood products may transmit the infection, especially concentrates of coagulation factors and fibrinogen, which have approximately 30% infectivity. Human albumin, plasma protein fractions, purified gamma globulin and hyper-immune globulin are unable to transmit the virus because they are pretreated by heat and alcohol. Thus no patient should receive blood or blood products unless they have been screened at source for HBsAg. In the US it has been found, not surprisingly, that blood from paid donors has a much higher incidence of HBsAg than blood from volunteer donors. Secondly an infected patient or a carrier of HBsAg may be dialysed in the unit without his or her antigen status being checked. There is then a danger of spread to other patients and staff.

All patients known to have chronic renal failure who might require dialysis should therefore be checked regularly prior to starting dialysis. Patients arriving unexpectedly with renal failure, either acute or end-stage, must on no account be dialysed in the main unit until they have been checked. The responsibility for ensuring that no one slips through the net is usually delegated by the director of the unit to the head nurse or her deputy. Emergency dialysis on a new patient should always be performed outside the unit and should be followed by an urgent request for HBsAg testing. This result should be available before the next dialysis and before the machine is used for a different patient. Other possible sources of entry are occasional visitors from other units (always inquire about the HBsAg test before accepting such a patient) and the acquisition of hepatitis by one's own patients if they visit other centers for dialysis. Check that the other center is free of hepatitis. The other potential source, which tends to be forgotten and is administratively difficult to deal with, is the cadaver kidney. If kidneys are retrieved and transplanted in the middle of the night, an emergency service for HBsAg testing must be available. If a transplanted patient develops hepatitis and subsequently rejects the graft, the carrier state poses a serious danger to the renal unit. Even with the most meticulous blood precautions an HBsAg positive patient will cause spread to other patients if dialysis is conducted in the main unit. Thus a positive patient must be dialysed in isolation and should preferably be trained as soon as possible for home dialysis. Transplantation of positive patients to remove the infection hazard from the dialysis unit may be dangerous to all staff involved with the patient's care and has not gained popularity as a way of solving the problem. This statement may be modified in future in centers where widespread vaccination of patients and staff has been carried out. But there is another factor to be considered. There is some evidence that renal transplantation may be dangerous for the asymptomatic healthy hemodialysis patient who happens to be a hepatitis B carrier. Even though the kidney transplant is a success, the liver condition may deteriorate and the patient may die of the complications of cirrhosis and portal hypertension 3−5 years later. One theory is that the immunosuppressive drugs given for prevention of rejection cause a loss of immunity to the hepatitis virus which consequently becomes more aggressive and damaging. This topic remains controversial and the results of transplanting HBsAg positive patients varies greatly from one center to another. Responsibility for dialysis of positive patients has to be accepted by all hemodialysis nurses and preferably by nurses who are antibody positive as a result of vaccination or subclinical infections which have recovered. Now that vaccination is widely available all staff have an obligation to have themselves protected. Antibody is detectable in most of those who have recovered from the disease and it remains positive for a long time. Some permanent immunity in such individuals almost certainly exists. The isolation facilities required for positive patients should be physically separate, though close to the main unit. Arrangements should be available for self-contained nursing of such a patient, together with separate entrances and exits for decontamination purposes, as well as negative pressure ventilation which extracts the air to the outside of the building.

All biological material from such a patient such as urine and feces and soiled dressings must be treated with antiseptic before being discarded. Special warnings must be clearly displayed on blood samples from the patient and these must be wrapped in waterproof bags separate from the requisitions. Hepatitis B immune globulin, whose effectiveness has now been proven by controlled trial, is now available for injection into any individual who accidentally receives inoculations or other exposure to HB positive blood. For maximum benefit the globulin should be given within 24 hours of exposure. Invasive investigations, operations and venepunctures in positive patients should be kept to a minimum. It is not feasible to keep separate operating rooms available for such individuals but operations can be scheduled for the end of the day when there is time to clean up carefully before the next day.

Dialysers should never be re-used in positive patients. Dialysers and blood lines should be flushed with antiseptic in the patient's own isolation area before they are discarded in waterproof bags.

If such a patient dies, special hygienic precautions should be taken in dealing with the body. Post-mortem attendants, pathologists and undertakers must be informed of the danger. An autopsy should only be performed after careful consideration and then only by an experienced pathologist.

The HBsAg positive patient who successfully performs home hemodialysis can be safely treated and observed, without risk to other patients and staff. If he reverts to negative he can be presumed to be non-infective and can then be placed back on the waiting list for renal transplantation. Some such patients who may still have a positive HB antibody have been found to become HBsAg positive again after transplantation. Is this another attack of hepatitis B? This seems unlikely in view of the patient's immunity. Or has the hepatitis B been reactivated by the renal transplantation and the immunosuppression? On the whole, it seems most likely to be a reactivation of a disease which was never completely eradicated, but remained in a latent phase. This phenomenon must be taken into account whenever transplantation is contemplated in a patient who is HBsAg negative, but has a positive antibody test.

A particularly difficult problem is the HBsAg positive patient who cannot be trained for home hemodialysis because of the lack of a suitable partner or adequate domestic accommodation. Such a patient may be suitable for CAPD. If neither of these can be arranged we have the prospect of long-term dialysis in hospital in isolation facilities. There may be an argument for collecting such patients from various hospitals and dialysing them in one regional center.

Blood precautions within the renal unit

New staff should be screened for HBsAg and HB antibody before starting work. This is mainly to demonstrate HBsAg negativity so that subsequent development of the HBsAg positivity will be seen to have arisen during the course of work. This may be important for compensation purposes. Whether an initial antigen positive state should be a bar to employment is highly doubtful. The danger of the carrier state in staff is controversial but has probably been overemphasized. Staff have not been shown to spread the disease to patients. The famous exception was that of a dentist, several of whose patients became positive. Study of his practice failed to reveal any faulty techniques and the mechanism of spread in this case remains speculative.

Any staff who develop a positive HBsAg after previously being negative should obviously be taken off work until they have been fully assessed medically, but if there is no clinical illness they should probably be allowed to continue as before. The presence of HB antibody, on the other hand, can be assumed to be a distinct asset since such individuals, by virtue of their acquired immunity, will be ideal for nursing the positive patient in isolation.

Hepatitis B 'e' antigen

The standard tests for detecting hepatitis B in its various forms are actually detecting hepatitis B 'surface' antigen—that is, the outer coat of the virus. It has been suggested that some individuals, who are HBsAg positive, are no longer actually infective because the virus itself has been killed and only the harmless surface antigen of the outer coat remains. It has been proposed that in order to detect live virus one has to detect antigen in the deeper structure of the virus. A technique now exists for detecting hepatitis B 'e' antigen, and positivity with this test is said to represent the presence of definitely live virus. There is some evidence, as yet tentative, which indicates that a positive 'e' antigen is associated with a worse prognosis because it demonstrates continuing invasion by live virus and active hepatitis. It also implies definite infectivity. The importance and reliability of this further refinement of diagnostic testing will no doubt become apparent in the next few years. The test is not yet generally available but the answers may be very helpful in a special case.

Non-A non-B hepatitis

For a long time nephrologists were mystified and concerned by the appearance in hemodialysis units of a condition associated with disturbed liver function tests and a negative HBsAg. This may occur as a single case or as an outbreak of several cases. The patients are seldom clinically ill or jaundiced and tests for other well-known causes of viral hepatitis, such as Epstein—Barr (EB) virus or cytomegalovirus (CMV), are usually negative. The condition bears no resemblance to hepatitis A and it usually disappears spontaneously in a few months. The explanation for this formerly enigmatic disorder lies in the now well-recognized entity which has come to be called non-A non-B hepatitis. Studies have shown that a virus or viruses, which are not A, B, EBV or CMV, can cause a mild hepatitis resembling hepatitis B. It seems to be primarily a post-transfusion hepatitis spread by the parenteral route, and it has an incubation period of 18–100 days. It may persist in a chronic carrier state. It is not often associated with chronic active hepatitis and only rarely does it cause fulminant hepatic failure. At present there is no direct serological test for this virus(es) and the condition will continue to be diagnosed by a process of exclusion. Its existence is another argument, if one is needed, for strict application of hygienic measures within the dialysis unit, even though there are no known cases of HBsAg positivity and even though there has been a full-scale vaccination program.

At present it is our policy when we have a case of presumed non-A non-B hepatitis to review carefully the drugs which the patient is taking, to exclude any which may be hepatotoxic, to advise the patient against drinking any alcohol, and to postpone renal transplantation until the liver function has returned to normal. The remainder of the hygienic precautions which have to be instituted in a renal unit are all based on common sense. The main thing to keep in mind at all times is that the blood or biological fluids of any patient at any time may be infected and are therefore potentially dangerous. Staff must wear suitable protective clothing, particularly long-sleeved gowns, when any procedure is being done. Disposable paper shoe covers prevent blood from being carried out on the footwear of staff and patients. Pull-on disposable vinyl gloves must be worn whenever there is a possibility of blood being spilled. Sterile gloves will of course be worn for the needling of fistulae. Removal of fistula needles is usually treated as a clean but non-sterile procedure. If any blood is spilled it should immediately be mopped up with strong hypochlorite solution. A strict routine of handwashing should be enforced. No eating, drinking or smoking should be allowed in any clinical area.

Needles, syringes and blood tubing must be disposed of in the proper containers. Each patient must have his or her own thermometer. Alternatively electrical thermometers with disposable plastic covers should be used. A separate, sterile, disposable isolator should be used to prevent blood from passing along blood lines to arterial and venous pressure monitors since blood entering a monitor could theoretically infect the next patient. These are obvious examples but each renal unit director will wish to review the blood precautions in the light of local practice. A detailed review of the code of practice should be carried out regularly, perhaps once a year, to check on the development of potentially dangerous habits or sloppy techniques. It may also be appropriate to change the code of practice in order to adapt to the demands of new knowledge. It is only by eternal vigilance that mistakes will be avoided. It might be argued that too much attention to the dangers of hepatitis will have an unsettling effect on staff morale. In our experience the staff tend to be efficient and confident if the problem is being taken seriously and if they know that care is being taken to protect them. Even if accidental exposure does occur to the blood of an infected patient, we now have a hyperimmune globulin which is of proven efficacy.

AIDS

The acquired immune deficiency syndrome (AIDS) is, at the time of writing, still a relatively remote threat to dialysis patients. Large numbers of such patients are still confined to a handful of large metropolitan centers such as San Francisco and New York where there are large communities of homosexuals. It is predicted, however, by the experts that AIDS will over the next few years become a problem of frighteningly massive dimension. The disease is already spreading to the heterosexual community by transfer to prostitutes. The fact that blood products can convey the disease is demonstrated by the widespread and tragic development of AIDS by hemophiliacs. Fortunately the virus has now been identified and serological tests are now available for identification of carriers. Plans are in place to screen all future blood transfusion to exclude the AIDS virus and this should effectively protect renal failure patients from infection by this route. At present our policy in dealing with AIDS in dialysis centers should be the same as that which we use to protect our patients from hepatitis B. However, there are some important differences between the two diseases.

● At present there is no known hyperimmune globulin to protect a health care worker who has become accidentally exposed to blood of an AIDS victim.
● At present there is no active vaccination available against AIDS.
● Unlike hepatitis B, which is usually not fatal, AIDS seems to be uniformly fatal ultimately once it has been acquired.
● Hepatitis B carriers can lead healthy and productive lives on dialysis.
● Patients who have AIDS in addition to end-stage renal failure always die within a short time, usually less than three months, despite receiving the best treatment, including regular dialysis.

Because of these considerations it has been suggested by some that to dialyse patients with AIDS is an unjustifiable risk with no long-term benefit to the patient. Nevertheless, medical and nursing teams are providing dialysis for such patients and it seems likely that many of us will be faced with this problem in the future.

The good thing about AIDS virus is that it seems to be much less infective than the hepatitis B virus. Relatively large doses of inoculum seem to be necessary to transmit the disease. Nurses who have received needle-stick injuries while attending AIDS patients have not developed the AIDS virus antibody; and as yet there is no report of AIDS developing in any medical, nursing or paramedical staff performing hemodialysis for patients with AIDS. There is a long tradition in the medical and nursing professions for dedicated care to patients suffering from dangerous and contagious diseases. Initial evidence indicates no sign of reluctance to uphold this tradition.

Hypertension

Hypertension and its complications of cerebral hemorrhage and heart failure used to be the main causes of death in patients on hemodialysis. Death from these causes has become rare since the importance of controlling hypertension has been fully appreciated. Control of blood pressure is now a constant preoccupation of both the doctors and nurses and a very high standard is demanded. Many patients reaching end-stage renal failure are on a variety of different hypotensive drugs. Within a short time many of the drugs can be stopped as the dialysis itself begins to control the hypertension. The aim should be to institute strict control of salt and water intake in the intervals between one dialysis and the next so that weight gain from this cause is kept to a minimum. Since most dialysis patients are what we call 'volume dependent' hypertensives and most of those who are well dialysed are also very good about restricting their salt and water consumption, these measures alone are enough to control blood pressure remarkably well in the bulk of the hemodialysis population. If patients are unable to control their fluid intake because they are uncontrollably thirsty, they may be receiving too much salt in their diets, or they may just be inadequately dialysed. Before accusing patients of being hopelessly undisciplined and lacking in self-control it is first necessary to look for an organic cause of excessive thirst. The commonest cause is inadequate dialysis. On many occasions we have seen patients achieve control of weight gain after we have increased their dialysis hours and/or the blood flow rate through the dialyser. When the predialysis urea and creatinine levels are brought down, the interdialytic weight gain is reduced. An unduly high dialysate sodium level may also provoke an unnatural thirst so it may be worth reducing the dialysate sodium concentration for that particular patient. With modern equipment this can be done individually for any patient. If these measures succeed in controlling weight gain but the patient remains hypertensive we have to resort to the use of hypotensive drugs. Of these, by far the most useful are the beta-blockers such as propranolol; twice daily dosage is enough. Their big advantage is that they do not tend to cause postural hypotension.

Traditional hypotensive drugs such as methyldopa are unsatisfactory in hemodialysis patients since they fail to control hypertension predialysis but cause marked postural hypotension postdialysis when salt and water have been removed. If a beta-blocker by itself is not enough one may have to add a vasodilator and for men with truly refractory hypertension one may be compelled to use the big guns such as minoxidil. This is not acceptable to most women because of the excessive hair growth which it causes.

There remains a small proportion of hypertensive dialysis patients who respond to volume depletion during dialysis by a paradoxical rise in blood pressure rather than a fall. This is almost certainly a sign of high renin production—the so-called high renin hypertensive. In such patients one can sometimes prevent this by giving an extra dose of a beta-blocking drug at the beginning of each dialysis. An even smaller group of patients will resist all these measures. Such patients may respond to an angiotensin inhibitor drug such as captopril but there may be a rare patient whose hypertension remains dangerously severe (refractory to all drug therapy) and in this case the only way to save the patient's life is to remove both kidneys. Bilateral nephrectomy to control hypertension is rarely necessary nowadays and should only be a last resort when all else has failed. This is because the anephric state is accompanied by severe anemia which leads to the necessity for regular blood transfusions thereafter until or unless the patient receives a kidney transplant.

One other approach to the control of resistant hypertension needs to be considered. Some people believe that hypertension responds to dialytic treatment which is designed to remove uremic substances of higher molecular weight, the so-called middle molecules. This can be done by using a highly permeable membrane such as the PAN (polyacrylonitrile) membrane in a dialysis system designed to cope with high levels of ultrafiltration or by performing hemofiltration, an alternative treatment described on p.283. There is still a fair amount of controversy as to the efficacy of hemofiltration in controlling refractory hypertension. The consensus is that it is of some value.

Anemia in patients on regular hemodialysis

Of all the problems which long-term hemodialysis patients have to put up with, chronic anemia stands out as being the most troublesome—mainly because we do not yet have very good remedies for it. Anemia, with hemoglobin levels as low as $70\,g/l$, is remarkably well tolerated by hemodialysis patients who seem to adjust to it, but it does undoubtedly account for tiredness, lethargy and loss of stamina, and always our aim should be to keep the hemoglobin as high as possible. If the hemoglobin falls much below 70 g/l, patients feel so tired that they will usually need blood transfusions. Young patients with good hearts tolerate anemia much better than older patients with bad hearts, especially those who have angina. Angina in dialysis patients, as in everyone else, is greatly aggravated by a fall in hemoglobin and improved by a rise in hemoglobin, so much so that we may be obliged in these patients to maintain the hemoglobin continuously above 80−90 g/l to keep them free of symptoms. Regular transfusions of 2−3 units of packed red cells may be the only way to do this. As in patients with chronic renal failure (not yet requiring dialysis) there is reduced red cell production by the bone marrow, partly due to the toxic effect of uremia on the bone marrow and partly due to lack of the renal hormone erythropoietin. Also, as in chronic renal failure, there is a shortened red cell survival time. Red cells, instead of surviving for their normal span of 120 days, are destroyed earlier, their premature demise being in proportion to the degree of uremia, which in turn is influenced by the adequacy or otherwise of the dialysis. In addition to these well-known causes there may be others which are peculiar to patients receiving long-term hemodialysis. An understanding of the main underlying causes as well as any additional causes helps to guide our management so that we can maintain the hemoglobin as high as possible. Let us then consider each factor in turn and work out a set of guidelines to help us to manage this problem as skillfully as we can.

Uremia

We know that uremia adversely affects every organ system in the body, and nowhere is this more important than in anemia. Adequate dialysis is fundamentally important and it has been shown that better control of uremia leads to higher levels of hemoglobin. Nowadays it has become fashionable to assess the adequacy of dialysis by urea kinetic modelling (see p.265) and undoubtedly it is an advantage to have a reliable and objective way of judging this, especially when we are so overcrowded with patients in our center hemodialysis units that everyone's time is being cut down to a minimum to make room for other patients. However, patients on home hemodialysis are not limited by such considerations and we have been impressed by the vigorous good health of some of our home hemodialysis patients who dialyse 6−7 hours three times per week compared to the 3−5 hours which is average for patients dialysing in the center. The other aspect of controlling uremia is the protein content of the diet. Most authorities recommend about 1 g of protein per kg of body weight per day. This represents adequate nutrition without pushing the predialysis urea levels too high.

The patient's remaining renal function and mass

If the patient has some residual renal function contributing to the control of uremia, this is a definite advantage, but more important even than this is the erythropoietin production from the 'end-stage' kidneys. Even though the kidneys are unable to maintain the patient without dialysis, they produce a variable but important amount of erythropoietin which helps the anemia. We know this to be true from erythropoietin assays and also from the fact that anephric patients (those who have had both kidneys removed) are always more severely anemic than those who have even one kidney remaining. Patients with polycycstic kidneys (large fleshy kidneys) nearly always have higher hemoglobins than other dialysis patients with equivalent degrees of uremia. This is almost certainly because such patients continue to produce large quantities of erythropoietin. Polycystic kidneys not infrequently cause trouble in hemodialysis patients either by bleeding or becoming infected but they should never be removed unless there is a powerful reason to do so such as recurrent, life-threatening infection, and then only the infected kidney should be removed leaving the other behind. Transplant surgeons sometimes press for removal of polycystic kidneys as preparation for a renal transplant. This should never be done except on clear-cut indications such as recurrent infection or massive size. If you do a bilateral nephrectomy in a patient with polycystic kidney disease on dialysis the hemoglobin may drop from 130 g/l to 50 g/l and this will reduce the patient from a state of vigorous good health to chronic severe disability. Thus one should always try to avoid the anephric state in a patient on long-term hemodialysis. You might argue that if the patient is having a transplant the hemoglobin is soon going to be normal anyway. But what happens if the transplant is cancelled for some reason or if it is at first successful but later fails? The patient is then back on dialysis with no kidneys and a hemoglobin of 50 g/l or less. Such patients may need transfusions every 3–4 weeks in order to remain active. This does not mean that bilateral nephrectomies should *never* be done but that they should be done only for very clear-cut and essential reasons.

Blood loss

All patients on hemodialysis have a certain minimal obligatory blood loss associated with the procedure (e.g. at the time of cannulation) and the residual blood left in the extracorporeal circuit at the end of dialysis. Also most patients have routine diagnostic blood tests once a month pre- and post-dialysis. Accidental clotting of the whole extracorporeal circuit will lead to a further large loss. The answer here is that we should be meticulously careful to avoid *any* unnecessary blood loss since repeated losses of small amounts are cumulative and become important in the long term. If severe anemia cannot be readily explained, one should always suspect the possibility of occult blood loss, especially from the gastro-intestinal tract. This can be recognized by finding occult blood in the stools. One then has to search for the source of bleeding. In recent years angiodysplasia of the colon has become increasingly recognized in older dialysis patients as a cause of recurrent serious blood loss. The diagnosis has become possible since development of improved visualization of the entire colon with the flexible fiber-optic colonoscope.

Hemolysis

Well conducted hemodialysis should not be associated with any significant hemolysis but we know from experience that minor episodes of hemolysis are very hard to detect unless one is suspicious and carries out appropriate testing. Occasionally outbreaks of severe, even life-threatening hemolysis have occurred in hemodialysis units for a variety of causes ranging from overheated dialysate to chemical contamination of the extracorporeal circuit. If hemolysis is suspected during an individual dialysis because the patient's appearance gives cause for concern or the blood returning to the patient looks odd in some way, it is a simple matter to take a blood sample and spin it down in a centrifuge. The appearance of the super-natant plasma in the centrifuge tube will give an immediate answer as to whether hemolysis has occurred or not.

Once we have excluded abnormal blood losses and hemolysis as a cause for anemia in our patient, we should make sure there are no deficiencies of hematinic factors. Vitamin B_{12} and folic acid deficiency can be excluded by simple blood tests. The best test in hemodialysis patients for determining the adequacy of iron stores is the serum ferritin. It should probably be checked in all long-term patients once every six months.

Hyperparathyroidism

It has now been demonstrated convincingly that a refractory anemia in dialysis patients may be due to hyperparathyroidism. This is usually an autonomous overactivity with hyperplasia of all four glands. The diagnosis will be suggested by the presence of a high serum calcium level even in the predialysis phase and a progressively rising alkaline phosphatase. The diagnosis can be confirmed by finding high levels of parathyroid hormone (PTH) even when the serum calcium is high. Total parathyroidectomy with a forearm implant of some parathyroid tissue is the best treatment. It will cure the bone disease and alleviate the anemia.

Possible ways of improving the hemoglobin level

The first rules which follow logically from what has already been said are:
1 Make sure the patient is very adequately dialysed.
2 Avoid any unnecessary blood loss.
3 Always try to preserve at least one kidney (preferably both) as sources of erythropoietin.
4 Use the serum ferritin assay to make sure that the patient is not iron deficient. Most patients on long-term hemodialysis need the equivalent of one 300 mg ferrous sulphate tablet per day, but it is not enough to give iron empirically. Experience has taught us that we must follow the serum ferritin level to be sure of giving enough iron as well as to avoid giving too much. It is now agreed that oral iron is as effective as parenteral iron in hemodialysis patients so there is no reason any longer to give iron by injection. Once we have done these four things and the patient is still symptomatically anemic, there is only one sure way to raise the hemoglobin and this is by transfusion of packed red blood cells.

Patients who are likely to get too much iron are those who receive very regular transfusions. They may develop a condition known as transfusion hemosiderosis. This mainly leads to excessive iron deposition in the liver and in cardiac muscle.

Blood transfusion is still a controversial topic and requires some knowledge of the dangers as well as the advantages.

The pros and cons of blood transfusion

A transfusion of packed red blood cells, best carried out during dialysis with blood crossmatched from a sample taken during the previous dialysis, is usually given 2−4 units at a time, and it will raise the hemoglobin about 10 g/l for each unit transfused. It will instantly relieve symptoms due to anemia and many patients on dialysis could not manage without it. The other advantage it has is that for some immunological reason, not as yet fully understood, it reduces the chances of rejection if the patient subsequently receives a kidney transplant. This is sufficiently well established that all patients being prepared for renal transplantation now receive an arbitrary number of blood transfusions whether or not they need them to correct anemia. This has become standard procedure. The only issue which remains to be settled is the optimum number of transfusions and this is likely to remain vague. What are the disadvantages of blood transfusions? Apart from the obvious comment that blood is an expensive commodity in short supply which should not be wasted, there are a number of other penalties or at least potential problems.

1 Every blood transfusion is a potential vehicle for the transmission of hepatitis virus. Screening all blood for hepatitis B can effectively eliminate this source, but there is as yet no marker for non-A non-B hepatitis and this can be a moderately serious illness. It is likely that cases of non-A non-B hepatitis are introduced into dialysis units fairly regularly by blood transfusions. There is also a theoretical danger of transmitting the acquired immune deficiency syndrome (AIDS) in this way. As yet there is no recorded case of this having happened in a hemodialysis patient but hemophiliacs have acquired AIDS from transfused blood products, so the risk is there, albeit exceedingly small.

2 Blood transfusions, especially in large numbers, lead to the development of cytotoxic antibodies in the transfused recipient. These are antibodies against certain foreign proteins such as the tissues of a potential kidney donor. If a patient on dialysis develops a high percentage of antibodies (reactive against a large percentage of potential donors) it will become progressively difficult to find a donor against whom he does not have antibodies. It is a golden rule of renal transplantation that one never transplants a kidney in the presence of a positive cytotoxic crossmatch test. On the other hand some people believe that development of these cytotoxic antibodies is useful in revealing those donors whose kidneys would be rejected anyway.

3 Some hemodialysis patients who are transfused regularly develop anti-red cell antibodies and these may make it progressively difficult to find compatible blood for them.

4 Finally, as has been said, there is the potential danger of transfusion hemosiderosis. Serum ferritin levels will give warning of this and will reveal those patients who already have large iron stores. These patients should not be given oral iron supplements.

Hypersplenism

This means development of an enlarged spleen which causes an increased destruction of all the main formed elements of the blood—red cells, white cells and platelets. Diminished numbers of all these types of cells is called pancytopenia. The condition is usually detected by being able to palpate the spleen in a patient on dialysis who has pancytopenia. If the splenic sequestration (removal and destruction) of cells is severe enough, the patient may benefit from splenectomy. However, splenectomy leads to an increased risk of developing pneumococcal infection which may be sudden, unpredictable and fatal. Now fortunately there is a pneumococcal vaccine available which is almost completely effective in preventing pneumococcal infection. It should be given prophylactically to all patients in whom splenectomy is planned.

Anabolic steroids

Androgens (male sex hormones) have been known for many years to have an effect in stimulating the bone marrow of patients with renal failure, probably by stimulating the production of erythropoietin in what remains of the kidney tissue still making erythropoietin. Unfortunately there is almost no detectable effect in anephric patients, who are the ones in most trouble from anemia. A controlled trial has shown that intramuscular injections of nandrolone decanoate or testosterone enanthate are more effective than oral fluoxymesterone or oxymethalone. These drugs should probably be reserved for patients who still have their (one or both) kidneys in place but who remain symptomatically anemic. Courses of treatment should probably be restricted to about six months to avoid side-effects and also because the benefit seems to persist for some time even after the drugs are stopped. Prolonged treatment with anabolic steroids for many years can lead to the development of tumors, especially adenomas of the liver.

Cobalt therapy

Cobalt in the form of cobaltous chloride, given orally, stimulates erythro-poiesis and raises the hemoglobin to a variable degree but it is generally agreed to be too toxic to be worth the risk. Cardiac toxicity in the form of a cardiomyopathy is the most worrying complication. It is therefore no longer used.*

---

*At the time of going to press we learn that synthetic erythropoietin will soon be available as an intravenous injection for patients suffering from the anemia of renal failure. Initial clinical trials have shown dramatic benefit with return to normal hemo-globins even in anephric patients. If these initial results are an indication of sustained future benefit, then this advance will revolutionize the quality of life of many thousands of patients.

Dialysis bone disease

Renal bone disease can be best understood by considering the abnormalities of vitamin D, calcium and phosphate metabolism present in patients with chronic renal failure.

Vitamin D metabolism

This fat-soluble vitamin is made available to the body to a large extent through the action of ultraviolet sunlight on certain cholesterol compounds of the skin and to a lesser extent by diet. Cholecalciferol (vitamin D_3) is produced in the skin and is then transported to the liver where it is turned into 25-hydroxycholecalciferol. This metabolite is then transported to the kidney where it is hydroxylated further to 1,25-dihydroxycholecalciferol. The diagram (Fig. 8.1) below shows the series of events.

1,25-dihydroxycholecalciferol is the most active and potent metabolite of vitamin D currently known. It is produced only by functioning kidney tissue. It acts on the intestine by promoting calcium absorption and it is essential for normal bone maturation and mineralization. Deficiency of this compound in children results in rickets.

In renal failure there is a block in the conversion of 25-hydroxycholecalciferol to 1,25-dihydroxycholecalciferol. Deficiency of this active metabolite is responsible for most of the bone problems we encounter in uremia. If chronic renal failure is not too advanced the block in vitamin D metabolism is not complete. There are now several vitamin D preparations available.

Vitamin D_2 (ergocalciferol) is the standard vitamin D preparation used in most centers. Its effect depends on the ability of the liver and kidneys to turn it into more active metabolites. Therefore its use in renal failure

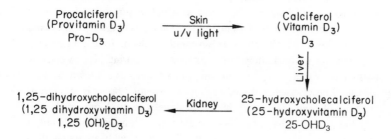

Fig. 8.1. The metabolism of vitamin D.

is rather limited. Nonetheless, it can be used in pre-dialysis renal failure patients where some conversion into more active compounds takes place. The dosage is of the order of 50 000—100 000 units orally daily.

DHT (dihydrotachysterol) is a synthetic vitamin D metabolite which is more active than ergocalciferol because it has some structural similarities to the active metabolite produced by the kidney. It can be used both in pre-dialysis and dialysis patients but its value again is limited.

1-a-OHD3 (1-alpha-hydroxycholecalciferol) is a synthetic vitamin D compound which has been specifically designed to by-pass the renal block encountered in uremia. It is a very effective drug and corrects both the malabsorption of calcium and the mineralization defects found in uremia. It has a short half-life and is, therefore, easy to use. The dose is 1—3 µg orally daily.

1,25-dihydroxycholecalciferol. This vitamin D metabolite has been synthesized and is now available commercially under the trade name of Rocaltrol or Calcitriol. It is very widely used in dialysis patients and the usual dose is about 0.25 µg daily. It is very effective in all patients with chronic renal failure and end-stage renal failure. It corrects the intestinal malabsorption of calcium, promotes healing of osteomalacic fractures and reverses the changes of osteitis fibrosa caused by secondary hyperparathyroidism.

Calcium and phosphorus metabolism

The skeleton is the biggest store of calcium and phosphate in the body. In situations where there is a tendency for the plasma calcium to fall, calcium is released from the skeleton to the circulation in an attempt to keep plasma calcium constant. This process is mediated by parathyroid hormone.

In renal failure, malabsorption of calcium, chronic metabolic acidosis and retention of phosphate all lead to a fall in serum calcium and this stimulates the parathyroid glands to secrete excess parathyroid hormone. This is known as secondary hyperparathyroidism. It is a physiological response but unfortunately in the process of restoring plasma calcium to normal it erodes the skeleton and the changes are known as osteitis fibrosa. The classical radiological sign of osteitis fibrosa is subperiosteal erosions of bone, best seen in the phalanges in an X-ray of the hands (see Fig. 8.2). But bone biopsy is an even more sensitive and reliable way of confirming the diagnosis. Nearly all patients who approach dialysis have a degree of secondary hyperparathyroidism, as shown by the results

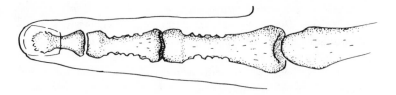

Fig. 8.2. Sub-periosteal erosions in osteitis fibrosa shown in an X-ray of the finger.

of bone biopsies. This in itself is not very dangerous but unfortunately as calcium is mobilized from the skeleton it occasionally gets deposited in arteries and soft tissues. Because of this complication an attempt is made to control this secondary hyperparathyroidism. In clinical practice one uses phosphate binders such as aluminum hydroxide to lower and control serum phosphate, thus removing one of the stimuli to secondary hyper-parathyroidism. It is worth noting that perhaps the best way to suppress osteitis fibrosa is to give active vitamin D such as 1-a-OHD3 or 1,25-dihydroxy vitamin D which rapidly corrects any secondary hyperparathyroidism present.

Clinical problems

(a) Pre-dialysis

Pre-dialysis renal patients do not usually have troublesome bone problems. There is a progressive secondary hyperparathyroidism in an attempt to maintain the serum calcium within normal limits but this usually does not produce many problems apart from occasional vascular and soft tissue calcification.

There are two well defined groups of pre-dialysis patients that require special care.

1 Growing children Children with chronic uremia tend to develop 'uremic rickets'. This is at a time when their vitamin D requirements are at a maximum and their failing kidneys cannot cope. The best treatment is adequate vitamin D replacement. DHT in a dose of 0.5 mg daily, or, better still, 1-a-OHD3 in a dose of 2 or 3 μg daily, is effective in improving the radiological and histological abnormalities. It is also important to correct any acidosis present, using sodium bicarbonate supplements. Aluminum hydroxide and other phosphate binders may be dangerous by lowering plasma phosphate too much.

   2 Patients with marked tubular problems and disproportionate metabolic acidosis Patients with ileal conduits, ureterocolic anastomosis, analgesic nephropathies and chronic reflux pyelonephritis tend to have marked metabolic acidosis. Perhaps for this reason they have a higher incidence of osteomalacic bone disease with fractures of bones, pain and muscle weakness. These patients develop bone problems when their renal failure is only mild. Muscle weakness, bone pain and fractures are not uncommon. Serum calcium falls and serum alkaline phosphatase rises sharply. Treatment is correction of the acidosis and adequate replacement of vitamin D. It needs to be continued for a long time. All patients treated with any of the vitamin D compounds must have their serum calcium checked regularly because if the calcium goes too high it will damage renal function.

(b) Patients on regular hemodialysis

Significant bone disease can now be avoided in the vast majority of patients on long-term hemodialysis. The main breakthrough came with the discovery of aluminum toxicity as the cause of most of the severe dialysis bone disease which we used to see years ago. It now seems clear that in the early days, when water for dialysis was not adequately purified by de-ionization or reverse osmosis, the aluminum in untreated water supplies crossed the dialysis membrane and gradually accumulated in the patient's body. As time went by it caused a progressive, vitamin D resistant osteomalacia. It usually started with pain in the feet, later spreading to affect other parts of the body. Muscles became stiff and weak and pathological fractures would start to occur, especially fractured ribs. Some patients became so bad that they were confined to wheelchairs. One of our early patients had such disintegration of his skeleton that his whole thoracic cage collapsed and he eventually died of cardiopulmonary failure. This should never happen again in the future. With adequate purification of water for dialysis aluminum toxicity of a degree to cause clinical symptoms or disability should never occur. A number of authorities have demonstrated undesirable amounts of aluminum being absorbed via the gastro-intestinal tract from aluminum containing phosphate binders. We ourselves had never seen a convincing case of aluminum toxicity from this cause until recently when we discovered that one of our patients had developed severe fracturing osteomalacia. She had several cracked ribs and severe back pain due to osteomalacia. The blood aluminum level was very high and large amounts of aluminum were found in her bone biopsy. She had never been exposed to aluminum in her dialysate and the assumption is that she must have acquired the toxicity from aluminum hydroxide which she had been taking orally in standard doses. She is now being treated with desferrioxamine to remove the aluminum from her body during each dialysis. Why some patients absorb toxic amounts of aluminum from the GI tract and others do not is still not clear but the lessons we have learned from this are:

1 Aluminum toxicity should be suspected in any patient developing vitamin D resistant osteomalacia while on dialysis if he or she is taking aluminum hydroxide regularly.

2 All patients taking aluminum hydroxide regularly while on dialysis should have the blood level checked from time to time, perhaps once every six months.

3 The search must continue for an alternative method for keeping down the serum phosphate level. Magnesium compounds can reduce phosphate absorption but magnesium causes troublesome diarrhea and if magnesium is absorbed in large amounts it can itself cause toxicity. High blood magnesium levels cause muscle weakness and eventually paralysis. This can be partially offset by lowering the magnesium concentration of dialysis fluid but then one has a balancing act in which the magnesium may also go too low. Low serum magnesium levels can cause cardiac arrhythmias. To put all this in perspective it should be acknowledged that most well cared for dialysis patients do not get any significant bone disease. The principles of correct management are as follows.

Firstly, the plasma phosphate is kept down (less than 2 mmol/l) in the pre-dialysis blood tests by adequate dialysis and by attention to restricting phosphate in the diet. Unfortunately phosphate is almost ubiquitous and the best one can do is to avoid high phosphate foods, especially some cheeses, such as cheddar. The next step is to use calcium carbonate, as much as 5 grams with each meal. This binds phosphate but may make the patient hypercalcemic and this may limit its use. Magnesium hydroxide may be tolerated in limited amounts but its use will be limited by its tendency to cause diarrhea. A mixture of magnesium hydroxide and aluminum hydroxide may be satisfactory and in many patients it seems necessary to give some aluminum hydroxide, but always the aim is to give as little aluminum as possible and only with meals which include phosphate. It is pointless, for example, to take aluminum hydroxide at breakfast time if breakfast consists of nothing more than a cup of coffee.

Secondly, the serum calcium is maintained at a level close to the normal range by administration of a vitamin D metabolite. Without vitamin D most hemodialysis patients are hypocalcemic. Dihydrotachysterol (DHT), 1-alpha-hydroxycholecalciferol and 1,25-dihydroxycholecalciferol are all effective and have their advocates. But one should stop short of making patients hypercalcemic before dialysis. The aim should be for the calcium to be slightly below normal before dialysis and somewhat above normal post-dialysis. In this way the median plasma calcium level, that is the average throughout the week, will be approximately normal. The alkaline phosphatase is also a good indicator of bone health. A high level is suggestive of either osteomalacia or osteitis fibrosa. Another cause of osteomalacia in patients on regular dialysis is the consumption of phenobarbitone and other anticonvulsants such as phenytoin sodium. These drugs interfere with vitamin D metabolism in the liver. They should therefore only be given if they are absolutely necessary. If they are needed by the patient it may be necessary to give extra vitamin D to make sure the patient has enough.

Autonomous hyperparathyroidism

It has been said already that various factors in chronic and end-stage renal failure combine to stimulate the parathyroids to produce parathyroid hormone (PTH) in large amounts. High levels of PTH lead to bony demineralization and a rise in the level of alkaline phosphatase. Skeletal X-rays, especially the hands, show the typical subperiosteal erosions. In order to suppress PTH one should try to maintain the serum calcium close to the normal range with a vitamin D preparation, keep the phosphate down as described above, and make sure the patient is well dialysed. Unfortunately this strategy may be frustrated if the parathyroids develop an autonomous overactivity which cannot be suppressed. This will become evident if it is seen that the serum calcium remains high even in the absence of vitamin D, the alkaline phosphatase rises progressively, and the serum PTH level is high even in the presence of a high serum calcium. Then you know that all four parathyroid glands have become hyperplastic and the only cure is a total parathyroidectomy. Under the same anesthetic a portion of one gland is implanted subcutaneously on the anterior aspect of the forearm. This will give the patient *some* intrinsic parathyroid hormone production but if it later becomes too much it is an easy matter to remove the excess from the new implantation site in the forearm. It is difficult and dangerous to go back into the neck a second time to remove a parathyroid remnant. The main danger is accidental section of the recurrent laryngeal nerve which will give the patient a permanently hoarse voice.

The operation of total parathyroidectomy and forearm implantation is almost uniformly successful if performed for the right reasons by a skilled surgeon. Very occasionally there is an extra parathyroid gland in a retrosternal position and this may necessitate a second operation to explore the area behind the sternum. Following total parathyroidectomy in a patient with severe osteitis fibrosa, there is usually a precipitous fall in serum calcium. This is because calcium starts rapidly entering bone in a process of remineralization. The serum calcium level has to be checked frequently and large amounts of calcium may have to be given intravenously for the first few days. Later the serum calcium level can again be maintained by giving one of the synthetic vitamin D metabolites.

If a patient has this syndrome of autonomous hyperparathyroidism while on hemodialysis it should be dealt with before the patient has a kidney transplant. After renal transplantation it has a tendency to get worse rapidly. You may then be faced with having to do an emergency total parathyroidectomy because of severe hypercalcemia in a patient on immunosuppressive drugs—not a good thing to have to do in the first few weeks after a transplant.

Fortunately all other forms of renal bone disease tend to improve rapidly after transplantation. The only bony complication which seems to be brought on by renal transplantation is a condition called avascular necrosis. This lesion affects mainly the head of the femur and the upper end of the tibia but it can also occur in one of the bones of the ankle. It is thought to be due to cutting off the blood supply to an area of bone supplied by one end-artery. Once the bone is devascularized it dies and becomes unusually dense or 'sclerotic' and it collapses to cause a long-standing painful condition complicated by osteoarthritis. When it affects the head of the femur it may be so painful that the diseased femoral head may have to be removed and replaced with a prosthetic one. Avascular necrosis of bone is associated with high steroid doses after renal transplantation. Now that steroid doses are being reduced, happily the incidence of avascular necrosis is declining. In our center we now hardly ever see it.

Pruritus

When pruritus occurs in patients with kidney disease it is usually generalized (all over the body) and it is usually due to uncontrolled uremia in patients who are approaching end-stage renal failure. When dialysis is started the pruritus rapidly gets better. If it does not get better it may mean that dialysis is not adequate. Certainly the vast majority of well dialysed patients do not have a problem with itching. However, as in all other areas of medical management, one should not jump to conclusions too hastily. It is important not to miss other causes such as drug eruptions, scabies, an occult candidiasis or even a contact dermatitis. Once these have been ruled out and the patient still has pruritus in spite of adequate dialysis (and good control of uremia) one should look for the possibility of soft-tissue calcification. This tends to occur when the product of serum calcium and serum phosphate is too high. Many a case of pruritus has been cured by bringing these down to normal levels. When all these causes have been eliminated one is left with coping with the problem. A few measures, although they can be credited with very little scientific rationale, may help in an individual case.

• Some patients claim to obtain relief from taking oral antihistamines such as hydroxyzine HCl 5–10 mg three times per day.

• Induction of sweating by saunas may be beneficial.

• Cholestyramine, which seems to benefit the pruritus from which jaundiced patients suffer, may occasionally be helpful in renal failure.

• The use of a bath oil to correct undue dryness of the skin may help a bit.

• Some authorities have advocated a low magnesium dialysate. We have tried this in some patients with resistant pruritus and found it to be singularly ineffective. What is more, there is a disconcerting tendency to cardiac arrhythmias in patients treated with a very low magnesium dialysate. The treatment in this case seemed to be worse than the disease.

We have never known a case of chronic pruritus that did not clear up when the patient received a successful kidney transplant.

Loss of sexual function

As the more serious and life-threatening problems in patients with renal failure are being effectively managed we are able to turn our attention to less life-threatening but nevertheless distressing symptoms such as loss of libido and sexual function. Unfortunately for male patients on hemodialysis, impotence is very common. Female patients frequently have amenorrhea and most of them have decreased libido. Perhaps because the male partner in any normal heterosexual relationship is the one who actually has to produce a performance by achieving an erection, it is the males among our dialysis patients who are most vocal in their complaints. And even they do not complain spontaneously because of their natural reticence. When asked most will admit that all is not well. What is known about the pathophysiology of this problem? We know that sexual function is a delicate mechanism at the best of times even in healthy people. Tiredness, lack of sleep, anxiety over one's work or one's bank balance, or simply fear of failure can all cause temporary impotence. Good sexual function thrives best in a well rested, relaxed and vigorously healthy body. Uremia adversely affects every organ system in the body and the reproductive organs are no exception. It has been shown that testosterone production is reduced in men on dialysis and the testes have a tendency to shrink progressively. Some patients respond to treatment with a male hormone preparation. Excessive prolactin production adversely affects potency and there is frequently excessive prolactin production in uremia. The drug bromocriptine, a prolactin antagonist, has been advocated for impotence in men on dialysis. In our experience there are no noticeable benefits but plenty of undesirable side-effects. Hypotensive drugs, except perhaps the beta-blockers, all interfere with potency, and many patients are regularly on antihypertensives.

Finally subclinical zinc deficiency is common in dialysis patients and zinc in trace amounts is necessary for normal testicular function. Our clinical impression is that some male patients benefit from zinc adminis- tration (e.g. zinc gluconate 10 mg orally daily) but it is by no means universally successful. It is probably worthy of a therapeutic trial in all males who show any interest in receiving help.

Recently it has been shown that organic impotence which becomes commoner as males get older may sometimes be due to narrowing of the arteries which supply the penis, with a consequent reduction in penile arterial pressure compared with systemic blood pressure. Impotence in these patients is more common in those who have arterial risk factors, namely diabetes, smoking, hyperlipidemia and hypertension. We know that chronic and end-stage renal failure are also arterial risk factors. Perhaps the premature atheroma of long-standing renal failure is an additional reason.

A successful renal transplant is very good for sexual function in both males and females, but contrary to popular belief not all males regain their prowess even after this. A return to normal should not be assumed or taken for granted. Patients may still have problems and may still need help. The management of impotence in these patients is highly specialized work and ideally all patients should receive the benefit of the best opinion if they need it. Happily the discussion of sexual problems with patients is no longer taboo. If it can be talked about openly but with sensitivity we have a chance to help patients who might otherwise not have the courage to ask.

Polyneuritis

Long-standing uremia sometimes leads to the development of a sym- metrical peripheral neuritis mainly affecting the feet and legs. Pins and needles and loss of sensation are later followed by loss of power with foot-drop. Loss of vibration sense is often the first sign. Nerve conduction studies are not only useful in detecting the early case but are also an excellent objective way of assessing progress when they are carried out serially. Development of polyneuritis in a patient with chronic renal failure may be an additional reason for starting dialysis as soon as possible because the longer dialysis is postponed the harder it will be to cure the polyneuritis by dialysis and/or renal transplantation. It has been observed that polyneuritis may deteriorate acutely when dialysis is first started but usually gradually improves thereafter if thoroughly adequate dialysis is continued. If there is no polyneuritis when regular dialysis is started there should certainly be no polyneuritis thereafter. If polyneuritis develops for the first time in a patient on long-term dialysis it is almost certainly a sign of inadequate dialysis. We used to see it in some patients on long-term intermittent peritoneal dialysis and it always improved when the patients were switched to a program of really adequate hemodialysis. It gets better even faster after a successful renal transplant.

Except in diabetics, polyneuritis is a relatively uncommon condition in most large renal centers. We think this is because patients start on dialysis earlier than they used to and dialysis is so much better than it used to be. Diabetics with renal failure are unfortunate in having two causes for polyneuritis—diabetes and uremia. These causes compound each other. Most diabetics by the time they reach end-stage renal failure have polyneuritis and some are so disabled that they can hardly walk. Renal transplantation is dramatically effective in improving the condition. Good blood glucose control is the other important aspect of management.

Polyneuritis can also be caused by deficiency of the vitamin thiamine. From this fact has arisen the notion that thiamine is good for polyneuritis and, since water-soluble vitamins including the B complex are removed by dialysis, it may seem logical to give extra thiamine to patients on dialysis who have polyneuritis. However, as far as we know there is no evidence that extra thiamine improves the polyneuritis of uremia unless there is a deficiency. All patients on long-term hemodialysis should receive daily supplements of the water-soluble vitamins, the B complex and vitamin C. Additional thiamine over and above this is probably quite unnecessary but it is also probably harmless.

Insomnia

Chronic renal failure in undialysed patients is usually associated with drowsiness and an increased requirement for sleep. These symptoms may continue once a patient is receiving regular dialysis but it is more common for patients on regular dialysis to complain of insomnia. They may have difficulty getting to sleep and may also be restless during the night, sleeping for only short periods, and then lying awake tossing and turning. The commonest cause for this insomnia is inadequate dialysis and it is often accompanied by the syndrome of restless legs. Sometimes this takes the form of nocturnal myoclonic jerks, a phenomenon that we have all experienced from time to time but which may become frequent and obtrusive in patients on dialysis. The first thing to ask oneself is whether the patient needs more dialysis and usually he does. However, if insomnia remains troublesome even in the presence of extremely adequate dialysis, one should wonder about the possibility that it may be caused by depression. Endogenous depression can occur in dialysis patients as much as in anyone else and it requires the same treatment. Tricyclic antidepressant drugs are very effective in patients on regular dialysis. A particularly useful drug in this group, partly because it is hypnotic in its effects, is trimipramine 25−50 mg taken at bedtime. All tricyclic antidepressants have a potential for causing cardiac arrhythmias so one has to be careful especially in patients with abnormal hearts. The best and most harmless straight hypnotics are the benzodiazepines such as diazepam (Valium), nitrazepam (Mogadon) and lorazepam (Ativan). The last of these is attractive because of its short duration of action and lack of hangover. Barbiturates have been largely abandoned all over the world as hypnotics and rightly so. They are particularly undesirable in patients on dialysis because they interfere with vitamin D metabolism and tend to last too long, making patients drowsy during the day. They have been known to cause a kind of cumulative toxicity because of lack of renal excretion. They should never be used in dialysis patients unless they are absolutely essential for anticonvulsant purposes.

Muscle cramps

Felt as an agonizingly painful spasm, most often in the calf muscles, but sometimes in the arch of the foot, muscle cramps are nearly always a sign of sodium deficiency. They occur during dialysis when sodium is being removed too fast and they commonly wake patients from sleep on the night after dialysis. There is an immediate compelling need to stretch the muscle to break the spasm. This can be done by a nurse or a spouse. Forceful dorsiflexion of the foot will overcome a calf muscle cramp. Prevention depends on avoiding sodium depletion. We have found that cramps have become less common since we raised the dialysate sodium concentration from 135 to 138 mmol/l. However, increasing the body sodium content may cause a rise in systemic blood pressure. Like everything else in renal failure, it is a delicate balancing act. If cramps are still troublesome even after correction of sodium deficiency, the best prevention is to take a tablet of quinine sulphate 300 mg. This should be given before dialysis if cramps tend to occur on dialysis or at bedtime if cramps tend to occur at night. One tablet a day is usually entirely effective and seems completely harmless. A deliberate overdose of quinine will cause blindness but this can be quickly and effectively reversed by hemodialysis.

Chronic subdural hematoma

Occasionally a patient on regular hemodialysis will begin to complain of persistent headaches, often on one side of the head, associated with periods of drowsiness and mental confusion, even stupor. The impaired level of consciousness may be fluctuating in type and often apparently aggravated by dialysis. In such a patient, particularly if he or she is elderly or hypertensive, one should suspect the possibility of a spontaneous subdural hematoma. The importance of diagnosing it accurately and quickly is that it is eminently treatable by a small neurosurgical operation to evacuate the clot. Diagnosis nowadays is made easy by the widespread availability of the CAT scanner (computer assisted tomography). If the condition is not suspected it may well cause sudden death on dialysis after a period of increasingly severe symptoms.

9

Management of Poisoning

Robert Uldall

A discussion of this topic in a textbook on renal nursing is justified by the fact that renal nurses are not infrequently involved in helping to save the lives of the most severely affected patients. The special techniques of hemodialysis and hemoperfusion are employed in a very small minority of all the poisoned patients for whom we have to take responsibility; but if we use these methods we should also have a good grasp of the simple methods which should be used first. For example we have no business to be carrying out hemodialysis for a severe case of aspirin poisoning until thorough gastric lavage has removed all the aspirin which may still be in the patient's stomach.

Similarly, we should not be so preoccupied with extracorporeal methods to remove a drug that in the meantime we allow the patient to die of inadequate ventilation. Overwhelmingly the most important impact that has been made on the morbidity and mortality of drug overdose has been achieved by simple methods of general medical support. Nurses may be involved in any of these procedures, from the most simple to the most complex.

Apart from one or two rare and dramatic examples, all poisons and overdoses of drugs are self-administered. An impressive reduction in the incidence of drug overdoses in children has been achieved in most advanced societies by the simple expedient of insisting on the use of childproof caps on all containers for tablets and pills.

Similarly the mortality from overdoses of sleeping pills has declined sharply since barbiturates have virtually disappeared to be replaced by the benzodiazepines. Benzodiazepines such as diazepam (Valium) and nitrazepam (Mogadon) are not harmless but they cause so little respiratory depression that successful suicide from overdoses of this group of drugs is rare.

The methods by which people attempt to commit suicide are largely dependent on availability. This is why coal-gas poisoning has become largely a phenomenon of historical interest, and glutethimide (Doriden), an extremely dangerous hypnotic, hardly ever causes death now because it is no longer used. Aspirin and aceteminophen (Paracetemol, Tylenol) are still widely used for suicidal purposes simply because they are readily available. The same applies to tricyclic antidepressants because so many people have them in their medicine cabinets. Simple household agents such as windshield fluid (methyl alcohol) and antifreeze (ethylene glycol) are also commonly used because every household has them.

However, because people at times of intolerable distress may ingest anything which comes to hand, we have to be prepared for a wide variety of agents. All over the world a series of Poison Information Centers have sprung up. These agencies are often a mine of useful information and the best of them provide a 24 hour service to give emergency advice by telephone.

In this short chapter we confine ourselves to practical tips on the main methods employed in the management of poisoning and an enunciation of some of the principles which help to determine which methods are likely to be useful in a particular case. Before we consider the special techniques it is worth emphasizing that a good deal of time may have to be spent on finding out as accurately as possible what the patient actually took and when. We should not be afraid of causing inconvenience to friends, relatives, the patient's pharmacist and the police in order to get an accurate description of what was actually ingested. Occasionally this may be impossible and we may have to depend on other clues. For example, blurred vision in the presence of a metabolic acidosis suggests methyl alcohol poisoning. There may still be time to save the patient's eyesight and his brain if the correct diagnosis leads to the correct treatment. Most urban centers now have a laboratory which provides a 24 hour service called a drug screen. Samples of blood and gastric washings are analysed for a wide range of common drugs and poisons. Once the drug or poison is identified it is often possible to obtain an accurate blood level. This in turn will help us to decide what measures need to be taken.

The techniques which have to be considered are:
1 Emetics to induce vomiting

2 Gastric lavage
3 Antidotes
4 Assisted ventilation
5 Alkaline diuresis
6 Exchange transfusion
7 Dialysis
8 Hemoperfusion

Emetics to induce vomiting

This method should probably be reserved for less serious cases of poisoning in children. On occasion it may be justified to give an emetic to a child who is wide awake and apprehensive rather than force him during an undignified struggle to accept a wide-bore stomach tube.

For all other cases we have to accept that gastric lavage is more efficient and more reliable and achieves more complete emptying of the stomach. Furthermore all emetics are toxic substances and it goes against logic to give a toxic substance to someone who is already poisoned.

Gastric lavage

As a general rule, all poisoned patients should have gastric lavage to remove from the stomach any unabsorbed remnants of pills or tablets. Obviously the chance of retrieving liquids, which will be absorbed very quickly, is much less than the chance of retrieving solids which stay in the stomach for a long time. Gastric lavage should *always* be performed in *every* case of aspirin poisoning regardless of when the aspirin was taken. Aspirin may be present in a solid mass in the stomach even 24 hours after ingestion.

There are some rules to be remembered when carrying out gastric lavage.
• Lavage requires a wide-bore, soft rubber tube inserted through the mouth—not a fine nasogastric tube. The lumen must be large enough for a whole aspirin tablet to be washed through it.
• There is no advantage in using anything other than warm water from the tap, unless the poison is lipid soluble, in which case castor oil should be present in equal quantities.
• The patient should always be prone with the head lower than the pelvis. This will discourage inhalation of vomit into the lungs. Suction apparatus should always be available.
• If the patient is unconscious or sufficiently obtunded that there is no

gag reflex, a cuffed endotracheal tube should be inserted before the stomach tube is put down. This will protect the airways.

• Never perform gastric lavage if a highly corrosive poison such as hypochlorite or mercuric chloride has been ingested. There is a danger of causing further damage to mucous membranes or even perforation of the esophagus.

• Always keep a sample of the gastric washings for chemical analysis.

• Once the washings are clear and you are sure the stomach is empty, put 50 g of activated charcoal into the stomach. This may adsorb significant amounts of the drug to prevent absorption into the bloodstream. The only exception to this would be if you are giving an antidote by the gastric route. There is no point in adsorbing the antidote.

Antidotes

In the majority of cases of drug intoxication there are no known antidotes but it is important to be aware of the few which may be life-saving. Table 9.1 shows the best known antidotes together with their indications for use.

The greatest danger from the opium group of drugs is suppression of respiration. One forgets that innocuous sounding drugs such as Distalgesic in UK and Darvon in North America contain dextropropoxyphene, which is an opioid. They have caused numerous deaths because they are so readily available and overdoses can so easily suppress respiration. Naloxone is almost magically effective in reversing this respiratory suppression. It should be given even on suspicion and may be helpful as a diagnostic test in cases of doubt.

The epidemic of deaths from acetaminophen overdoses in the UK is largely the result of the wholesale substitution of this drug for aspirin. To some extent the same thing has happened in North America. Death occurs from liver necrosis about three days after ingestion. *N*-acetyl cysteine prevents liver damage if it can be given within 8−15 hours of the ingestion. After this it is usually too late. In the form of 'Mucormist' it can be given orally or intravenously. It is logical to use charcoal orally to adsorb the drug and Mucormist intravenously to prevent liver damage.

One of the most tragic forms of poisoning is that caused by methyl alcohol, present in many freely available household agents such as windshield fluid, fondue fuel, paint diluent, and several others. This alcohol is relatively harmless, having the same intoxicating effects as ethyl alcohol, until it is metabolized by the liver to formaldehyde and formic acid.

Table 9.1. Well-known poisons and their antidotes

Drug or poison	Antidote
Opiates morphine heroin pethidine pentazocine propoxyphene codeine	naloxone (Narcan)
Acetaminophen paracetamol tylenol	*N*-acetyl cysteine (Mucormist)
Methyl alcohol Ethylene glycol	ethyl alcohol
Mercuric chloride	dimercaprol (British anti-lewisite BAL)
Iron (ferrous sulphate, gluconate, fumarate, etc.) Aluminum	desferrioxamine (Desferal)
Copper	penicillamine
Lead	ethylene diamine tetracetic acid (EDTA)
Cyanide	amyl nitrite sodium nitrite sodium thiosulphate cobalt edetate

Formaldehyde is exquisitely toxic to the optic nerves, causing blindness, and to the cerebral hemispheres, causing brain destruction. The breakdown of methyl alcohol by the liver can be completely prevented by prior or simultaneous ingestion of ethyl alcohol since the alcohol dehydrogenase system of the liver has a 20 times greater affinity for ethyl alcohol than for methyl alcohol. Many alcoholic derelicts roaming the streets of large urban centers all over the world know that they can safely supplement their drinking with small amounts of 'methylated spirits' provided that they always keep drinking plenty of proper booze as well. Although most deaths from methyl alcohol are deliberate suicide, accidents have happened when irresponsible and ignorant people have used this agent without knowledge of what it can do. Ethyl alcohol will keep such patients safe until the methyl alcohol is either expired by the lungs (70%), excreted by the kidneys (30%), or removed by dialysis. Ten millilitres of methyl alcohol, unprotected by ethyl alcohol, is enough to cause complete and permanent blindness. Many patients could be saved if the value of this antidote were more widely known. Ethyl alcohol is an equally effective antidote in cases of poisoning by ethylene glycol, the main constituent of most commercial preparations of radiator antifreeze. Ethylene glycol is also a simple intoxicant until it is broken down by the liver to oxalic acid. Oxalic acid in high concentrations damages the renal tubules and can cause acute and even permanent renal failure. Again the correct treatment is alcohol plus hemodialysis. The ethyl alcohol blood level can be maintained during dialysis by putting ethanol into the dialysate in the concentration which is optimal to protect the patient.

Space does not allow discussion of all the possible antidotes but hospital emergency departments should have all the main antidotes easily available and this kind of information prominently displayed.

Assisted ventilation

In cases of poisoning the adequacy of ventilation is not closely related to the level of consciousness. Some drugs paralyse respiration at an early stage and some patients seem more susceptible than others, so keep a close eye on the breathing. If breathing stops give artificial respiration—either mouth to mouth or with an airway and an Ambu bag if this is available. The patient will need an endotracheal tube and a ventilator. The adequacy of ventilation should be assessed by arterial blood gas estimation since it is very hard to judge clinically.

Alkaline diuresis

The majority of drugs and poisons are removed from the body at least to some extent by way of the kidneys. The excretion of certain drugs, especially phenobarbitone and salicylates, can be significantly speeded up by making the urine alkaline. This is the basis of alkaline diuresis.

To carry out alkaline diuresis the patient must have an intravenous infusion erected as quickly as possible. An indwelling bladder catheter is an essential requirement so that the urine flow rate can be accurately measured and the pH continually monitored. The choice of electrolyte solution is an individual matter for the medical staff. The aim used to be to provide a balanced combination of sodium chloride and water to produce a urine flow rate of at least 500 ml/hour for an average adult. If alkalinization of the urine is intended sodium bicarbonate is incorporated into the regimen. A commonly employed scheme is 0.9% sodium chloride, 5% dextrose and 2.4% sodium bicarbonate used in cyclical rotation.

Intravenous mannitol was traditionally used to obtain a good diuresis but has been shown to have no advantage over furosemide which is considerably safer. Mannitol may occasionally precipitate pulmonary edema by causing undue plasma volume expansion. Furosemide can be injected into the tubing at intervals. If the patient's cardiovascular state gives cause for anxiety it is probably wise to have a central venous pressure catheter in place. This simple device, which measures the pressure in the right atrium of the heart in centimetres of water, provides warning of impending overhydration and serves as a guide to the rate of infusion that the patient will tolerate. As the diuresis proceeds the patient may become hypokalemic from urinary potassium loss so that potassium may have to be added to the infusion. The main indications for alkalinization of the urine are for salicylate poisoning and poisoning with phenobarbitone. Excretion of both these drugs is assisted by making the urine alkaline. The urine should be tested periodically with indicator paper to make sure that a pH between 7 and 8 is being achieved. When the patient begins to improve the rate of infusion can be slowed down. A urine culture should be taken before the bladder catheter is removed. There are certain forms of drug overdosage for which forced diuresis is positively unwise or should only be used with great caution. Examples are the tricyclic antidepressants. These are inclined to cause arrhythmias, and forced diuresis carries the risk of precipitating pulmonary edema. The conservative approach to treatment should be employed in these cases. It is important to be aware that overdosage by tricyclic antidepressants may cause sudden death from arrhythmia even days after the patient has come out of coma. There are some good studies now purporting to show that alkalinization is more important than a high urine flow rate for increasing the excretion of phenobarbitone and salicylate. The massive diuresis which was formerly so fashionable may in fact not be necessary. For some drugs, such as amphetamines, which are weak bases, urinary acidification can be used to enhance excretion.

Exchange transfusion

The indications for exchange transfusion in the treatment of poisoning are very few indeed. One outstanding example in which it may be lifesaving is in the treatment of arsine poisoning. Arsine is a colorless, odorless and deadly poisonous gas which is liberated into the atmosphere whenever metals contaminated by arsenic come into contact with strong acids. Such accidents happen occasionally in industrial chemical processes. The arsine becomes bound to hemoglobin in a complex which is not readily dialysable. Large amounts can be removed by exchange transfusion.

Such patients will require hemodialysis for their associated renal failure and it is convenient to make use of the same vascular access (femoral or subclavian catheter) to carry out the exchange transfusion first. Exchange transfusion is also useful in cases of incompatible blood transfusion (also a form of poisoning) and in cases of massive hemolysis of red blood cells from whatever cause.

Dialysis

Dialysis tends to be reserved for very severe cases of poisoning in which there is danger of death or serious organ damage in spite of attention to conservative medical support and the techniques already mentioned. However, dialysis should only be contemplated if it is known or can be predicted that substantial amounts of the drug can be removed by this method. Fortunately there is now quite a lot of information available on which drugs or poisons can be removed by dialysis, and even if we do not have immediate access to this information we can probably work it out from first principles. Hemodialysis is generally much more efficient for the removal of poisons than peritoneal dialysis. The exception is infants and young children in whom peritoneal dialysis is relatively more efficient than in adults though still not as efficient as hemodialysis. However, peritoneal dialysis is easier to perform in very young children, unless a hemodialysis unit specializing in very small children is easily within reach. The following points should be considered.

Solubility in water

It seems obvious but dialysis through a semipermeable membrane depends on the substance being soluble in water. A notoriously dangerous hypnotic called glutethimide (Doriden) caused many deaths by suicide. It could not be removed by dialysis because it was fat soluble and not water soluble.

Protein binding

In order for a drug to be dialysable, it must not be significantly protein bound. Proteins are far too large to go through a semipermeable membrane so the drug will not pass through either.

Molecular weight of the substance

Substances of low molecular weight (500 daltons or less) are easily dialysed whereas substances of high molecular weight will not pass through the membrane. This rule has become less rigid with the introduction of new membranes such as polyacrylonitrile (PAN) which are much more permeable to larger molecules. However, the same principle applies. One still needs to know roughly the molecular weight of the substance and the permeability characteristics of the membrane used for the dialyser.

Distribution of the drug or poison in the various water compartments of the body

The drug lithium carbonate, widely used in the treatment of mood disorders, especially manic-depresive psychosis, illustrates some of these points well. High blood levels of lithium are extremely dangerous since they may cause permanent neurological damage in the form of ataxia and intellectual deficit. Lithium has a low molecular weight, is water soluble, not protein bound and is extremely well dialysed. However, dialysis removes it very fast from the extracellular fluid compartment and there is a delay while it diffuses out of the cells. If dialysis is stopped too soon the blood level may rebound to toxic levels as the drug comes out of the cells. This may necessitate a repeat dialysis. Examples of drugs which should be removed by dialysis as fast as possible in order to prevent organ damage are:

Drug	*Toxic effect*
methyl alcohol	optic nerves and brain
ethylene glycol	renal damage
quinine	blindness
lithium	neurotoxicity

Vascular access for hemodialysis in cases of poisoning should as a rule be done through femoral catheters (see p.217). A double-lumen femoral catheter is better than a single femoral catheter and an arm vein. This is because femoral catheters are very secure whereas a patient who gets restless on starting to wake up may thrash about and dislodge the cannula in the arm.

Hemoperfusion

It has been known for a long time that charcoal would adsorb drugs. It was ingested or put into the stomachs of people who had been poisoned in order to bind the poison and render it harmless.

Some years ago some ingenious medical innovators got the idea that if blood containing poisonous drugs were passed through a column of charcoal the charcoal would adsorb the drugs out of the blood. This indeed proved to be the case and the first experiments of perfusing blood through charcoal were performed. Activated charcoal turned out to be extremely active in removing a variety of drugs from the bloodstream if heparinized blood was perfused through it. When this was tried on a clinical basis two serious problems were discovered. Firstly, the tiny fragments of charcoal tended to be carried along in the bloodstream and ended up as minute emboli in the lungs of the patient. Secondly, it was discovered that the patient's platelet count dropped dangerously low because platelets also got adsorbed on the surface of the charcoal. For a while the technique was abandoned but later a way was found to coat the charcoal with a very thin layer of acrylic hydrogel. This effectively prevents any serious platelet adherence and also stops the charcoal embolization.

Charcoal hemoperfusion is now an established technique which turns out to be greatly superior to hemodialysis for the removal of certain poisons. For example, hemoperfusion is very effective in removing short- and medium-acting barbiturates which are not well removed by hemodialysis. It is also very effective for removing glutethimide which, being lipid soluble and protein bound, is hard to remove by hemodialysis. Some dramatic results have also been achieved with such drugs as methaqualone (Mandrax) and acetaminophen. There do not seem to be any special dangers associated with hemoperfusion and no real contra-indications though for salicylates and water soluble poisons with low molecular weight which are not protein bound we would still prefer to do dialysis. The charcoal column achieves dramatic results within the space of two hours—often more so than could be achieved with hemodialysis in a much longer time.

The extracorporeal circuit shown in Fig. 9.1 merely perfuses heparinized blood into the bottom of the column and this emerges from the top to go through a bubble trap before returning to the patient. The column comes from the manufacturer primed with saline and it is very important not to let any air get into it. Air gets trapped in it, reduces the area of the active surface and greatly reduces the efficiency. Hence the need to fill the arterial line complete with saline before starting the extracorporeal circulation.

The other point to remember is that you need fairly large doses of heparin since heparin seems to be adsorbed on the column.

At present hemoperfusion is reserved for very severe cases of poisoning in which the clinical condition is deteriorating in spite of the best conservative supportive measures. For example, if the patient has unresponsive hypotension in spite of adequate fluid administration, a high central venous pressure and good ventilation, hemoperfusion should prob-

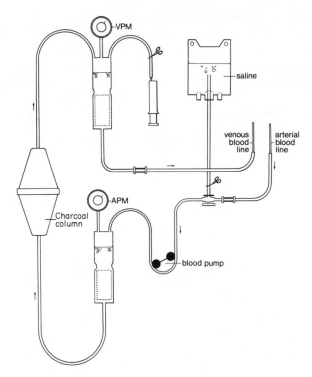

Fig. 9.1. Hemoperfusion cicuit. Charcoal hemoperfusion for poisoning.

ably be carried out. Often blood pressure will improve within a short time of starting therapy.

An advance which proved even more effective than activated charcoal is an amberlite resin mounted in a column (called XAD4). Clinical trials in special centers have shown quite dramatic results. They have greater adsorptive capacity than charcoal and can be used for many hours without having to be renewed.

In the present state of knowledge the charcoal and resin columns are definitely for one use only. There is no question of regenerating them and using them again. They are very expensive. It is unlikely that they will ever be needed in large numbers because they are not intended to be used except in the small percentage of the most severe cases of poisoning.

An interesting and perhaps important use for hemoperfusion is in the management of poisoning by the weed-killer paraquat. This substance kills by inducing a progressive pulmonary fibrosis days after the initial ingestion. Only small amounts are in the bloodstream at any one time. If one removes it by hemoperfusion the blood level rebounds as the drug comes out of the tissues when the treatment is stopped. It is therefore necessary to keep on repeating the hemoperfusion at least every day and perhaps twice a day in order to prevent the fatal lung damage. This extremely tedious treatment seems to offer the only hope in an otherwise uniformly fatal outcome.

10

Renal Transplantation

Carl Cardella and Elizabeth Wright

Regular dialysis in hospital or home has proved itself to be an acceptable means by which many people who would otherwise be dead continue to lead useful lives. In the best centers the chance of surviving for several years with this treatment is very high. Unfortunately the degree of rehabilitation which is achieved is very variable and sometimes quite poor. Strength, vitality and stamina are seldom completely normal. Dependence on the machine, besides being very expensive, is often a continuing source of frustration and anxiety. For such a patient a successful kidney transplant offers a chance to lead an almost normal life. Within weeks of the operation the patient will notice a dramatic return of strength and the hemoglobin will rise rapidly to normal. He/she will be able to eat and drink normally with no dietary restrictions. He/she will recover the ability to do hard manual work, run for a bus, engage in sexual activity, and sleep without hypnotics. Once established in a stable state the patient only requires to take regular oral anti-rejection therapy and attend the out-patient department perhaps once every one or two months. The quality of life is similar to that of a well-controlled diabetic, the only difference being that injections are not required—only tablets.

In the past, transplantation was characterized by a high mortality rate but over the years this has decreased substantially. At the present time the mortality for a young transplant candidate should be less than 5% at one year. This mortality rate is probably still slightly greater than that on dialysis but the difference between the two has decreased substantially over the years. As a result of this decrease in mortality more and more patients are seeking transplantation not only because of the quest for a better quality of life but because the risk in seeking this better quality of life is substantially lower than in the past.

Historical background

Transplantation of simple tissues such as the skin has been practiced for centuries and the first successful corneal graft was performed in 1852. Transplantation of whole organs such as the kidney was held up until a way could be found to join blood vessels. This was finally done at the beginning of this century by a French surgeon called Alexis Carrel who used an over-and-over everting stitch with a fine needle and silk suture.

Fig. 10.1 is redrawn from the original by Carrel in 1902. The same basic method is in use today though the materials have been considerably improved.

During the first half of this century surgeons performed transplantations of kidneys and other organs in laboratory animals. They found that an organ removed from its normal position in an animal and implanted in a different position in the same animal (an autograft) often functioned well for many years. In contrast to this, an organ transplanted into another animal of the same species, an allograft, although it functioned well for a few days, then became swollen and apparently inflamed and even finally completely destroyed. Transplants performed between animals of different species (heterografts) were often destroyed within hours rather than days and hardly functioned at all. Later it was found that organs could be exchanged between identical (uniovular) twins or between different animals of the same highly in-bred strain, and these survived in a healthy state, just as though they were autografts.

We now know that the rejection of transplanted organs is an immunological phenomenon in which antibodies formed by the host react against the foreign tissue or antigen and an inflammatory reaction results. In addition lymphocytes and other small round cells from the host enter and invade the graft causing further inflammation and destruction especially in relation to blood vessels. When this reaction occurs in a kidney the first parts to be affected are the capillaries supplying the tubules. There is a cellular infiltration and edema in and around the tubules. The glomeruli tend to be affected much later. There is also a late and rather slowly developing kind of chronic rejection seen in patients on immunosuppressive therapy in which the arteries and arterioles

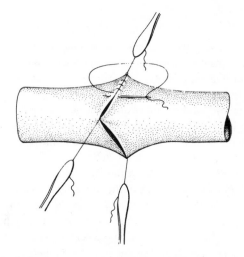

Fig. 10.1. Method of end-to-end vessel anastomosis. Redrawn from the original by A. Carrel.

supplying the kidney become progressively narrowed by successive layers of fibrin laid down in the lumen.

The rejection phenomenon effectively prevented the clinical application of transplantation except in a few operations carried out between identical twins, the first of which was performed in the Brigham Hospital in Boston in 1954. The first attempts to suppress the rejection phenomenon were by means of total body irradiation designed to paralyse the reticulo-endothelial system. In 1959 the first successful renal allograft was accomplished by this method. It was highly dangerous because during the period of bone marrow suppression the patient succumbed to overwhelming infection. Later when the bone marrow recovered, the graft was frequently rejected. The few initial successes were perhaps mainly to a fortuitously high degree of tissue compatibility between donor and recipient.

It was the discovery of immunosupressive drugs, azathioprine (Imuran) and prednisone, that finally made transplantation a realistic form of treatment with an acceptable rate of success. In the last few years the results have improved as a result of more effective immunotherapy, improved patient management and the effect of HLA matching, particularly for the DR locus.

Kidney donors

Since the advent of modern renal transplantation, kidneys have been used from four main sources; namely living related donors, living unrelated volunteer donors, primates (chimpanzees and baboons), and human cadavers. Heterografts taken from the monkey family were very quickly abandoned because, as one would expect, the genetic dissimilarity between donor and recipient was so great that extremely rapid and severe rejection occurred which was almost uninfluenced by immunosuppressive therapy. For a short time unrelated volunteers in the form of convicts serving life sentences in a State Penitentiary in the USA were given the opportunity to donate kidneys; but the results of these operations were no better than with unrelated cadaver kidneys. Matters were brought to a head when one of the prisoners escaped with his visitors in the early post-operative period! This resulted in a general agreement to avoid using unrelated healthy volunteers except under some very exceptional circumstances such as emotionally related volunteers; for example a husband giving a kidney to his wife. Even this type of unrelated living donor transplant remains very controversial.

Transplantation from living relatives, though considered by some authorities to be ethically unjustified, is still practiced in many centers and has consistently given the best results. Transplants between siblings and from parent to child are the most commonly performed, though occasionally donations from uncles, aunts or cousins have been very successful. The most consistently successful have been the sibling transplants where there is an identical match demonstrated by tissue typing techniques. The selection of living donors is a serious responsibility for medical staff, who have to be sure that the donor is a true volunteer and is not under pressure from other members of the family. If there is any doubt about complete willingness on the part of the donor the operation should not be done. This is the reason why most people feel that sons and daughters should not be allowed to donate to parents, since they may feel under an obligation from a sense of duty. Many potential donors can be ruled out at once by virtue of age, occupation or known medical disability, but if they are apparently healthy they should be checked for compatibility of ABO blood groups. Certain occupations such as the Armed Services, the Police and the Fire Services are a bar to kidney removal because the danger of injury would have a restricting effect on the donor's subsequent career. The Rhesus factor can be ignored. If donor and recipient are ABO compatible an appointment can be arranged for tissue typing tests. If tissue typing shows a good enough match (opinions still vary as to the degree of incompatibility which can be accepted) the potential donor must undergo a thorough history, physical examination and complete investigation designed to demonstrate that he or she has an entirely normal urinary tract and no significant disability in any other system. For example, essential hypertension or chronic bronchitis would certainly be a bar. If the donor passes all the tests the final investigation is a renal arteriogram to demonstrate the anatomy of the renal arteries. The kidney which is to be donated should have a single renal artery for ease of anastomosis. Arteriography requires admission to hospital with 24 hours bed rest after the procedure because it involves femoral artery puncture to inject the contrast medium.

Many patients with end-stage renal failure do not have a suitable living related donor able to provide a kidney. For such patients a kidney from a corpse is the only alternative. For practical purposes this means we have to consider any young person dying in hospital as a possible kidney donor. Conditions such as hypertension, septicemia, active tuberculosis, disseminated cancer or any disease of the urinary tract would make the kidneys unfit to be used. A previous history of known infective jaundice is a probable contra-indication and a positive hepatitis B test is a complete contra-indication to use of the kidneys for fear of transmitting hepatitis—especially dangerous in any patient on immunosuppressive drugs. Patients with severe head injury, cerebral glioma or subarachnoid hemorrhage tend to be ideal kidney donors, but there are many other causes of death in which donation of the kidneys could be considered. We have for example carried out some very successful transplants using kidneys from patients whose brains have been destroyed by methanol intoxication.

Cadaver kidney retrieval

First, the consultant in charge of the case must give permission for the patient to be considered as a potential donor. Next, the permission of the relatives must be sought for removal of the kidneys after death, if death should occur. By law the next of kin must sign a form of consent. In the case of an entirely sudden and unexpected death which occurs quickly it is very hard to approach relatives for permission when they are in a state of shock over the bereavement. Many of us hesitate to seek permission under these circumstances and the oppoortunity to use kidneys may be unavoidably lost. In contrast, if the patient remains in coma for several days the next of kin has a chance to get adjusted to the disaster and may even spontaneously offer the kidneys as an opportunity to do some good for someone else. Many countries have now adopted the idea of a donor consent card. This is the card which people carry, sometimes attached to the driving licence, in which they state their willingness to donate their organs after death. The legal force of this signed donor consent form prior to death is often dubious. In most instances the physicians involved with the organ retrieval still seek the consent of the next of kin. This is done to avoid any turmoil in a grieving family. The physicians in charge of the kidney retrieval program always attempt to have the next of kin in agreement with the wishes of the patient to be a donor.

Once permission for kidney removal has been obtained blood is taken from the patient for tissue typing, hepatitis B antigen testing and cytomegalovirus testing. Both these viruses are capable of being transmitted to the recipient with sometimes devastating results. The current trend is for computers to store the tissue typing data of the large numbers of potential transplant recipients who are on regular dialysis. The tissue typing information of the potential donor is then fed into the computer, which selects the recipients with the greatest degree of similarity with that of the donor. The larger the number of potential recipients the greater is the chance of an identical match. It is a great help if one knows in advance of death where the kidneys are going and for whom they will be used. Medical staff and patients can then be alerted and certain preparations made. If death seems imminent the transplant team will wish to have a sterile pack of surgical instruments ready nearby as well as cold solution for perfusing the kidney. When death occurs it should be certified by two physicians, one of whom may have been the original doctor taking care of the patient. Only when both physicians are satisfied that the patient is dead are members of the transplant team allowed to remove organs. In the past kidneys were removed outside the operating room but this is no longer justified because of the risk of infection and inadequate facilities to remove the organs safely. The operation is now performed in the operating room under sterile conditions with an anesthetist in attendance. Nearly all donors are on ventilators, and it will have been ascertained that without the ventilator there is no spontaneous respiration. It will also have been decided by the patient's own doctors that there is no prospect of recovery and that it is appropriate to discontinue artificial ventilation and allow the patient to die. Under these circumstances and only after very careful thought and full discussion, the kidney retrieval is carried out as an elective procedure in an operating room. Ventilation is continued until everything is ready in the operating room. The abdomen is prepared, the instruments are ready, and the cold perfusing solution is at hand to perfuse the kidneys as soon as they are removed. The operation proceeds and the kidneys are removed, perfused and placed in cold storage. The length of time to remove the kidneys varies according to the surgeon performing the operation but the total time required is usually between 15 and 30 minutes. The period of time in which the kidneys are warm in the body but without circulation, that is after the renal artery has been clamped, is called the warm ischemia time. The period in which the kidneys are perfused and on cold storage is called the cold ischemia time. Some additional warm ischemia time is inevitable while the kidneys are being inserted into the recipient.

At the time of harvesting the kidneys, mannitol is the only drug that is routinely given. This is an osmotically active agent which increases diuresis and can prevent acute tubular necrosis in some animal models. In the past, drugs such as heparin, phenoxybenzamine, Largactil, corti-costeroids and others have been used but they are of no proven benefit and are usually not part of current donor management protocols.

The concept of brain death and the heart-beating donor

Once it has been decided by the donor's physicians that irreversible damage has occurred in the brain, the patient can be said to have 'brain death' or be 'neurologically dead'. Brain death is a clinical diagnosis and is defined as cerebral death (permanent loss of consciousness) plus permanent loss of spontaneous respiration, control of blood pressure, cranial nerve reflexes and withdrawal from pain. Usually, but not always, the spinal reflexes may also be lost. A diagnosis of brain death is frequently assisted by the electroencephalogram but this is not absolutely necessary. Usually two flat EEGs several hours apart are evidence of brain death. Falsely flat EEGs have been recorded after drug overdose and hypothermia. It is only after brain death has been determined that the patient can be taken to the operating room for organ removal.

Storage and transport of kidneys

Kidneys removed from the body must be cooled as quickly as possible. It is probably unwise to use kidneys with a warm ischemia time in excess of about 30 minutes. Cooling lowers the metabolic rate and protects against ischemic damage. Various cold perfusion solutions are used and research is still continuing to find the perfect one. Cooling is done by gravity infusion through a cannula in the renal artery. If there are two renal arteries the surgeon tries to take a cuff of aorta from which both the arteries arise. Both arteries are perfused, and the cuff makes it much easier to perform the arterial anastomosis.

Once they are cooled the kidneys are placed in separate bags of cold perfusion solution, double wrapped in another sterile sealed bag and placed in separate insulated containers for transport to their destination. The containers should be carefully labelled left and right kidney. Each container should have attached to it a cyclostyled data sheet giving clear information from the surgeon who removed the kidneys about the ana-tomical features of the blood vessels and ureter, as well as the exact warm ischemia time, and the ante-mortem state of the donor. Any drugs which were given to the donor before death should also be recorded. This information is invaluable for the surgeon at the hospital where the recipient will receive the transplant. By this time it is hoped that it will have been decided where the kidneys will be sent and which patients are to receive them. Once the surgeon has removed the kidneys and satisfied himself that they are cooled, he should turn his attention to obtaining lymph nodes, usually from the mesentery. Lymph nodes and/or a piece of the spleen must be sent with each kidney to allow the receiving center to perform a cytotoxic antibody crossmatch test. The transplant will not be done if this test is positive.

Storage of the kidney on a perfusion machine

Kidneys can be stored with or without a perfusion machine. Without a perfusion machine they are maintained in the flushing solution that was administered just after removal. The temperature at which they are stored is about 4°C. The kidneys are protected by plastic and maintained in an ice slush until used. The maximum length of time that such kidneys can be stored before implanting into the recipient is about 48 hours although longer times have been recorded. The incidence of acute tubular necrosis increases with very prolonged cold storage times. An alternative method for storage of kidneys is via a perfusion machine. There are several of these machines available and essentially they all provide the same function which is to perfuse the kidney with an oxyge-nated solution and maintain it at low temperatures. The machine requires a pulsatile pump and a refrigeration unit. It is fairly costly to purchase and maintain. It is much more cost efficient to use cold stored kidneys. It is, however, more convenient for the surgeon to use machine perfused kidneys. Preservation time tends to be longer with machine perfused kidneys and the incidence of acute tubular necrosis tends to be lower than with cold stored kidneys maintained for an equivalent period.

This perfusion is a highly specialized procedure, the details of which need not concern us here. It is enough to know that by this means kidneys can be stored if necessary for two or three days before they are transplanted. They can be transported long distances by air or road and transplanted at a time which is convenient. The other advantage of perfusion is that it allows one to test the kidney to assess the degree of ischemic damage. Such parameters as perfusion pressure and flow rate as well as the pH and the lactate content of the perfusion fluid give a fairly accurate prediction of the viability of the organ. This is extremely useful if one is in doubt about the amount of damage which has been inflicted by ischemia.

Tissue typing

The allograft rejection phenomenon depends on the difference between antigens in the donor and the recipient. These antigenic differences may be due to tissue specific antigens or to antigens which are more widely distributed throughout the body and are referred to as transplantation antigens or human leukocyte associated antigens (HLA antigens). These antigens are carried on most cells including lymphocytes and platelets but their distribution in tissues varies considerably. The HLA antigens are the most important antigenic determinants of the allograft rejection phenomenon and they are determined by genetic information derived from the sixth chromosome. On this chromosome there are at least five regions which contribute to antigenic sites on the plasma membranes of cells. These five sites, called the HLA sites, are referred to as the HLA A, B, C, D and DR loci and give rise to corresponding antigens on the cell surface. For each genetic locus there are two antigens expressed on the cell surface. Clinically significant HLA antigens are of the HLA A, B, D and DR series. Since the immune response between donor and recipient depends on the differences in these antigens, the aim of tissue matching is to reduce the differences and thus decrease the immune response of the recipient to the donor kidney. The effect of matching can best be seen in living related donor transplants where results, currently and historically, have been significantly better than those of cadaveric grafts. In the case of sibling transplantation there is a 25% chance that both donor and recipient will be identical. If this is the case, one can expect virtually 100% graft function at the present time. For cadaveric donors, however, the incidence of HLA identity is very small and to achieve this would require a large organ donor pool. At present, with the number of antigens which are known, it seems that we need a pool of several hundred recipients to be sure of finding a good match for each particular donor.

The transplant antigens are, of course, carried on the kidney cells but it is not yet feasible to test for the kidney antigens directly. Fortunately the same antigens seem to be shared by the peripheral blood leukocytes. Tissue typing depends on detection of the antigens in the leukocytes by seeing if they react against certain known antisera which contain high concentrations of antibodies against them. The details of the technique need not concern us but suffice it to say that it is a difficult and time-consuming method. In all tissue typing laboratories it is performed by specially trained technicians. Blood or tissue for typing must be taken into fresh containers provided by the laboratory, and for patients on regular dialysis samples should be taken before rather than after dialysis, because blood from a fully heparinized patient is not satisfactory for the test.

The significance of HLA typing in renal transplantation has been clarified over the last few years. At the present time it appears that matching for the B and DR loci provides optimal graft survival. Thus, if both antigens at the B locus and both antigens at the DR locus are matched between donor and recipient, the chance of graft success is substantially higher than if there is mismatch at either of these loci. Matching for the A locus does not appear to have a great influence on graft survival.

Thus, the criteria for proceeding with transplantation are ABO compatibility and a negative crossmatch using recipient sera and donor cells. If two or more matches occur at the B and DR loci then preferential selection would take place and priority would go to the recipient showing the best match with the donor.

The cytotoxic crossmatch test is of fundamental importance. In this test the recipient's serum is tested for antibodies against the donor lymphocytes. Donor lymphocytes may be obtained from spleen, lymph node or peripheral blood. Since large numbers of lymphocytes are required, it is advantageous to have either spleen or lymph node from the donor and this is usually taken from the donor at the time of kidney retrieval. The test measures the presence of complement-dependent cytotoxic antibodies and a positive test is indicated by the presence of dead cells in the preparation. If the percentage of dead cells exceeds 10% then this is taken to be a positive crossmatch. It is a contra-indication to transplantation if this positive crossmatch was obtained on sera taken on the day of surgery. If a positive crossmatch results from sera taken months prior to the time of the transplant, this is not necessarily a contra-indication to transplantation provided that the serum taken on the day of transplant does not contain these antibodies.

These antibodies can be directed against T or B cells. T cells express the HLA A, B and C series antigens in high concentration whereas B cells express the DR antigen in very high concentration. Thus, at the present time it is important to separate T and B cells in order to determine whether the patient has antibodies against T or B cells, since this will influence the decision. Antibodies against T cells on current serum are a contra-indication to transplantation whereas antibodies against B cells are not necessarily so. It is clear that, if the patient has antibodies against T cells at the time of transplantation, a hyperacute rejection will result, and the graft will be lost immediately. If, on current sera, there are antibodies against B cells but none against T cells, most authorities consider this a permissible situation. However, there have been one or two cases of accelerated rejection reported. It is not clear yet whether this is related to true B cell antibody. Thus, ideally a patient should have a negative crossmatch against T cells on serum taken on the day of transplantation. If this is the case, rejection in the first few hours after transplantation is avoided but rejection in the weeks that follow transplantation could still occur since it may take several days for the immune response to the graft to occur.

Preparation of the recipient

In the early days of renal transplantation grafts were sometimes performed in patients who were uremic, emaciated and perhaps infected, in a heroic attempt to save life. The results tended to be uniformly disastrous. We have learned by our experience. Dialysis is used to save life and improve the patient's general condition. Transplantation should only be attempted when the patient's general condition is good. The reason is that immuno-suppressive therapy, which has to be given after the operation, reduces the patient's resistance to infection as well as his powers of wound healing, making him vulnerable to all kinds of complications. The lesson which has been learned in other forms of surgery must be strongly re-emphasized for transplant surgery. A patient in good general condition before operation stands a better chance of surviving the operation itself. The points which should receive special attention are as follows.

1 The patient must be well dialysed, usually several weeks or months of hemodialysis, preferably three times a week, or if he is on peritoneal

dialysis he should be well rehabilitated on this form of treatment. If a cadaver kidney becomes available for such a patient he should be fit to receive it at short notice. Dialysis may still be necessary prior to the operation.

2 He should be well nourished. A diet containing 1 g of protein per kg body weight with an adequate calorie content is commonly used to make sure that patients do not come to operation in an emaciated state.

3 He should be active and rehabilitated.

4 He should be free of any infection, especially in the urinary tract.

5 In order to prevent post-operative chest complications smoking should be strongly discouraged.

6 Care will have been taken by medical staff to ensure that the patient has an anatomically normal lower urinary tract so that there will be no difficulty in bladder emptying. Cystoscopy may have to be carried out in doubtful cases. If the bladder is grossly abnormal and cannot be used for transplantation it may be possible to fashion an ileal conduit or loop, into which the ureter of a transplanted kidney can be placed at a later date. If the patient has a history of chronic pyelonephritis, with or without renal calculi and free vesico-ureteral reflux, it may be deemed necessary to remove the infected kidneys and ureters in a preliminary operation. This will serve to protect the transplanted kidney from infection transmitted from the infected upper tracts.

7 The blood pressure must be well controlled. It is now rare for bilateral nephrectomy to be required in order to control blood pressure. The available antihypertensive drugs are sufficiently potent to allow optimal blood pressure control prior to the transplant procedure.

8 Bilateral nephrectomy is rarely required except when infection involves both kidneys. In the case of polycystic kidneys unilateral nephrectomy is sometimes required in order that the new transplant can be placed in the pelvis. Occasionally polycystic kidneys are so large that they extend into the pelvis and there is inadequate space to do the new transplant. If polycystic kidneys have been repeatedly infected then they are usually removed prior to transplantation. In the absence of infection and significant bleeding, polycystic kidneys are no longer routinely removed. In fact it is a great advantage to the patient on dialysis to have at least one kidney still in place. If the transplant fails and the patient has to return to dialysis in an anephric state, the anemia is likely to be chronically disabling.

9 Splenectomies are no longer done routinely prior to the transplant. Early data suggested that splenectomy did have a beneficial effect on

graft outcome but it is clear with the available new immunosuppressive drugs that this is not a routine procedure for transplant recipients. Splenectomized patients have a significant incidence of spontaneous and life-threatening pneumococcal infection. This can be prevented by inoculation with a polyvalent pneumococcal vaccine. If splenectomy is planned for some special reason it is sensible to give the pneumococcal vaccine at least four weeks before the operation. This should provide reliable and permanent protection.

10 In the case of recipients of living donor kidneys whose operation is being performed electively, therapy can be started with Imuran, usually five days before operation.

11 It has now been clearly established that pre-transplant blood transfusions have a beneficial effect on graft outcome. The mechanism of this effect is unclear. The optimal number of transfusions has not been established but most centers now give between two and five units prior to transplantation. The risks of transfusion include transmission of viruses which cause hepatitis, cytomegalic infection and possibly acquired immune deficiency syndrome (AIDS).

12 Several routine bacteriological and laboratory tests are done prior to operation. These include routine stool culture. Occasionally parasites such as *Strongyloides stercoralis* can be present in the bowel and this may lead to life-threatening complications in the post-transplant period. If found to be present it must be eradicated before transplantation is contemplated. Baseline liver function, electrolytes and blood gas studies are commonly performed.

13 All patients being considered for transplantation should have had a recent hepatitis B antigen test. Most authorities now agree that a positive test means no transplant because of the risk of progressive liver disease (either hepatitis or malignancy) in the recipient. All health care workers should receive hepatitis B vaccine in order to be protected from acquiring hepatitis from a patient or carrier.

14 Finally, it is a great advantage to keep a brief summary of all the essential information about every potential transplant recipient in an accessible file where it can reliably be found in the middle of the night. Blood group and tissue typing data, and whether or not there are any known cytotoxic antibodies, what operations the patient has had previously, and the state of his blood vessels—these are all valuable facts to have at one's fingertips before the patient is sent for to come into hospital. All this information can be summarized as a standard form on one or two sheets of paper.

15 Perioperative antibiotics are commonly used to reduce the incidence of post-operative infection.

Pre-operative contact with the transplant ward nursing staff

When a patient is admitted to a transplant ward prior to the transplant, there is usually very limited time before the operation and a lot to be done. The patient is usually excited and apprehensive about the procedure, and also anxious in the presence of strange nursing staff. Transplant nursing staff should understand and respect this anxiety and do their best to learn as much as possible about the patient, his or her dialysis method, and the previous drug treatment. Remember that most of these patients are very knowledgeable about dialysis and often have a close bond with their former physicians and nurses. This is natural and you should not feel threatened by it. Learn as much as you can about the patient while making the preparations for surgery. Does he or she still have a significant daily urine output? If the patient is normally anuric (only a few drops every two days) then you know that any urine produced after surgery is coming from the new kidney. Does the patient have any other associated disability such as diabetes, labile hypertension, a tendency to go into heart failure when fluid overloaded, or a chronic peptic ulcer? All these problems could cause difficulty in the post-operative period and we should try to anticipate and prevent them. Explain to the patient the need for such things as skin preparation, pre-operative medication, peritoneal dialysis fluid culture (in PD patients) and the need for closed bladder drainage after surgery. Reassure the patient about post-operative pain medication and explain to the diabetic how the post-operative blood glucose control will be handled. Make sure the patient knows the names of the new doctors who will be looking after him and if possible encourage the patient's own dialysis nurse(s) to visit in the post-operative period. Prepare the patient for the possibility of rejection episodes and how they will be handled, and about the possibility of dialysis being required temporarily until the transplanted kidney starts to function. Explain what monitoring and observations will be needed after surgery and what tests and diagnostic procedures such as radio-isotope scanning and percutaneous renal biopsy may be required. Long-term dialysis patients are much more medically aware than the average population and may be considerably more demanding. The kidney transplant is a crucially important event in the life of a dialysis patient. Try to let the patient see that you understand this and let him believe that everything possible will be done to make it a

success. The questions patients ask may be quite searching and sophisticated. If you do not know the answers do not be embarrassed but find
someone who does. Excellent communication of this kind will give the
patient confidence and ensure his or her best cooperation in what may be
a difficult exercise for everybody.

The surgical operation

Experience has shown that the best position in which to place the kidney
is in one or other iliac fossa outside the peritoneal cavity. The main reason
for this position is the problem of the blood supply of the ureter. The
ureter receives its blood supply from three main sources: a branch from
the renal artery, branches from the posterior abdominal wall, and a vessel
coming up from the bladder. When a kidney with its ureter is removed
for transplantation, only the branch coming from the renal artery is left
intact. This is capable of vascularizing the first 15 cm or so of the ureter,
beyond which the blood supply is deficient. Thus the surgeon only has a
15 cm length of ureter available for anastomosis. Hence the kidney must
be close enough to the bladder for this short length of ureter to reach.
The other obvious advantage of the iliac fossa position is that it is very
superficial and the kidney can be palpated thereafter through the abdominal wall whenever it has to be examined.

Fig. 10.2 shows a diagram of the operation which is most commonly
performed. The artery is anastomosed end-to-end with the internal iliac
artery which has been ligated, divided and turned back to meet the renal
artery. If the recipient's internal iliac artery is unusable for some reason,
such as the presence of severe atheroma, the donor renal artery can be
placed end-to-side on the external iliac artery. If there are two donor
renal arteries on a patch of aorta, the patch can be sewn in place on the
external iliac. A potential disadvantage of using the internal iliac artery
for anastomosis to the donor renal artery is that one thereby reduces
blood flow to the pelvis. In fact if both these arteries are used one after
another in successive transplant operations (in the event of failure of the
first) there is a high chance of permanent impotence in males due to
inadequate arterial supply to the penis to sustain an erection. The renal
vein is anastomosed end-to-side with the external iliac vein. The ureter
is anastomosed to the bladder through an oblique tunnel which under-
mines the bladder mucosa. This is designed to prevent vesico-ureteral
reflux. Some operators prefer to join the donor ureter end-to-end with
the recipient ureter and others anastomose the recipient ureter to the

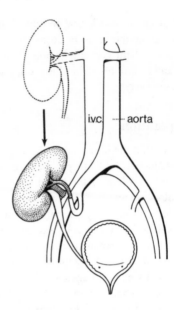

Fig. 10.2. The operation of renal transplantation.

donor renal pelvis. Both these procedures are less common than the uretero-vesical anastomosis. It is usual for a left kidney to be placed in the right iliac fossa and vice versa, because this is the way that the blood vessels and ureter lie in the most convenient position for anastomosis, but either kidney can, if necessary, be placed on either side. The kidney does not need to be stitched in place but finds its own position when the abdominal wall is closed. During the operation and just before the anastomosis is opened the patient is usually given some intravenous mannitol to assist the initial function of the kidney. It is also common practice to give a dose of intravenous prednisone during the operation. An indwelling Foley catheter is placed in the bladder before the patient returns to the ward. If the kidney has had a short period of warm ischemia (and this should certainly be the case with a kidney removed from a living donor in an adjacent room) there will be an almost immediate flow of urine accompanied by visible ureteric peristalsis when the anastomosis is opened. It is less usual for cadaver kidneys to function immediately. It is often helpful to take a biopsy from a cadaver kidney at the time of operation because the extent of possible damage to the kidney may be in doubt.

Post-operative care

With the completion of a successful operation in a well-prepared patient who has been given a well-matched kidney it may be tempting to assume that the battle has been won and that the rest will be straightforward. Unfortunately this is not so. The first few post-operative weeks can be an anxious time during which the interested nurse will really come into her own. In transplantation, perhaps more than in any other form of medical treatment, a successful outcome depends on the cooperation of a large number of individuals and departments, each with different skills. The chief ward nurse plays a central role in helping to coordinate all these separate services for the benefit of her patient. Good communication is essential, especially between medical and nursing staff. For example, the immunosuppressive therapy will be ordered separately for each patient every day and will depend on the renal function as well as the hematology results. It may be necessary to change the orders more than once in 24 hours. This could easily lead to confusion unless medical and nursing staff work closely together and have a foolproof system of charting the drugs which are ordered.

The aims of the post-operative period can be summarized as follows.

- Promote wound healing and rehabilitation of the patient.
- Diagnose and treat rejection.
- Prevent severe uremia.
- Avoid toxicity from immunosuppressive drugs.
- Diagnose and treat infections early and adequately.
- Deal with any other complications.

It will be seen from this list that there are a lot of things to think about. There is not a big margin for error. A small mistake may have far-reaching consequences, so we have to pay meticulous attention to detail.

It will be useful at this point to say something about immunosuppression—the drugs and other methods which are used to suppress rejection.

Imuran

Imuran (azathioprine) is a derivative of 6-mercaptopurine. Until recently Imuran was the basic mainstay of immunosuppressive therapy which all transplant recipients must take indefinitely and if possible without interruption. The guiding principle in the first few months is to give the biggest dose that the patient can safely tolerate. Toxicity first becomes apparent in the form of leukopenia (lack of white blood cells) and then, usually later, thrombocytopenia (lack of platelets). Occasionally thrombocytopenia occurs first. For this reason when patients are first on Imuran their hemoglobin, white blood cell count and platelets are checked every day. The differential white cell count is also important because disproportionate depletion of the polymorphonuclear leukocytes is dangerous in terms of making the patient susceptible to infection. Unfortunately reduction of the dose when leukopenia first becomes apparent does not always result in an immediate rise in the white cell count. Instead there may be dangerous leukopenia and thrombocytopenia for up to two weeks. For this reason doses must be carefully judged according to a prediction of what each patient will tolerate. A healthy patient with normal renal function can usually take 3 mg/kg/day. One has to walk a tightrope between toxicity on one side and rejection on the other. If rejection occurs the dose is not normally increased because this leads to danger of toxicity. Other drugs are used to suppress acute rejection episodes.

Imuran should never be stopped unless there is dangerous bone marrow suppression or the graft has failed and has to be removed. An exception to this is the development of cytomegalovirus (CMV) infection (see p.361). After the first few months the dose is often reduced slightly to one which we know the patient will safely tolerate. In the early postoperative period nurses can help by making sure that the hematology results are always available for the medical staff to see at the time that the drugs are being ordered. She will also draw attention to any results which give cause for anxiety, though naturally it is the duty of the medical staff to look at these results and act accordingly. If medical and nursing staff are both vigilant there will be less chance of important information being overlooked. For example, many hyperkalemic cardiac arrests have been averted by nurses acting promptly after becoming aware of a high serum potassium level in their patients.

Prednisone

Prednisone is the second main immunosuppressive drug and also the drug which is used in large doses to suppress episodes of threatened rejection. It is common to use prednisone from the first day of operation though the dosage varies from one center to another. In general, lower baseline doses are used than in previous years. Always the aim should be to use the minimum to prevent rejection. Some transplant teams like to withhold prednisone until signs of rejection appear. As soon as a threatened rejection becomes apparent the steroid therapy is immediately increased. The most popular regimen for treating rejection is large doses of intravenous methylprednisolone (Solumedrone) for at least three consecutive days. The dose is usually geared to the patient's body weight, depending on local policy. When rejection comes under control the dose is fairly rapidly lowered to a maintenance level. It is worth remembering that prednisone in high doses produces a leukocytosis (high white count), which may mask the leukocytosis of infection and may, for a while, spuriously elevate the white count of a patient who is developing Imuran toxicity.

Dyspepsia induced by prednisone is not at all uncommon and antacid therapy has almost become a routine in transplant patients post-operatively. Certainly any patient with a known duodenal ulcer is highly vulnerable after transplantation because of the steroids, so much so that transplantation may be considered unwise until definitive surgical treatment of the ulcer has been carried out. Surgical treatment has become almost a rarity since the advent of such drugs as cimetidine and ranitidine which are so miraculous in suppressing gastric acid secretion. If steroid therapy has to be continued in high doses for a long time there is a serious danger of aggravation of bone disease. In patients who have a very successful result from transplantation with very little sign of rejection, one aims to reduce the steroids to a non-toxic dose as soon as possible, but experience has shown that it is unwise ever to stop the steroids completely. Even 5 mg per day of prednisone seems to provide a protective effect against rejection and this small dose should be continued indefinitely.

Cyclosporine

Cyclosporine is a new drug which is produced from two forms of fungi. It may well replace azathioprine as the mainstay immunosuppressive drug for renal transplant patients. It can be used either alone or with prednisone but it does have several side-effects. Its major side-effect is nephrotoxicity. This may be acute and is especially a problem in the early post-transplant period when the kidney has already suffered damage from ischemia. A combination of the ischemic insult and cyclosporine toxicity can cause lack of function in recently transplanted kidneys. The other form of nephrotoxicity is chronic, characterized by fibrotic changes in the kidney. This can lead to an increase in serum creatinine and eventually renal failure. The challenge with cyclosporine will be to keep the dose sufficient to prevent rejection but not high enough to cause renal damage. Many units avoid the use of cyclosporine in the early post-transplant period because of its acute nephrotoxicity. The other side-effects of cyclosporine include gum hypertrophy, hirsutism, hypertension and neurological abnormalities. The major change in immunotherapy in the last ten years has been the introduction of cyclosporine to immunosuppressive regimens. The long-term effects of cyclosporine in terms of renal damage are not yet known but some experts are so worried about this aspect that they stop the drug after a few months, replacing it with the old faithful combination of Imuran and prednisone. Triple therapy consisting of all three drugs in reduced dosage is also being studied.

Graft radiation

Graft radiation is no longer used by most transplant centers. Controlled trials indicate that it has no value.

Polyclonal anti-lymphocyte serum

The value of this product has now been clearly established. It is very effective in treating transplant rejection and can replace intravenous Solumedrol therapy. These anti-lymphocyte preparations include serum or the globulin fraction of serum or purified fractions of immunoglobulin. Generally the polyclonal preparations contain both IgG and IgM and react with a broad spectrum of lymphocytes including T cells, B cells and monocytes. It must be given intravenously and is often associated with a febrile reaction in the first 12 to 24 hours. If this reaction occurs it is important to reduce the rate of infusion so that the patient can tolerate the drug without systemic toxicity. After the first 24 hours systemic toxicity is uncommon and the drug can be given in full doses. Other complications of the drug include serum sickness and acute anaphylaxis but these are rare. The drug is very potent and reduces the number of peripheral T cells. This predisposes to viral infections such as herpes or cytomegalovirus infection. Anti-lymphocyte serum can only be used for a short period of time and it is commonly used in the first 7 to 10 days to prevent rejection or at a later time to treat rejection.

Monoclonal antibodies

These are second generation anti-lymphocyte products. They differ from the polyclonal preparations in that they are specific monoclonal antibodies directed against specific lymphocyte subsets. They are produced in mice and have the advantage of being uniform without the biological variations seen in the polyclonal preparation. They have a disadvantage in that their spectrum of activity may not be as great as the polyclonal preparation. It may, in fact, be necessary to use several monoclonal preparations in order to achieve the effect that is seen with the polyclonal preparation.

Cyclophosphamide

The only role of cyclophosphamide in transplantation at the present time is to replace azathioprine in patients who are unable to take the azathioprine because of toxicity. The dose of cyclophosphamide varies between 1 and 2 mg/kg/day. The major complication is leukopenia and thrombocytopenia. Hemorrhagic cystitis is rare in transplant patients on cyclophosphamide perhaps because of the large diuresis and therefore dilute urine that these patients have at night.

Other drugs

Heparin and anti-platelet drugs have been used by various investigators over the years either to prevent or reduce the impact of rejection. None of these agents has a well defined role in transplantation and they are no longer used.

Plasma exchange

Plasma exchange or plasmapheresis, which has been mentioned earlier in relation to treatment of antibody-mediated diseases such as Goodpasture's syndrome, has a strong theoretical justification in the prevention of antibody-mediated transplant rejection, so-called humoral rejection. We have studied its effect very extensively and conducted one of the largest controlled trials ever undertaken to test its value. The result came out in favor of plasma exchange but the benefits were not as significant as had been predicted from our initial clinical impressions, which is so often the case when any treatment is subjected to a proper controlled trial. We still sometimes use plasma exchange for a few days in cases of biopsy-proven humoral rejection, especially when the patient is not responding to more conventional treatment.

Prevention of infection

The use of immunosuppression in the post-operative period is bound to increase the risk of infection in a patient who is already at risk because of uremia. Precautions usually taken for prevention of infection, apart from the routine cultures from the patient, are:

• Meticulous bedside nursing care with particular attention to oral hygiene and cleanliness of the genitalia.

• Throat and nasal swabs from all personnel concerned in the patient's clinical care.

• Institution of barrier nursing in the early post-operative period or at any time when the patient is particularly at risk, e.g. because of leukopenia.

Carriers of resistant staphylococci in the throat or nose may have to be excluded from contact with the patient until the organism has been eradicated. Policy with regard to barrier nursing varies from one unit to another, but certainly proper facilities should be available for full barrier nursing in single cubicles in special cases.

All these measures to prevent infection are greatly dependent on good nursing leadership and discipline. Every nurse must take pride in seeing that they are carried out, and may at times have to remind the doctors to obey the rules!

One remarkable advance in the prevention of infection in transplants, originating in Minneapolis and now widely used elsewhere in North America, is the use of trimethoprim-sulpha to prevent *Pneumocystis carinii* infection. This protozoal infection of the lungs may be rapidly fatal in immunosuppressed patients if it is not diagnosed and treated promptly. It can be entirely prevented by daily administration of trimethoprim-sulpha (Septra, Septrin, Bactrim) and many transplant centers now keep their patients on it throughout the first year.

In a similar vein prophylaxis with INH should be given to transplant recipients who are at risk of developing TB. This may also be continued throughout the first year.

Post-operative management is greatly influenced by whether the kidney begins to function immediately or not. In our experience the majority of kidneys from living donors have excellent early function, while many cadaver kidneys, because of an unavoidable period of warm ischemia as well as perhaps several hours of cold ischemia, have delayed function for up to two or three weeks due to ischemic tubular damage.

The presence of good early function makes management so much simpler that this type of case will be described first.

The case with good initial renal function

The patient will probably arrive back from the operating room with a visible flow of urine into the catheter drainage bag. The first thing to do is to get an immediate baseline of all the main observations including temperature, pulse, blood pressue, respiration and urine flow rate. Central venous pressure measurement may also be useful as a guide to the rate of intravenous fluid administration. Urine flow should be measured hourly at first. Clear orders will be required from the medical staff about analgesics, intravenous fluids and immunosuppresive drugs. An accurate fluid intake and output chart is an obvious essential requirement. All urine should be kept to be sent to the laboratory at the end of each 24 hour period. Daily serum creatinine estimations are important in assessing progress and for detecting rejection. Initially the urine is often blood-stained from bleeding at the site of the uretero-vesical anastomosis. There is a tendency for clots to form which may block the catheter. This, in our experience, has been the commonest cause of a sudden cessation of urine flow during the first 24 hours. The difficulty can be overcome by irrigation of the bladder in a sterile manner with saline or aqueous chlorhexidine solution to get rid of the clots. Remember to ask the patient whether he has any skin allergy to chlorhexidine before using this in the bladder or you may cause a painful allergic cystitis. The medical staff will wish to be called if there is any sudden drop in urine output or any other disturbing change in vital signs. Early institution of deep breathing and coughing can help to prevent chest infections which are so common in the early post-operative period. If the patient develops anuria or oliguria which is not due to clot obstruction of the catheter, other more serious causes will have to be considered by the medical staff. Of these the commonest will be acute rejection, a condition which may occur as early as 24 hours after operation.

Diagnosis of acute rejection

In some ways acute rejection is like acute appendicitis—signs of a general constitutional disturbance as well as signs of local discomfort and tenderness over the graft. In most cases of acute rejection some or all of the following features will be apparent. The patient begins to feel unwell and often looks unwell for no obvious reason. Frequently his temperature shoots up to 39°C or more, he may develop an increase in heart rate and there may be an acute rise in blood pressure. Simultaneously or shortly after this there is a fall in urine output and renal function. The most characteristic local sign is enlargement of the kidney. This may seem to be about twice its previous size. It may also be painful and tender. The pain and tenderness is surprising in view of the fact that the renal nerves have been cut. Perhaps the pain is mainly due to inflammation of the tissues surrounding the kidney. In patients with clear urine there is often an increase in proteinuria and on microscopy there may be an increase in lymphocytes. If all these signs are present the medical staff will have no difficulty in diagnosing rejection. Often only a few signs will appear. It is then a matter of experience and judgment to decide whether rejection is occurring or not. In general we tend to treat rejection on suspicion because the risk of neglecting rejection is greater than the risk of high doses of immunosuppressive drugs. Most rejection episodes adequately and promptly treated respond within 24–72 hours with a disappearance of symptoms and signs. The patient suddenly feels well again, the temperature and blood pressure return to normal and there is a rapid improvement in urine output. More severe rejection episodes may take longer to respond and may require more vigorous therapy. If there is any serious doubt about the diagnosis a renal biopsy should give the answer. Renal biopsy is technically easy to perform in transplanted kidneys because of their superficial position, but the danger of complications, especially bleeding, has discouraged the use of renal biopsy as a routine. We have found it very helpful in doubtful cases. The slides can generally be made available for examination in 24 hours.

Other causes of sudden loss of renal function

Acute rejection is not the only cause of sudden loss of renal function in the early post-operative period. Renal artery thrombosis with total infarction of the graft occurs occasionally and will be accompanied by complete anuria (as opposed to oliguria) if the patient has no urine coming from his own diseased kidneys. The kidney will also feel soft and indefinite on examination. If there was previously an audible renal artery bruit this will disappear. Diagnosis can be confirmed by a renal scan and if necessary by a renal arteriogram, and the patient will have to go back to the operating room to have the kidney removed.

Urinary extravasation occasionally occurs due to a leak in the ureteric anastomosis. Pain and swelling around the kidney will be due to urine in the soft tissues surrounding the kidney and this may leak out through the suture line of the abdominal wound. These leaks can usually be treated conservatively by re-insertion of the indwelling catheter if this has been removed. Some of them will then dry up. Occasionally the patient may have to be taken back to the operating room to have the leak repaired. Urinary extravasation has been one of the major causes of surgical failure of grafts. Fortunately with improved techniques of ureteric implantation it is becoming less common.

Acute fulminating pyelonephritis in the transplanted kidney may occasionally mimic acute rejection. Pus in the urine and a positive culture may give the clue to diagnosis, but in one of our patients the correct diagnosis only appeared when we saw the renal biopsy.

The case with poor initial function

In contrast to the patient with good initial renal function, the patient who has oliguria due to ischemic renal damage presents us with several additional problems of management. The first and most obvious will be the need for regular hemodialysis until renal function picks up. This leads to the danger of bleeding from heparin. If possible a clear day should be allowed to elapse after operation for hemostasis to occur before the first post-operative dialysis. During the first hemodialysis heparin should be kept to a minimum and guided by coagulation tests. Because the patient is oliguric he should be treated like any other patient with acute renal failure by appropriate fluid restriction.

Peritoneal dialysis can be resumed in the post-transplant period providing the peritoneal membrane has not been entered inadvertently during the surgery. If this has happened the patient should be converted to hemodialysis until the peritoneal membrane is healed. Peritoneal dialysis can be continued on an either intermittent or continuous basis in order to maintain the patient in normal fluid and electrolyte balance.

The next big problem about the oliguric patient is the difficulty of diagnosing acute rejection. A fall in urine output is one of the most reliable signs of rejection. This sign will not be available to help us because urine output is already negligible. Furthermore, although it may be possible by using other signs to diagnose rejection in the oliguric patient, it may be almost impossible to be sure that the rejection has been adequately suppressed by treatment. Renal biopsy may be helpful but there is the additional risk of bleeding from heparin at the next dialysis. In recent years renal scans have shown themselves to be of some value in the transplant with oliguria. Various isotopes can be used to provide a variety of important information. A technetium scan will provide information about intrarenal blood flow. A ^{131}I hippuran scan will give information about excretory function. By means of the scan we may be able to diagnose rejection even though the patient is oliguric.

Thirdly, the oliguric patient will be less tolerant of Imuran and it is harder to judge the maximum tolerated dose. The dose will have to be increased judiciously as renal function recovers.

Fourthly, the cadaver recipient tends to be in poorer health than the living donor recipient due to the fact that the operation is done as an emergency and there is less time to correct anemia and abnormalities of hydration.

These factors, combined with the persisting uremia after operation, make the patient more prone to infective complications.

The final factor which has tended to militate against success in the cadaver case has been the greater degree of immunological incompatibility which usually exists between donor and recipient. Hence there is a greater tendency to rejection and greater difficulty in controlling it. In view of all this it is perhaps not surprising that the survival figures for cadaver grafts have not up to now been as good as for living donors. It is to be hoped that with better tissue typing in larger pools of dialysis recipients, as well as better kidney preservation techniques, the results from cadaver renal transplants will improve to such an extent that the use of kidneys from healthy related volunteers will become unnecessary and unjustified. At present this seems a long way off.

Infective complications

Sealed bladder drainage is usually discontinued after about a week but, despite meticulous catheter technique, urinary infections are distressingly common. Frequent urine microscopy as well as daily urine cultures on all patients will ensure that infections are recognized early. Antibiotic therapy is effective in dealing with these, but in some patients, especially females, infections are inclined to recur at intervals for the first few months. Chest infections once treated are unlikely to recur unless the patient has a bronchitic tendency or persists in smoking cigarettes. The other extremely common infection is candidiasis or 'thrush'. It is usually seen in the mouth as adherent white patches and it may progress down the gastro-intestinal tract to cause troublesome diarrhea. It can be eradicated very successfully with nystatin or Fungilin or a combination of the two, but the treatment should be continued for a full three weeks to make sure it does not recur.

Finally, transplant recipients on heavy immunosuppression may occasionally fall victim to unusual pathogens in unusual sites which are not generally encountered in healthy people. These so-called 'opportunistic infections' may be acute or chronic and may become apparent quite late, even after good rehabilitation has been achieved. They will present the physician with puzzling diagnostic problems and may be hard to eradicate. This is one of the reasons why we like to reduce the dose of immunosuppressive drugs after the first few months and again after a year or two when the tendency to rejection should have become progressively less.

One of the most distressing infections falling into this category, and deserving special mention, is cytomegalovirus (CMV) infection. CMV is ubiquitous but tends only to affect immunosuppressed individuals. The heavier the immunosuppression and the more drugs being used, the greater is the likelihood of CMV. The infection is characterized by a high swinging temperature, a toxic state, and profound prostration in the absence of any other detectable cause. Patients lose their appetites, rapidly lose weight, and become severely depressed. After an interval there will be a rising titer of antiviral antibody demonstrated. Nowadays we tend to treat this condition on clinical suspicion. The correct management is to stop the Imuran and reduce the prednisone to a maintenance level. This intervention requires courage and confidence but nearly always results in progressive recovery after an interval of anything from 2 to 6 weeks. Remarkably the kidney hardly ever seems to be rejected during the time that the Imuran is withdrawn. It is as though the CMV itself has anti-rejection effects. Before this policy of withdrawing the immunosuppression was instituted patients not infrequently died during an attack of CMV infection. Now they nearly always recover. We are now so aware of the danger of CMV that all potential transplant recipients are tested routinely for CMV antibodies. An antibody negative patient is never given a kidney from a donor who is a CMV carrier.

Uncontrollable rejection

In the majority of successful renal transplants the tendency for rejection is only seen in the first few post-operative weeks. The one or two rejection episodes are quickly suppressed and thereafter the patient remains in a stable state on a safe and easily tolerated regimen of immunosuppressive therapy. Those with a more troublesome rejection tendency may require more prolonged and vigorous anti-rejection therapy, but may still have a very good long-term result. There is a minority in whom uncontrollable rejection occurs either early in the post-operative period or as a late slowly progressive phenomenon. The danger is that in our attempts to control rejection we may overdo the immunosuppressive drugs and so make the patient vulnerable to an overwhelming infection. Alternatively death may occur from uncontrollable bleeding due to thrombocytopenia. There is no virtue in saving the graft if in so doing we succeed in killing the patient. It would be far better to decide at an earlier stage to sacrifice the kidney in order to keep the patient alive. The patient can be returned to regular dialysis and actively rehabilitated to await the chance of a second transplant at a later date. The decision to abandon a kidney is a difficult one to make. The patient's disappointment will be so acute that he may find it hard to continue the struggle and face the prospect of going through the whole process a second time. Maintaining the patient's morale as well as his physical condition under these circumstances may require a great deal of patience and devotion. It is also important for the peace of mind of the other dialysis patients to demonstrate that patients with failed transplants can be successfully returned to regular dialysis.

An interesting and tragic late form of rejection, often seen a year or more after an apparently successful transplant, shows itself in the development of heavy proteinuria (of nephrotic proportions). A renal biopsy will show mainly glomerular changes. This is a form of humoral or antibody-mediated rejection and has come to be called 'transplant glomerulopathy'. No treatment has as yet been shown to make any difference to the outcome which is always ultimately complete failure of the graft.

Transplants in small children

If a child has passed puberty the technical problems of dialysis and transplantation are really no greater than those in an adult, apart from emotional and psychological factors.

For the very small pre-pubertal child it is a different situation entirely. Hemodialysis and transplantation are difficult for various reasons. This subject is tackled by Dr Alan Watson and his colleagues in the final chapter of the book.

Renal transplantation in diabetics

Transplantation has been attempted more frequently and with greater success in diabetics in recent years. Diabetics are also doing much better on dialysis. They did very badly on intermittent peritoneal dialysis but they can now be treated very well with hemodialysis, at least for limited periods while waiting for a kidney transplant, and some of the older diabetics are doing extremely well on CAPD. If transplantation is planned, dialysis should be started early, before uremia is too far advanced, and transplantation should be done as soon as possible after the patient is well and stabilized on dialysis. The patient's blood vessels are likely to be atheromatous and this will increase the difficulty of the vascular anastomosis. The operation and the prednisone therapy will both serve to make the diabetic state unstable so that frequent measurement of blood sugar will be required in the post-operative phase. Diabetics are peculiarly prone to infections of all kinds and these will have to be treated early and vigorously. If the operation is a success there tends to be a particularly gratifying improvement in the polyneuritis from which most of these patients have been suffering. Diabetic retinopathy also tends to be arrested or at least its progress is slowed to some extent. The best transplant centers are now achieving results in diabetics as good as those in non-diabetics. The prognosis in diabetics is, however, not determined by the incidence of rejection and renal failure but by the frequent presence of serious vascular disease. Diabetics survive their renal failure, only to die later of myocardial infarctions. Aggressive programs of aortocoronary by-pass have not so far had much impact on this problem. Those who manage to avoid heart attacks have a distressingly high incidence of peripheral arterial disease leading to the need for amputations in some cases. However, these setbacks should not in any way discourage us from trying to help diabetics with renal failure. Instead they should inspire us to provide better management of diabetes at an early stage, paying close attention to proper care for all systems with a network of well-coordinated experts. It may be that more meticulous blood pressure control as well as more perfect glycemic control will reap rewards in the future in terms of less vascular complications.

Long-term follow-up

Patients can be discharged from hospital once the wound is soundly healed, renal function is relatively stable, and the drugs are at a safe dosage level which the patient can readily tolerate. It is good practice to insist that the patient knows the names of the drugs as well as the exact dose and strength of the tablets. The possible consequences of discontinuing therapy should be made quite clear. Out-patient reviews may be necessary every two or three days at first with gradually lengthening intervals between visits. At each out-patient visit a physical examination, full blood count, urine culture and full series of renal function tests are normally performed. The patient is usually instructed to contact the unit at once if he feels at all unwell so as to arrange to be examined by one of the transplant team. Later on at least part of the responsibility for his care may be accepted by his own doctor. A return to full-time working should not be long delayed in a successful case. The patient may need a push to get started. Occasionally a tense, fluid-filled swelling insidiously develops around the kidney in the first few months following the operation. Aspiration may reveal lymph, and, if so, one can confidently diagnose a lymphocele. This complication can be dealt with by surgical drainage into the peritoneal cavity.

There are now many reports of successful pregnancies in renal transplant recipients. There are two potential risks in pregnancy in transplant patients. The first concerns aggravation of renal function. The second concerns a possible danger to the fetus because of immunosuppressive drugs or problems of delivery of the fetus through the pelvis which is narrowed by the presence of a transplanted kidney. Women who already have a family would be well advised to undergo sterilization at the time of the transplant or whenever the opportunity presents itself. Long-term oral contraceptives are not advisable because transplant patients may already have a thrombotic tendency which is likely to be aggravated. The advice one should give to a married woman who badly wants a child will depend on various factors including her age, blood pressure and level of renal function, but it may be justified to let her go ahead once she is fully aware of the risks. Very careful planning is essential.

Late complications (of transplantation)

Bone disease

Classical renal osteodystrophy with osteomalacia and osteitis fibrosa as previously described resolves rapidly after successful renal transplantation, provided the renal function obtained is satisfactory. The restored vitamin D metabolism with normal production of 1,25-dihydroxycholecalciferol appears to be responsible for the improvement in renal osteodystrophy. Osteomalacia rapidly improves within the first 12 months and by the end of the year it is found in only a very small minority of patients. In these patients one usually finds another added cause for the persistence of osteomalacia. Malabsorption, gastric surgery, and the use of anticonvulsants and barbiturates are occasional causes for this kind of post-transplant osteomalacia. Osteitis fibrosa and secondary hyperparathyroidism also improve after renal transplantation, but the rate of resolution is slower and clearly this depends on how large the parathyroid glands were before transplantation and also on the function of the transplanted kidney.

There are two new developments to be found after renal transplantation. The first one is the development of osteoporosis. This is in fact the result of the excessive steroid therapy which patients receive in an effort to ensure that the kidney grafts are not rejected. Osteoporosis is not usually troublesome, but in some patients it is accompanied by skeletal fractures and pain.

The second complication that develops after renal transplantation is *avascular necrosis of bone*. This is a most troublesome complication and the incidence in most series used to be something between 10 and 30% of all transplanted patients. Subarticular joint surfaces are affected and the bone crumbles away. This leads to acute pain and the gradual destruction of the joint surface leads to secondary osteoarthritis with severe pain and lack of mobility. Any joint can be affected, but this condition affects particularly the hip joint and the knees. The explanation is still not clear. Excessive steroid therapy may predispose to it, but other factors play a part too. Treatment is still not satisfactory. Patients are advised to restrict weight bearing and occasionally reconstructive orthopedic surgery is carried out. Perhaps because of improved immunosuppression, avascular necrosis has become relatively rare in recent years.

Cataracts

The high dosage of steroids which patients receive during the first few months after a transplant is probably the cause of the high incidence of cataracts which these patients tend to develop. Patients attending the transplant clinic should have a regular examination by an ophthalmologist. The development of cataracts can be anticipated and observed. The patients can be reassured about their failing vision and operations can be carried out when the time is right.

Renal artery stenosis

If a patient has normal blood pressure after a successful transplant and then subsequently develops progressive hypertension, one should always be suspicious about the possibility of renal artery stenosis. The suspicion becomes almost a certainty if there is also an increasingly loud bruit audible on auscultation over the graft where none existed before. The narrowing, which can be demonstrated by renal arteriography, is nearly always at the anastomosis of the donor renal artery with the recipient vessel. Surgical correction or by-pass of this stenosis is horrendously difficult because of the inflammatory fibrosis in the area caused by the presence of the foreign organ. Except in the most outstandingly skilled hands, operation nearly always results in loss of the graft. Some cases have been helped by transluminal angioplasty, and we have found that most cases respond to long-term therapy with warfarin and dipyridamole (Persantin). Perhaps this condition is a form of localized vascular rejection with fibrin and platelets laid down in the area of maximal turbulence.

Long-term prognosis

Long-term survival for transplant recipients depends on complete suppression of the rejection process as well as avoidance of such complications as the late development of glomerulonephritis in the graft. Many patients who received their grafts in the early 1960s are at present leading normal lives with normal renal function. There seems no reason why they should not remain healthy for many more years, though it is perhaps too soon to predict a normal life expectation. As improvements in matching and immunosuppression reduce the number of patients with uncontrollable rejection one hopes that long-term survival will be achieved in the vast majority of transplant recipients. With currently available immunosuppressive drugs one year graft survival is about 75% and five year graft survival is about 50%. The first year mortality in young patients without any systemic disease or coronary artery disease is less than 5%. In the presence of coronary artery disease, significant lung disease or diabetes the mortality increases but in all high risk groups it is less than 10%. The spectrum of patients suitable for transplantation has increased considerably over the years. It is not uncommon to transplant patients in their 60s and even in their 70s. As yet there has been no success in the over 80s! Furthermore patients with severe coronary artery disease which has been successfully stabilized are also transplant candidates. Patients with stabilized chronic obstructive lung disease are now also considered for transplantation. Obviously the presence of a risk factor increases the chance of a serious complication and this must be explained to the patient.

It is the practice of all transplant units at the present time to ask for informed consent from patients who are about to consider transplantation as a method of treating their end-stage renal failure. This allows the patient to make an informed decision about the various modalities of treatment available. Unfortunately the numbers of patients able to benefit from long-term support for end-stage renal failure is likely to overwhelm the facilities available to treat them for many years to come. Our preoccupation with expanding these facilities should not distract us from the even more important job of improving methods for early treatment and prevention of kidney disease.

11

Dialysis and Transplantation in Children

Alan R. Watson, Annette Vigneux and Janet Willumsen

Pediatric dialysis and transplantation programs involve children of all ages, from neonates weighing less than 1 kg to mature adolescents. The management of children with renal failure requires a great deal of technical skill and adaptability. It is essential to have experienced nurses participating in a team approach geared to the medical, nutritional and psychological needs of children.

Many of the general principles and techniques of dialysis and transplantation discussed in previous chapters also apply to children. This chapter emphasizes the aspects of treatment that are unique to, and particularly important in, the care of children.

Development of the kidney

The newborn infant's kidney is immature and contains only 17% of the cells found in an adult kidney. The remainder of the cells develop by six months of age. The kidney then continues to grow by increasing the size of the cells. The newborn kidney has the same number of nephrons as the adult, but they function differently, mainly because of the resistance to blood flow within the kidney. The glomerular filtration rate (GFR) at birth averages only about $20\,ml/min/1.73\,m^2$. This increases to $80\,ml/min/1.73\,m^2$ by six months of age and reaches the normal adult rate in the second year of life. The newborn infant tends to have a higher blood urea and phosphate level and a lower plasma bicarbonate concentration. Very immature infants, between 28 and 32 weeks gestational age, are particularly prone to excessive salt loss in the urine, and this is also a feature in children who are born with obstructions to the urinary tract.

Advances in the intensive care of neonates over the past decade have resulted in increased interest in the development and physiology of the newborn kidney. Increased use of obstetrical ultrasound has led to intrauterine detection of fetal abnormalities such as hydronephrosis or cystic kidneys. Although it is uncertain at present whether surgery on the fetus *in utero* might prevent or reduce subsequent renal damage, it is an advantage to be forewarned about the need for possible surgery soon after birth.

Metabolism

The infant's metabolic rate is much more closely related to body weight than the adult's. In combination with high insensible water losses, increased fluid and energy demands, and the inability to regulate water intake it is not surprising that metabolic derangements can develop rapidly in infants and small children.

It should be noted that surface area calculations are often used in pediatrics for the administration of appropriate fluids or medications. The surface area can easily be calculated from nomograms using standard height and weight measurements.

Blood pressure

Blood pressure rises steadily throughout childhood and normal values for both sexes at all ages are readily available in pediatric textbooks. The upper normal limit at birth is usually 100/65 mm Hg; this rises to 135/90 mm Hg by 14 years of age. Automatic blood pressue or Doppler ultrasound machines are particularly useful for taking blood pressure in the small child. The cuff bladder should encircle at least 3/4 of the circumference of the arm with a cuff that is at least 2/3 of the length of the upper arm in width.

Acute renal failure

Acute renal failure (ARF) seems to occur much less commonly in children than in adults. The incidence and causes vary from country to country depending upon referral practices and the socio-economic status of the population. Poor conditions increase the incidence of diarrheal illnesses, causing dehydration and acute tubular necrosis (ATN) as well as infections which can result in post-infectious glomerulonephritis.

Oliguria in children is usually defined as a reduction in urine output to less than $300 \, \text{ml/m}^2/\text{day}$, but in neonates the critical value is less than $0.6 \, \text{ml/kg}$ body weight/hr. High output failure also occurs in children.

Causes of acute renal failure in children

The main causes are:
1 renal hypoperfusion, e.g. dehydration, septicemia, hemorrhage;
2 hemolytic uremic syndrome (hemolytic anemia, thrombocytopenia, azotemia);
3 glomerulonephritis;
4 bilateral pyelonephritis;
5 obstructive uropathy, e.g. posterior urethral valves; and
6 nephrotoxic poisons, e.g. antibiotics.

Management of acute renal failure

Children, especially infants, are often acutely ill and there is a need to diagnose and treat the metabolic derangements simultaneously. Some causes are obvious but it is important to enquire into prodromal illnesses, such as diarrhea and sore throat, which might precede hemolytic uremic syndrome and post-streptococcal glomerulonephritis respectively. Oligohydramnios in pregnancy may be a clue to an underlying kidney problem such as hypoplasia or dysplasia in a newborn infant. Ultrasonography, when performed by an experienced radiologist, considerably improves diagnostic accuracy and has been particularly helpful in ruling out urinary obstruction.

If a prerenal cause for the ARF is suspected, volume expansion using blood, albumin or normal saline in a dose of $10-20 \, \text{ml/kg}$ body weight over $60 \, \text{min}$ should be undertaken. Frusemide $2 \, \text{mg/kg}$ or mannitol $0.5-1 \, \text{g}$ per kg body weight iv may then be given to induce a diuresis.

In established ARF, fluid intake will be restricted to $300-400 \, \text{ml/m}^2$ in 24 hours, i.e., insensible water losses, plus the previous day's output. It is important to remember that the fluid intake must be increased by 12% for each $1°C$ rise in temperature over normal body temperature. The child must be weighed accurately at least once daily. In a diuretic phase it may be necessary to weigh the child two or three times a day so that fluid orders can be adjusted.

Drug therapy

Hyperkalemia, acidosis and other electrolyte or metabolic disturbances are managed as previously described using medication in doses appropriate to the child's size, as shown in standard pediatric texts. Severe acute hypertension may be controlled by giving diazoxide, 2.5 or 5 mg/kg body weight as a rapid infusion over 2—5 min. Alternatively, nitroprusside infusion may be used but this necessitates monitoring in an intensive care setting. Other antihypertensive drugs employed include propranolol, hydralazine and methyldopa. Young children are particularly prone to convulsions which can usually be controlled by a slow intravenous infusion of diazepam 0.2 mg/kg body weight.

Nutrition

The increased metabolic and energy demands of children with ARF are difficult to meet without the help of an experienced dietitian. The dietitian regulates the calorie content of low solute humanized cow's milk preparations for infants and provides high calorie feeds for children who will cooperate with oral feeding. It is difficult to maintain adequate nutrition with intravenous feeding regimens because of the high fluid volumes involved. Early dialysis may be indicated in children with acute renal failure because without adequate calorie intake children may lose up to 1% of their body weight per day. Other reasons for early dialysis in children are as detailed for adults.

Dialysis therapy

Peritoneal dialysis is usually considered the treatment of choice for ARF in children who do not have intra-abdominal problems. The technique is generally available, relatively safe, and better tolerated in the face of hemodynamic disturbances. Although peritoneal dialysis is only about 20% as efficient as hemodialysis in adults, it is about 50% as efficient in small children due to the higher ratio of peritoneal surface to body surface area. However, ultrafiltration may be difficult to achieve, especially in small children.

Hemodialysis must be contemplated when peritoneal dialysis cannot be used or must be abandoned, and in certain situations such as poisoning where hemodialysis or hemoperfusion may be preferentially required. Local facilities and technical expertise will determine the method of vascular access which may be accomplished acutely using central venous catheters.

Peritoneal dialysis in acute renal failure

The principles of peritoneal dialysis in acute renal failure are the same as those in adults, except that the conscious child is sedated with either intravenous diazepam or an intramuscular mixture, such as chlorpromazine, promethazine and meperidine, which is currently used at our center. Ideally two nurses should be in attendance, one specifically to allay the child's anxiety in the absence of the parents.

The child may need catheterization to ensure that the bladder is empty. The midline subumbilical position or lateral abdominal site is chosen for the introduction of the catheter. Since a younger child cannot tense the abdomen, 30 to 50 ml/kg body weight of warmed dialysate is introduced before the cannula is inserted.

Special stylet peritoneal catheters for children are commercially available. In neonates and very small children the technique may be adapted using a guide wire introduced via a 16 gauge intravenous cannula which is then removed and replaced by a chest drain or Shaldon catheter.

Dialysis exchanges are usually performed hourly using 40 to 60 ml/kg body weight in infants and small children and 30 to 40 ml/kg in older children up to a maximum of 2 litres per cycle. Dialysis solutions with a glucose concentration of higher than 4.25 g/l should be avoided because of the risk of hyperglycemia and excessive ultrafiltration. In patients with severe lactic acidosis, bicarbonate-containing dialysis solutions may have to be substituted.

Although dialysis exchanges are traditionally done manually, peritoneal cyclers are available which can deliver dialysis volumes of 100 ml to 3 litres. It is essential that such automatic cycling systems record fluid input and output accurately. If accuracy cannot be guaranteed the child must be nursed on a bed scale to ensure precise and continuous observation of weight changes and fluid balance.

Hemodialysis in acute renal failure

Vascular access can be difficult to obtain and maintain, particularly in small children. Peripheral arterial venous shunts of appropriate size for small children have been developed and are usually placed under general anesthetic. The radial artery and cephalic vein is the preferred site in older children but in smaller children and infants more proximal sites such as the brachial artery and cephalic vein or the profunda femoris artery and saphenous vein may be used.

Acute hemodialysis of newborn infants can be performed by catheterizing the umbilical vessels. Some centers use Shaldon type cannulas inserted into the femoral veins on a daily basis. In larger children, two cannulas can be inserted in the same femoral vein but in patients weighing less than 40 kg one cannula should be used in each femoral vein. The femoral vein is a useful route for emergency hemodialysis, particularly in the unconscious patient. In the intensive care situation, we have employed subclavian (Uldall) catheters, using the Seldinger technique, for short-term hemodialysis via the femoral vein and obtained adequate blood flow and urea clearance with a single-needle system. In large adolescent patients it is also possible to use double-lumen catheters in the femoral vein.

Experience with percutaneous placement of central venous catheters into the subclavian vein in children is limited. We have found that it is difficult to place such catheters in children under 12 years of age using local anesthetic. Femoral catheters are generally left in place only very briefly but a properly tunnelled and maintained subclavian catheter can be left in place for much longer (one 15-year-old male in our unit had a subclavian catheter for six months without incident). Surgically implanted jugular catheters have now become the acute access method of choice and will be discussed later.

The technique for hemodialysis in ARF is essentially the same as that for chronic renal failure. Dialysis should be initiated at an early stage whenever possible. Daily treatments of short duration may be necessary to avoid too rapid correction of metabolic abnormalities and to cope with the catabolic state.

Children have comparatively little vascular reserve and therefore it is essential to monitor the patient's vital signs and blood pressure with frequent weighing on a sensitive bed scale. The new gen ation of dialysis machines with ultrafiltration control has helped considerably in this respect. A rapid fall in plasma osmolality leading to an intracellular water shift and the dialysis disequilibrium syndrome can be prevented by using a variable sodium dialysate concentration or an infusion of mannitol (1 g/kg body weight) throughout the entire hemodialysis treatment. In patients who are being ventilated or have severe metabolic disturbances, bicarbonate may be substituted for acetate in the dialysate. If a single-needle dialysis system is employed the dose of heparin should be carefully adjusted using activated clotting times.

Continuous slow ultrafiltration

Continuous slow ultrafiltration, as described for adults, can also be employed in children. However, consideration must be given to the extracorporeal volume involved in the system and the rate of fluid removal. The technique is likely to be successful only if there is good arterial access.

End-stage renal disease in children

End-stage renal disease (ESRD) is not as common in children as in adults. Acceptance rates into renal replacement programs range from three to six new cases per year per million child population (age group 0–15 years). However, data from the European Dialysis and Transplant Association (EDTA) Registry show that in 1983 the number of children starting dialysis ranged from 0.4 to 8 new cases per million child population in the various participating countries. The variable incidence may reflect differences not only in the economic development of various countries but also in commitment and availability of facilities and trained personnel to provide care for children with ESRD.

Although the techniques of intermittent peritoneal dialysis and hemodialysis have been in clinical use since the late 1950s, it was a decade later before long-term dialysis programs for children were initiated in a few specialist centers. Some authors expressed strong reservations about the psychological trauma of dialysis and transplantation in children and there were various technical difficulties in hemodialyzing very small children for prolonged periods. As a result very few children under two years of age or weighing less than 10 kg were accepted for hemodialysis. Improvements in techniques of vascular access, increased technical and clinical expertise in transplantation in small children, and the advent of continuous ambulatory peritoneal dialysis (CAPD) have resulted in an increased number of patients under five years old commencing treatment. However, the question of starting treatment for ESRD in very small infants can still present an ethical dilemma. It must be appreciated that growth failure in the first two years of life will not be reversed by treatment in future years. Recent reports of neurological and developmental handicaps in children who developed chronic renal failure in the first year of life suggest that, if treatment is to be commenced, it should be early, comprehensive and aggressive.

Causes of end-stage renal disease in children

The causes of ESRD are shown in Table 11.1. Hypoplasia and dysplasia of the kidney and such hereditary renal diseases as cystinosis are much

Table 11.1. Causes of chronic renal failure in children

Causes	% of cases
Glomerular disease	34
Malformation of urinary tract and pyelonephritis	22
Hereditary—familial • Medullary cystic disease • Cystinosis • Polycystic disease • Alport's syndrome	16
Renal hypoplasia or dysplasia	11
Other causes • Wilms' tumor • Lupus • Oligomeganephronia	12
Uncertain	5

more important causes of renal failure in children than in adults. Knowledge of the primary renal disease is important because the speed of progression toward end-stage renal disease depends upon the etiology. Hence, the prognosis given to the child and parents varies. Children with underlying conditions such as hypoplasia usually progress slowly, whereas those with very active glomerulonephritis may develop ESRD very quickly. Some glomerular diseases have a high recurrence rate in the transplanted kidney and this may affect the timing of transplantation in individual cases. A genetically transmitted disease necessitates genetic counselling, and possibly investigation of family members.

Treatment facilities for children with end-stage renal disease

Ideally, children with chronic renal failure should be cared for in pediatric centers where specific attention is paid to their overall growth and development. The basic staff requirements for such centers are a pediatric nephrologist, nurses experienced in dialysis of children, a dietitian, a recreation therapist and a social worker. In addition it is necessary to have access to pediatric surgery, urology, child psychiatry and a hospital school. Centralization of pediatric facilities may require children and families to travel long distances for assessment and treatment but this may be preferable to the occasional treatment of children in adult centers where techniques may be inappropriate and psychological problems are more likely to arise.

Pediatric nephrologists generally agree that a renal transplant is the best treatment for children with ESRD, as it offers the best form of rehabilitation. In fact, children may not be accepted into a long-term dialysis program without a clear understanding that transplantation is the ultimate goal. Commencement of dialysis is therefore combined with active preparation for eventual renal transplantation. Specialized pediatric centers that encourage transplantation appear to have reduced patient mortality. With patients who live considerable distances from the pediatric center, transfer to intermediate care in adult units has been helped considerably by the advent of continuous ambulatory peritoneal dialysis (CAPD). This technique is replacing home hemodialysis in many countries and is now our dialysis therapy of first choice.

Indications for long-term dialysis

The indications for initiating dialysis in a child depend as much on clinical status as on biochemical criteria. Therapy is generally commenced when the GFR is less than $5\,ml/min/1.73\,m^2$, which usually coincides with a serum creatinine level of $900\,mol/l$ ($10.17\,mg/dl$) in older children and $\leq 500\,mol/l$ ($5.65\,mg/dl$) in small children with a reduced muscle mass. Other indications are persistent nausea, anorexia or reduced activity, especially if combined with growth failure, uncontrolled hypertension, severe anemia, acidosis, hyperphosphatemia and hyperkalemia which cannot be controlled with diet or exchange resins. As in adults, heart failure, uremic pericarditis and uremic neuropathy or encephalopathy are definitive and late indications for dialysis.

Intermittent peritoneal dialysis

Until the advent of CAPD in 1978, intermittent peritoneal dialysis (IPD) was considered a viable dialysis option, particularly in children who still had some residual renal function. It can be performed on an in-patient basis or, in rare cases, at home using an automatic cycler and hourly exchanges for up to 20 hours twice a week. Although patients appeared to do well initially in 40 hours a week of IPD, many required transfer to hemodialysis as their endogenous renal function decreased.

Continuous ambulatory peritoneal dialysis

Continuous ambulatory peritoneal dialysis was introduced in 1978 and has enabled many children to have home dialysis therapy with all its attendant benefits. Although the technique was adopted in 70% of new pediatric patients in Canada in 1983, the equivalent figure from Europe was only 17%.

CAPD techniques

The techniques of catheter insertion, catheter care, training and monitoring procedures have been described elsewhere. However, three points that are particularly relevant to children require emphasis.

(1) *Catheters.* The variation in the sizes of pediatric patients requires that a range of catheters (Fig. 11.1) be available to the surgeon who performs the operation, which is usually done under general anesthetic. Our own preference is for single cuff catheters as children can have very little subcutaneous tissue and double cuff catheters tend to erode easily. We believe that the best way to reduce leaks after catheter insertion or one-way failure is to place the catheter in the paramedian position and ensure that there is good inflow and outflow of peritoneal fluid through the catheter before the child leaves the operating room.

(2) *Dialysis volumes.* The dialysis volume per exchange after catheter insertion is gradually increased over 4 to 5 days to the final CAPD volume of 30 to 50 ml/kg body weight or 1200 ml/m^2. We endeavor to use the currently available bag sizes of 300 ml to 3 l but special orders can be custom-made to the required volume. If a smaller volume is required, a simple scale can be used to measure the volume instilled from the bag.

(3) *Dialysate composition.* With increasing experience, peritoneal dialysis solutions may be modified to overcome problems such as hyponatremia, hypermagnesemia and hypocalcemia. Dialysis solutions containing amino acids in place of glucose are being considered to combat protein losses into the dialysate.

Training

We train our patients as in-patients over a 10 to 14 day period. Where facilities are available, training could also be carried out on an out-patient basis. A CAPD pediatric nurse is assigned to the family during this time. At least one parent and patients themselves who are over 12 years of age and have the necessary manual dexterity and psychological aptitude are taught to do bag changes. Whenever possible, fathers as well as mothers should be involved in the training process so that they are not excluded from the child's ongoing care.

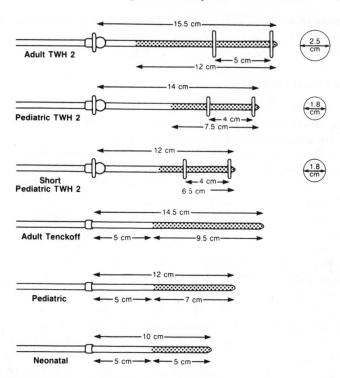

Fig. 11.1. Range of peritoneal dialysis catheters used for long-term peritoneal dialysis in children.

Advantages of CAPD

CAPD has several major advantages. First, it allows greater freedom and improved school attendance as the child visits the out-patient clinic only once a month after he or she has been stabilized on dialysis. The increased school attendance and peer group interaction should have great benefits psychologically and socially. Since CAPD is a continuous procedure, fluid intake and diet are less restricted and this is especially important for adolescents who may have poor compliance with a strict diet. Another benefit is the child's active participation in his own treatment which has psychological advantages over the usually completely passive hemodialysis situation. In addition, the cost of maintenance CAPD is below that of in-center hemodialysis and families and agencies are saved the expense and time of transporting children back and forth from the hemodialysis unit at least three times a week.

CAPD can be used on a reasonably long-term basis to allow patients who have lost a first tansplant to delay consideration of a second in order to regain their health, complete a vital school year, or make necessary psychological adjustments. It is also used in children whose kidney failure is due to a severe acute glomerulonephritis, e.g. SLE, until the inflammatory process has subsided.

Disadvantages of CAPD

The morbidity associated with placement and maintenance of the peritoneal catheter has been reduced with experience and newer catheter designs, but exit site and tunnel infections are still a significant problem, affecting 25% of patients. The incidence of peritonitis in our center is one episode every 11.6 patient months. Only one patient has required transfer to hemodialysis on a temporary basis for this complication. In contrast to the adult experience, peritonitis has not been a cause of CAPD failure in children. The long-term consequences of CAPD on nutrition and growth in children are still being evaluated. The protein losses in younger children may be very significant with time. Furthermore, a technique which demands four bag changes every day with meticulous aseptic technique has led to considerable strain on families and patients. This must be anticipated and programs devised to alleviate the problem. With our younger patients, we have tried to prevent the burnout phenomenon by offering short patient admissions either to our own unit or to the local hospital to relieve the parents. This involves training additional nurses.

Monitoring of CAPD patients

We have found that having a CAPD nurse provide telephone contact on a regular basis with the patients gives invaluable support that is particularly appreciated during the first few confidence-building weeks at home. When they are stable, the children are seen in the clinic at monthly intervals. Each visit involves a transfer set change in a clean area, routine biochemical monitoring and evaluation by the pediatric nephrologist, dietitian and social worker. The dialysis transplant coordinator is also involved if organization of blood transfusions and preparation for transplant are required. An assessment of bone development is carried out every three months along with X-rays and parathyroid hormone blood levels. Close dietary supervision is maintained using home dietary records, and the patient's nutritional status is assessed using skin fold thickness and mid-arm circumference measurements in addition to height, weight and head circumference measurements.

Exit site problems and peritonitis are treated as described previously. We have found children in diapers to be at no greater risk for peritonitis and we have even looked after one child with a temporary defunctioning colostomy for 12 months who had only one bout of peritonitis. CAPD has not proved to be a significant risk factor for transplantation but children with peritonitis are taken off the transplant waiting list for two weeks while the peritonitis is treated. A mild exit site infection is not a contra-indication to transplantation but the catheter may well be removed at the time of renal transplant. Otherwise catheters are left in place until the child is discharged from hospital following the renal transplant, as some children have a tendency to develop post-operative ascites which can be drained through the peritoneal catheter.

We encourage our children to exercise and swim. To facilitate swimming we are currently using an ostomy flange attachment over the catheter exit site onto which the ostomy bag containing the CAPD tubing and empty dialysis bag can be snapped in a 'tupperware-like' arrangement.

CAPD is successful in children only if close attention is paid to the logistical difficulties involved in providing facilities, and possibly trained nursing support, at school for the midday bag exchange. The involvement of community resources requires a great deal of coordination and effort.

To maximize growth in small children so that transplantation may be feasible, we have often combined CAPD with aggressive feeding regimens using nasogastric or gastrostomy tube feeds. This helps to prevent some of the time-consuming struggles between parents and anorexic infants.

Continuous cycling peritoneal dialysis (CCPD)

CCPD may well play an increasing role in helping to prevent the 'burn-out' associated with CAPD, especially in families with young children and adolescents who are likely to be on dialysis for some time. Although this technique reduces the number of connections by at least 50%, the reported peritonitis rate appears to be the same as for CAPD and at the same time it is more costly.

Long-term hemodialysis

Nurses who work in adult units often feel anxious when confronted by a child who requires hemodialysis. If a child cannot be treated in a pediatric center, medical staff with pediatric training should be readily available for all emergencies that may arise. The child's size and comprehension will be important factors in tailoring the dialysis treatment to his or her needs.

Vascular access

The creation of an AV fistula is feasible in most children and has been reported in infants weighing less than 10 kg. However, fistulae take much longer to mature in children and there may be the additional problems of high output congestive failure and unequal limb growth. Adolescents who are very conscious of their body image may be troubled by the appearance of a large fistula.

Nurses accustomed to working in adult units may be reluctant to cannulate young children. We do not employ injections of local anesthetic prior to the needling (usually with 16 or 17 gauge needles). Although a local anesthetic spray gives some psychological support, we have found the best way to calm the child is by having a parent or nurse talk to and reassure him or her throughout the procedure.

As in adults, the preferred site for an AV fistula is at the wrist, but other sites may be used such as the saphenofemoral loop and PTFE grafts in the forearm. Although the carbon button method of painless vascular access sounds ideal for children, it should be borne in mind that hemodialysis is a short-term measure before transplantation and therefore such a procedure does not seem justified.

Since an AV fistula may not work or may take a very long time to mature in the younger child, an AV shunt may be substituted. However, the shunt carries a higher risk of clotting and infection.

Central venous catheters

From our experience with central lines for total parenteral nutrition and chemotherapy, we have developed a central venous (WBW) catheter of either 1.57 or 2.65 mm internal diameter which is placed into the external or internal jugular vein, usually under general anesthetic (Fig. 11.2). The catheter is fixed in the neck using a small silicone rubber grommet and tunnelled subcutaneously onto the anterior chest wall where the exit site is covered with a non-adhesive gauze dressing beneath a larger sterile semipermeable dressing. When not in use, the catheter is filled with the appropriate volume of heparin solution (1000 iu/ml) and clamped securely. If the catheter is not being used for regular dialysis, it is flushed with heparin solution once a week. In addition, the catheter exit site is inspected and redressed at least once a week.

The WBW catheter is similar to the Hickman catheter used in other units except that there is no dacron cuff to anchor the catheter and therefore it can be removed more easily at the bedside by gentle traction. The advantages of the central venous catheter include:

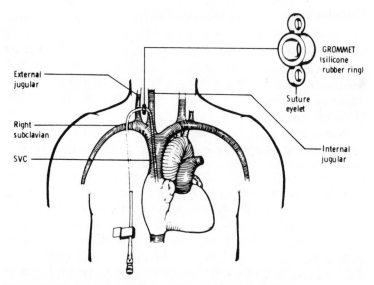

Fig. 11.2. WBW catheter. Diagram of catheter inserted in external jugular or internal jugular vein and emerging from skin exit site on anterior chest wall.

- a vascular access which is available for immediate use;
- no needling and therefore fewer psychological problems;
- no destruction of blood vessels;
- availability of both arms during dialysis for schoolwork, eating and play, as well as blood pressure monitoring, etc.; and
- the multipurpose nature of the catheter that can be used for total parenteral nutrition (TPN), iv infusion of fluids and medication, blood withdrawal for sampling, CVP monitoring and plasma exchange therapy.

Disadvantages of the central venous catheter

One important disadvantage of the central venous catheter is intermittent blood flow. The catheter is placed preferentially at the superior vena cava/right atrium junction. Since it has a single end hole, it may occlude in contact with endothelial surfaces. The patient's position may have to be altered. We have adjusted several catheters at the bedside by simple traction. A second disadvantage is the risk of catheter-associated sepsis when the catheter has multiple uses. Strict catheter care protocols must be followed to avoid using the catheter simply as an intravenous line. We have had very few clotted catheters using the intermittent heparin flush protocol. Suitable single-access technology must be available to minimize recirculation problems.

Central venous catheters were designed for acute vascular access but, so far, three patients in our unit have had them in place for more than six months. Although the AV fistula is still regarded as the gold standard for vascular access, the central venous catheters may suffice for relatively long periods while the child awaits a renal transplant and also provide acute access for CAPD patients who need to stop peritoneal dialysis temporarily.

Monitoring the child on dialysis

Although two stable adolescent patients may have only one nurse, younger children are nursed on a one-to-one basis. The younger the child, the more frequent the need for physical assessments during dialysis and these should include weight, heart rate (cardiac monitor if necessary), blood pressure (automatic blood pressure machines are now available and less disruptive) and level of responsiveness. Since young children cannot express themselves, undue restlessness, staring eyes, twitching or vague symptoms such as stomach complaints should alert the nurse to possible hypotension or disequilibrium.

The use of single-needle dialysis may require constant monitoring and adjustment of the equipment to ensure adequate stroke volumes and consequently dialyser clearances.

Dialyser and blood lines

A generally accepted rule for pediatric dialysis is that the extracorporeal blood volume (dialyser and blood lines) should not exceed 10% of the child's blood volume. This is calculated using the formula blood volume = 80 ml/kg body weight. For example,

20 kg child × 80 ml = 1600 ml blood volume
10% of 1600   = 160 ml

Therefore, 160 ml is the total blood volume that should be in the extracorporeal blood circuit during dialysis. If this volume is exceeded, the dialyser and blood lines can be primed with blood or albumin solution.

It is important that the dialyser and blood lines for each individual patient be carefully selected to achieve a safe, efficient dialysis. Factors to take into consideration include:
● priming volume of the dialyser,
● having a low compliance dialyser (the increased extracorporeal blood

volume accommodated by a large compliance dialyser may lead to hypotension),
- knowing the ultrafiltration rate of the dialyser in ml/mmHg/hr (however, this is now a less serious problem with controlled ultrafiltration machines; a range of dialysers suitable for infants up to adolescents is illustrated in Table 11.2),
- dialyser membrane characteristics such as biocompatibility.

Blood lines must also be tailored to the size of the child; the range of sizes available is illustrated in Table 11.3. Some flexibility is always required when dealing with mixing and matching of accessories to meet the needs of specific patients. An experienced dialysis technician is invaluable in this respect.

Single-needle dialysis

Single fistula needles with single-needle machines have found increasing acceptance in recent years and we currently use them whenever possible in our patients to avoid the psychological and physical impact of repeated fistula needling as well as the creation of fistula stenoses. Vascular access via femoral, subclavian and jugular catheters has increased the demand for this welcome technological advance.

Ultrafiltration and dialysis disequilibrium

Even with accurate bed scales and very close monitoring, children are notoriously prone to developing hypotension because of their size and low circulating blood volumes. The advent of dialysis delivery systems with accurate ultrafiltration control has been a major advance in the management of children. Every unit involved with the care of children should strive to have the most modern available technology rather than relying upon physical measurements of weight loss. In children who are hypoalbuminemic, fluid removal may require the concomitant infusion of 25% albumin infusion (0.5−1 g/kg).

Dialysis disequilibrium can be prevented at the start of dialysis by restricting the urea clearances to 2 ml/min/kg body weight (calculated from the published characteristics of the selected dialysis membrane). Urea clearances can be progressively increased over the next few dialysis sessions to 3−4 ml/min/kg. Disequilibrium can also be prevented by using a high initial sodium dialysate with a gradual reduction in the sodium level to normal serum levels towards the end of the dialysis

Table 11.2. A selection of dialysers suitable for use in a pediatric unit*

Dialyser	Priming volume (ml)	Compliance ml/100 mmHg	Effective surface area (m²)	Type of dialyser	Ultrafiltration coefficient (ml/mmHg/hr)
Mini minor—Gambro	20	6	0.20	Plate	0.4–0.6
Excel .3p—Asahi	30	0	0.30	Hollow fiber	1.4
Lundia minor—Gambro	33	10	0.41	Plate	1.2–1.6
PPD .8—Cobe	45	25	0.80	Plate	2
Taf .6—Terumo	48	0	0.60	Hollow fiber	2.2–2.4
Disscap .8—Hospal	52	0	0.80	Hollow fiber	2.7
Nephross Lento—Organon Teknika	57	0	0.70	Hollow fiber	2.8
Lundia 10-2N—Gambro	60	10	0.80	Plate	2–3
Biospal 1200 S—Hospal	60	2.3	0.50	Plate	18
HF 70—Cobe	65	0	0.70	Hollow fiber	2.8
Lundia 10-3N—Gambro	72	13	0.80	Plate	3–4
Biospal 1800 S—Hospal	75	27	0.70	Plate	25
CDAK 3500—Cordis	85	0	0.90	Hollow fiber	3.0–3.3

*Data supplied by manufacturers.

Table 11.3. Blood lines suitable for pediatric hemodialysis

Blood tubing	Arterial volume (ml)	Venous volume ml	Total volume ml
Dravon blood line—Cardiovision			
S3086 Art. S3087 Venous	4.1	11.5	15.6
Pediatric blood lines—Gambro			
Art 367-A3 Venous 414-AX	12	21	33
Dravon blood line—Cardiovision			
S-3088 Art. S3089 Venous	28	22	50
Pediatric blood lines—Gambro			
Art. 402-A6, Venous 412-AX	28	28	56
18-490—Cobe (for use with Centry)	37.5	30.5	68
BSM2—Single pump—Hospal			
A36P, PV7	38	46	84
D9-510 Cobe	35	50	85
BSM2—Double pump—Hospal			
A36P V28P	38	74	112

*Data supplied by manufacturers.

treatment. Some delivery systems incorporate an optional automated variable sodium dialysate.

Other strategies to prevent disequilibrium include the infusion of 25% mannitol using 1 g/kg body weight over the treatment period. The dialysate flow can also be reduced from the traditional 500 ml/min to lower values when initiating dialysis therapy. Very rarely do we need to consider increasing the dialysate glucose concentration to 500 mg/dl (28 mmol/l) or even higher to circumvent rapid osmolar changes.

Composition of the dialysate

Children were included in the original report of acetate intolerance. It has been suggested that they are one group in whom bicarbonate dialysis should be considered in order to meet the increased buffering capacity needed for growing bones. Recent innovations have provided equipment to deliver bicarbonate buffered dialysate on a routine basis. However, like others, we have recognized few instances of true acetate intolerance and we do not advocate the routine use of bicarbonate dialysis except in very young children and patients who are hemodynamically unstable or on ventilators in the intensive care unit.

Children may become catabolic very quickly and the potassium concentrations in the dialysate bath may have to be kept very low, with checks on serum levels during the dialysis session.

Frequency of dialysis

Young children, particularly those who are anephric may require daily dialysis to prevent excessive fluid shifts when less frequent dialysis is performed. In addition, the need to provide an adequate nutritional intake may produce fluid overload and hypertension if daily fluid removal via dialysis is not carried out. Stable patients usually receive dialysis for 3 to 4 hr thrice weekly depending upon their native renal function, clinical status and biochemical values. Urea kinetic modelling may help to define the need for dialysis times in individual cases. The use of high flux dialysers in the adolescent has allowed shorter dialysis times when incorporated with delivery systems that have accurate ultrafiltration controls.

Heparinization

The use of single-needle dialysis is accompanied by low dose systemic heparinization. As a rough guide, 100 iu/kg body weight of heparin is administered during each dialysis and individual doses can be adjusted using activated clotting times.

Blood sampling

One advantage of dialysing children in pediatric centers is that the laboratories are normally geared to using small amounts of blood. Blood samples should be restricted to a minimum at all times. A simple rule is not to take more than 0.1 ml of blood per kg body weight for each dialysis; for example, the maximum sample for blood testing from a 20 kg child is 2 ml (20 kg × 0.1 ml = 2 ml).

Drug therapy in ESRD

During hemodialysis sedatives are not given routinely, but low doses of diazepam may be required for the occasional patient who is agitated during the initial few sessions.

Propranolol and hydralazine are the usual drugs employed to control hypertension in children. Occasionally 'second line' drugs such as prazosin and minoxidil are used. Captopril has also been used successfully, but the requirement for increased antihypertensive therapy suggests either poor compliance with drug or fluid intake or the need for native nephrectomy.

The use of aluminum hydroxide compounds to control serum phosphate levels in dialysis patients has recently received a great deal of attention. This is particularly true in children because of possible long-lasting effects of aluminum on brain and bone development. We have subsequently stopped the routine use of these compounds and have tried instead to control serum phosphate levels by dietary means and the use of alternative phosphate binders such as calcium carbonate. During hemodialysis high flux dialysers may be used to help to increase phosphate clearances, and aluminum levels in the dialysis water should be low.

Diets and growth in children with ESRD

A dietitian is an essential member of the pediatric dialysis team because of the focus on growth in patients with high energy requirements combined with the problems of anorexia, food refusal and adolescent rebellion. Loss of height in the first two years of life will rarely be regained and in our unit very young patients are supplemented using nasogastric or gastrostomy tube feedings. Energy supplements are often prescribed for all age groups and regular assessments using home dietary records and nutritional parameters, such as skin fold thickness, are performed.

The dietary intake of phosphate and calcium may have a direct bearing on the development of renal osteodystrophy which in turn affects growth. Although dietary restrictions are generally less with CAPD than with patients on hemodialysis, the diet must be phosphate restricted in both, in order to avoid the use of aluminum-containing phosphate binding agents.

In addition to careful and regular assessments of height and weight, the head circumference, of infants in particular, should be recorded. Bone age is frequently delayed in respect to chronological age and so are puberty and sexual maturity. These should all be recorded. Developmental assessments should be carried out in the younger child.

Psychological support and play therapy

Every opportunity should be taken to interact with the child and his or her parents and provide reassurance to the family at all times. The nurse will help to reinforce the dietitian's instructions and encourage the child to carry on with school work which will be supervised by the teachers attached to the unit. The nurses are in an ideal situation to make the dialysis experience enjoyable rather than traumatic, to try to maintain and improve compliance, and to bring to the attention of the medical staff any physical or emotional problems which may arise.

We feel the introduction of nursing methods such as primary nursing care, where an individual nurse is assigned to a patient and his/her family throughout treatment, have helped considerably in this respect. Parental involvement with younger children in the dialysis unit is always encouraged. However, since older children need to be allowed to move out of the protective family environment in order to mature into adults, too much parental involvement at this stage may have to be discouraged. Children need to vent their feelings and frustrations as much as adults do and it is appropriate to allow them to cry as an expression of their emotions. The whole tone of the unit depends upon the nurses creating a friendly, empathetic atmosphere in which the children can continue their emotional and scholastic development. Close liaison with the medical social worker and occasionally with the child psychologist and psychiatrist is also necessary.

Play is the work of children. Play therapy organized by the recreational or occupational therapist is used as an educational tool to encourage self expression. It helps to allay anxiety. We frequently use doll models when explaining the procedures a child is likely to encounter and we encourage them to practice the techniques on the dolls (Fig. 11.3). Older children and adolescents may have a problem with 'body image' in relationship to fistulae, cannulae and scars and this aspect needs to be considered and discussed.

Management of any child with ESRD requires a major team effort. It has been our experience that increasing use of the multidisciplinary approach results in fewer psychologically disturbed children, and this undoubtedly has been a major benefit of dialysing children in a pediatric environment.

Renal transplantation in children

Dialysis therapy is seen as only an interim measure in children until transplantation becomes possible. Transplantation offers the best opportunity for overall rehabilitation because it frees the patient from dialysis routines and dietary restrictions thus allowing greater participation in school and peer activities. Many centers have now developed the technical expertise to transplant children of all ages and sizes after they have developed ESRD. However, renal transplantation is by no means a magic

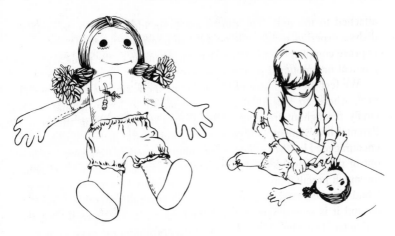

Fig. 11.3. (a) Doll with WBW catheter in place.
(b) Child practicing CAPD technique with a doll.

cure-all and, although results in older children are comparable to those in adults, they have not been so successful in young children. Transplantation in children weighing less than 10 kg remains fraught with problems, and, with the advent of CAPD, it may be more appropriate to maintain these children on dialysis with aggressive feeding regimens to increase their growth until they are big enough to make transplantation technically easier.

In view of the difficulties associated with transplantation, it is essential that families be prepared. They must appreciate that a transplant is only one form of therapy. If it fails, the child must usually be returned to dialysis.

Pre-operative management

The cause of the child's chronic renal failure has some bearing on the preparation for a renal transplant. Congenital urinary tract problems such as posterior urethral valves require expert assessment by a urologist. All surgery on the urinary tract must be performed before the child is placed on a transplant waiting list. Children whose bladders are not adequate to receive the transplant ureter and the large urinary volumes may require a bladder augmentation procedure such as attaching a portion of the patient's colon to the bladder. Although patients have been successfully transplanted using an ileal conduit which drains onto the surface of the abdomen, it is preferable to use or enlarge the patient's own bladder and allow the patient to use long-term intermittent self-catherization.

The transplant team may decide to remove the kidney(s) and ureter(s) from children who have vesico-ureteral reflux which poses a high risk of infection in the post-transplant period. Hypoplastic or dysplastic native kidneys, which in young children commonly put out large volumes of dilute urine, may also be removed before or at the time of transplant to reduce the risk of clotting in the blood vessels of the transplanted kidney if the child becomes dehydrated. Severe hypertension on dialysis is another indication for removal of kidneys either before or at the time of renal transplantation.

Children whose kidney failure is due to a severe acute nephritis or rapid glomerulosclerosis may be maintained on dialysis until the inflammatory process has subsided.

Pre-operative teaching

Pre-operative teaching should be carried out by a designated nurse, supported by a nephrologist, surgeon and social worker. It is essential to use methods of teaching which are appropriate for the child's developmental age. The child must be taught to expect the numerous intravenous lines and catheters which will be in place when he wakes up in the intensive care unit. It is surprising how many children vividly remember the nasogastric tube or urinary catheter when they later recount their experiences.

Donor selection

Murray performed the first successful renal transplant in 1954 using an identical twin as a living donor. However, it was not until the 1960s that renal transplantation was used in the treatment of children with end-stage renal disease. The transplant program at the Hospital for Sick Children in Toronto was started in 1969 and since then more than 200 transplants have been performed; only 5% of them have been from living, related donors despite the advantages discussed previously. In some centers in the United States, living, related donors are involved in up to 40% of transplants. Very few centers ever accept a kidney from a minor for living related transplant and, although parents are often highly motivated to donate kidneys to their children, there may be a major discrepancy in size between the adult parent and the young child. This should not be seen as an absolute contra-indication to the transplant. The kidney may be placed intra-abdominally rather than extraperitoneally in the iliac fossa, which is the usual approach.

In the effort to obtain small kidneys for small children, donors of all ages have been considerd, including anencephalic babies. However, because the results have been very disappointing some centers do not recommend using donor kidneys from children under 1 year of age. On the other hand, an older child's kidney can be placed in an adolescent or young adult.

Preparation of the recipient

Most centers now follow the recommendation of five transfusions in the pre-transplant period. The question of histocompatibility matching and cytotoxic antibodies has been discussed elsewhere.

It goes without saying that a child should be in the fittest state possible to receive a kidney transplant and should also be in the right psychological frame of mind. Children who are on the transplant recipient list and develop peritonitis on CAPD are not given transplants until the infection has been eradicated. Exit site infection of a chronic peritoneal catheter is not a contra-indication to transplantation. The catheter may be removed at operation, although it is normally removed when the child is going home after transplantation at 3−4 weeks.

Operative procedure

The surgical operation in children is similar to that described for adults, with the kidney being placed in the iliac fossa location. Children who are not yet walking may not have large enough iliac vessels, and in such instances the vascular anastomosis may be made directly to the vena cava and aorta. Surgeons have been reluctant to transplant adult kidneys into children weighing less than 10 kg because there may be associated hypotension, large volume diuresis, and cardiac embarrassment from the large kidney. However, the intra-abdominal placement of adult kidneys into infants is feasible if the problems are anticipated.

Post-operative care

Our patients are managed in the pediatric intensive care unit for 24−48 hours and if no problems arise are then transferred to the renal ward. However, in small children who have received a large donor kidney, we have adopted a policy of electively ventilating them to prevent pulmonary edema from a fairly liberal fluid input regimen.

Routine monitoring of the patient on the ward consists of vital signs and accurate fluid balance sheets. The urinary catheter is removed at the earliest opportunity but is usually left in place until the patient's condition is stable towards the end of the first week, and antibiotic coverage is administered during that time. If the peritoneal cavity has not been opened, oral feeding may commence within 48 hours. Total parenteral nutrition may be necessary if a child has had an intra-abdominal operation or there are complications.

Separation anxiety is one of the major traumatic aspects of transplantation for children, especially if they are isolated in adult units. An open door policy of visiting by close relatives should therefore be encouraged and parents may be involved in the care of their child, which helps to reduce anxiety levels in child and parent. Again the attitude and involvement of the nursing staff and recreational therapist are very important.

Immunosuppressive therapy

Prednisone and azathioprine remain the standard immunosuppressive regimen, with azathioprine being administered in a dose slightly higher than that used for adults, approximately 3 mg/kg body weight. Intravenous methylprednisolone is administered for the first week at a dose of 3 mg/kg body weight (maximum 120 mg). Thereafter the prednisone is tapered rapidly so that in most cases by the end of three weeks the child is down to 20–30 mg of prednisone daily. A number of steroid regimens have been suggested, but, in order to encourage post-transplant growth in our patients, we try to change them to alternate day prednisone at the earliest opportunity. If there are no rejection episodes, this is usually accomplished by three months post-transplant, but in many units the process may take 6 to 12 months.

Additional immunosuppression may be given to high risk patients in the form of antilymphocytic serum, but usually this treatment is reserved for acute rejection episodes which do not respond to bolus doses of methylprednisolone. There is increasing experience with the use of cyclosporin in children as well as adults. Although this drug has a steroid-sparing effect, its potential to damage the kidneys may negate its benefits in the long run. The diagnosis and treatment of acute and chronic graft rejection are essentially the same as those described for adults. The addition of plasma exchange treatment for acute rejection has been used in our institution, but with questionable benefit. High doses of medication, particularly steroids, employed in the post-operative period may induce acute personality changes in children. This danger must be recognized. Every attempt must be made to provide the child with as much human contact (and play or distraction therapy) as is appropriate for the child's clinical condition and level of functioning.

Rehabilitation

If a transplant is successful, rehabilitation prospects with full school attendance and vocational training are excellent. However, psychosocial adaptation may be poorer and noncompliance with immunosuppressive therapy can be a real problem. Even with an early switch to alternate day prednisone therapy, the child may remain stunted in growth if the allograft function is not very good and the bone age already advanced.

Conclusions

Although there are many similarities in the dialysis and transplant management of children and adults, a number of points are unique to the management of children. We have stressed the effects their stage of physical and emotional development will have on the therapy offered. There have been a number of exciting advances in the past few years which have helped considerably in the management of children on dialysis. These include advances in vascular access and the technology of ultrafiltration control, variable sodium, bicarbonate dialysis and the use of single-needle machines. The advent of CAPD in 1978 was a tremendous boost for home dialysis therapy with all its attendant benefits, especially for patients living some distance from a pediatric center. Wider acceptance of the technique is still needed. Renal transplantation remains the optimum therapy for children with ESRD and it is hoped that improved matching techniques and the development of non-nephrotoxic cyclosporin-like compounds will help to make transplantation even more successful in the future.

Suggested reference sources

Pediatric Kidney Disease. C. Edelman, Jr. (editor). Boston, Little Brown and Co., 1978.
End Stage Renal Disease in Children. R.N. Fine & A.B. Gruskin (editors). Philadelphia, W.B. Saunders, 1984.
Replacement of Renal Function by Dialysis. W. Drukker, F.M. Parsons & J.F. Maher (editors). Amsterdam, Martinus Nijhoff, 1983, pp.514–536.

Appendix 1

Dietary Information

Jean Pettit

Five main constituents of the diet normally have to be taken into account when planning diets for patients with kidney disease and renal failure. These are fluid (water), protein, sodium, potassium and phosphorus. As an aid to nurses and patients we have included lists of foods containing large proportions of these nutrients and the approximate amount per normal serving or basic unit. The lists can be used as a guide to warn patients what to avoid and may provide explanations for undesirable gains in fluid or electrolytes or rises in serum urea.

When we speak of foods as being 'high' or 'low' in certain nutrients, various criteria are employed. Obviously, serving size is of major importance. For instance, 100 g of pepper contains 32 mmol K^+ whereas 100 g of tomato contains only 6.3 mmol K^+. One should think that pepper would be considered much higher than tomato; but the amount of pepper one would use at a meal would probably be no more than a quarter of a teaspoonful, or 0.5 g, which contains 0.2 mmol K^+, whereas one medium tomato weighs 150 g and contains 9.5 mmol K^+. Therefore we consider tomato to be high in potassium but we do not worry about pepper.

Because intake is totally dependent upon the amount of food eaten, the contents of the various nutrients have been quoted as units/serving size or basic unit. Amounts are specified in both imperial and SI units.

Normally when restricting fluid we do not calculate for water content of most foods. Only those items which are fluid at body temperature (e.g.

gelatin desserts, custard) or from which water or juice can easily be squeezed (e.g. grapefruit, watermelon), and of course those foods which are frankly fluid, are usually counted. As a rule, patients get extra fluid from water consumed without realizing it, perhaps when they clean their teeth and swallow that mouthful afterwards or with their medications, which they consider part of their medication rather than a fluid. Perhaps, however, there is an excessive intake of foods with a high fluid content. These may be found in the tables following.

Although protein is present in varying quantities in almost all foods with the exception of pure sugars, fats and alcohol, the most concentrated forms of protein are found in those of animal origin, such as meat, milk, eggs, fish, poultry and cheese. With the exception of milk, these contain on average 7 g protein/25 g of product (8 g/oz). Milk, on the other hand, contains approximately 1 g protein/28 ml (1 fluid oz) or 8 g protein/225 ml (8 fluid oz). In general, breads, grains and vegetables contain an average of 2−3 g protein per serving (one 25 g slice or 125 ml [4 fluid oz]). There are, however, exceptions, the more common of which will be listed in the supplement that follows.

It is very difficult to compile a complete list of high sodium foods, as various sodium compounds are added to most of our processed, prepared and convenience foods for a multitude of purposes, and are constantly being altered and added to. A few of these will be listed in the supplement; but generally speaking, if a food is processed, it is high in sodium. At one time one could say that if a food was salty it contained a large amount of sodium. But this is no longer the case, as many of these sodium compounds do not have a 'salty' taste. Therefore it is very important to read labels and avoid foods containing MSG (monosodium glutamate), soy sauce and any other sodium (Na^+) compounds.

According to various nutrition textbooks, the normal potassium intake in North America varies between 50 and 120 mmol/day. When we speak of a 'low' potassium diet, we are thinking in terms of 45−65 mmol/day. Potassium is found in almost all foods, though in higher concentration in some. In certain categories, such as meats, there is little difference in the potassium concentration from one kind to another. Therefore an average potassium value is used. But in fruits and vegetables the potassium may vary from 1 to 10 or more mmol/serving (125 ml or 4 fluid oz) and it is these that are utilized in controlling potassium intake. However, it is important to remember that quantity affects the total amount of potassium consumed. For instance, many patients believe that if a food is 'low' or 'moderate' (i.e. 'allowed') they can eat as much of it as desired. But, if two or three times the amount specified is ingested, the amount of potassium consumed can soon add up to an excessive intake. It is also important to remember that, as the protein intake increases, so also does the potassium. The items listed in the supplement will be mainly those that are considered high for their category.

Phosphorus is another nutrient that is found almost universally, although it is highest in protein-rich foods, especially milk, cheese, nuts and organ meats. To date we have not been able to achieve a low phosphorus diet (<700 mg/day) with adequate protein which would be palatable on a long-term basis. Following the phosphorus restriction we give, it is possible on an 80 g protein diet to hold the phosphorus intake to 1000–1200 mg (31–37 mmol) per day, rather than 1600 mg (50 mmol) or more, depending upon the food choices. In developing the restricted phosphorus diet, the criterion used was the ratio of phosphorus to other nutrients, particularly protein. The graphs in Fig. A.1.1 should demonstrate the thinking. Some high phosphorus foods, such as milk, eggs and cheese, are very difficult to eliminate from the diet. Therefore they are limited rather than totally restricted. In North America we have another problem with phosphorus. It is added to almost all processed foods in one form or another. Watch for the words phosphorus (P) or phosphate on package labels. In addition to the graphs, other high phosphorus foods have been included in the supplement. Some of these are not normally restricted in the renal diet because of the many other restrictions; but if a patient eats them excessively he must be given a limit.

Finally, it should be remembered that commercial food production is constantly changing and evolving. New and exciting foods are being packaged and preserved for speed and convenience. Remembering that most of these contain one or more of sodium, potassium and phosphorus it is wise always to read labels. Modern legislation, because it insists on accurate description of container contents, is on our side.

These graphs give a quick visual indication of the amount of phosphorus in various forms of protein foods.

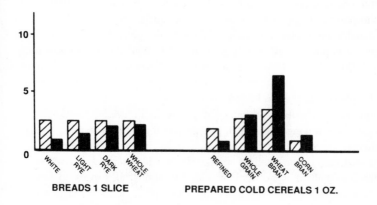

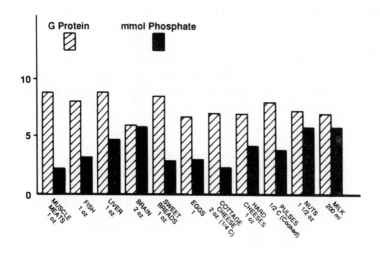

Fig. A1.1. Bar graphs showing phosphate and protein values of various foods.

Foods high in fluid content

Food	Amount		Water g (ml)
apples	1 medium	150 g	128
cantaloupe	1/4 medium	100 g	91
cherries	15 large, 25 small	100 g	80
grapefruit	1/2 medium	100 g	88
grapes	1/2 cup	80 g	65
oranges	1 medium	150 g	129
raspberries	3/4 cup	100 g	84
strawberries	1 cup	150 g	135
watermelon	1 cup cubes	200 g	185
cucumber	1/2 cup, sliced	73 g	70
lettuce, iceberg	1 cup chunks	74 g	70
lettuce, romaine	1 cup chunks	37 g	35
summer squash	1/2 cup, cooked	100 g	95
tomato	1 medium	150 g	140
aspic	2 tbsp.	28 ml	25
gravy	1/4 cup	57 ml	55
sauces	1/4 cup	57 ml	54
cereals, cooked	1/2 cup	118 ml	103
cornstarch pudding	1/2 cup	125 g	95
baked custard	1/2 cup	130 g	100
ice cream	1/2 cup	67 g	42
jello (jelly)	1/2 cup	120 g	101
milk	1 cup	244 g	218
popsicle	1 average	88 g	59
sherbet	1/2 cup	96 g	64
soups	1 cup	227 ml	211 (194-222)
sour cream	2 tbsp.	24 g	17
yoghurt, plain	6 oz	170 g	145

Some foods rich in potassium

	Amount		mmol K
Beverages			
Bovril concentrate	1 tbsp.	15 ml	6
Marmite concentrate	1 tbsp.	15 ml	13
Horlick's malted milk	2 tbsp.	30 ml	4
Ovaltine	2 tbsp.	30 ml	4
milk, cow's	1 cup	225 ml	8
milk, goat's	1 cup	225 ml	10
Breads			
Boston brown bread	1 slice	44 g	3
bran bread	1 slice	34 g	2
bran muffin	1 average	40 g	4
dark rye bread	1 slice	32 g	4
malt bread	1 slice	23 g	2
raisin bread	1 slice	25 g	2
whole wheat bread	1 slice	25 g	2
Cereals			
whole grain	1 oz	28 g	2−8 (avg. 3)
bran	1 oz	28 g	3−12 (avg. 7)
Flour or grain			
oats, raw	1/4 cup	37 g	3
soy flour	1/4 cup	24 g	10
whole wheat flour	1/4 cup	30 g	3
Cheese			
Norwegian mysost	1 oz	28 g	11
salt-free	1 oz	28 g	5−6
Fruit			
apricots, fresh	3 fruit	106 g	8
apricots, dried	10 halves	35 g	12
avocados	1/2	100 g	15
bananas	1 med.	114 g	12
currants, dried	1/4 cup	36 g	8
dates, natural & dried	5 fruit	42 g	7
figs, dried	2 fruit	37 g	7
guavas	1 fruit	90 g	7
kiwi fruit	1 med.	76 g	6
mango	1 med.	207 g	8
cantaloupe	1/4 fruit	133 g	11
casaba (melon), cubed	1 cup	170 g	9
honeydew melon, cubed	1 cup	170 g	12
nectarine	1 med.	136 g	7

Some foods rich in potassium—*cont'd*

	Amount		mmol K
orange	1 med.	131 g	6
orange juice	1/2 cup	120 ml	6
papaya	1/2 fruit	152 g	10
passion fruit juice	1/2 cup	120 ml	9
persimmon, Japanese	1 fruit	168 g	7
plantain, cooked	1/2 cup slices	77 g	9
pomegranate	1 fruit	154 g	10
prickly pears	1 fruit	103 g	6
prunes, dried	5 fruit	42 g	8
prune juice	1/2 cup	120 ml	9
raisins	1/4 cup	41 g	8
rhubarb, raw	1 cup diced	122 g	9
sapodilla	1 fruit	170 g	8
sapotes	1/2 fruit	112 g	10
soursop	1/2 cup pulp	120 ml	8
sugar-apples	1 fruit	155 g	10
tangerine juice	1/2 cup	120 ml	6
Nuts			
Brazils	4 med.	15 g	3
cashews	6–8 nuts	15 g	2
chestnuts, fresh	2 lg, 3 sm	15 g	2
coconut, dried	1/4 cup	22 g	3
filbert (hazelnuts)	10–12 nuts	15 g	3
peanuts	1/4 cup	38 g	7
pecans	1/4 cup	27 g	4
pistachios	1/4 cup	31 g	8
Soups			
canned, ready-to-eat (except beef noodle, turkey noodle, onion, chicken gumbo, chicken noodle, chicken rice)	1 cup	225 ml	3–15 (avg. 7)
Spices			
curry powder	1 tsp.	2 g	1
paprika	1 tsp.	2 g	1
turmeric	1 tsp.	2 g	1
Sweets			
brown sugar	1 tbsp.	15 ml	1
chocolate, bittersweet	1 oz	28 g	4
chocolate, milk	1 oz	28 g	3
chocolate, semisweet	1 oz	28 g	2
maple syrup	1/4 cup	60 ml	4
molasses, light	1/4 cup	60 ml	18

Some foods rich in potassium—*cont'd*

	Amount		mmol K
Supplemental feeds			
Compleat-B	1 bottle	250 ml	9
Ensure	1 can	235 ml	7
Flexical HN	1 can	235 ml	8
Isocal	1 can	235 ml	8
Meritene	1 can	295 ml	13
Sustacal	1 can	235 ml	10
Enrich	1 can	235 ml	9
Vegetables			
artichoke, globe, cooked	1/2 cup	84 g	7
beans, white, cooked	1/2 cup	85 g	9
beans, red, cooked	1/2 cup	87 g	8
beans, lima, fresh, cooked	1/2 cup	84 g	9
beans, lima, dried, cooked	1/2 cup	100 g	16
beet greens, cooked	1/2 cup	100 g	9
breadfruit, cooked	1/2 cup	110 g	14
chard, Swiss, cooked	1/2 cup	83 g	7
chick peas, cooked	1/2 cup	81 g	8
blackeye peas, cooked	1/2 cup	84 g	8
dandelion greens, cooked	1/2 cup	100 g	6
leeks	2–3, 5 inches	70 g	6
lentils, cooked	1/2 cup	100 g	6
mushrooms, fresh	10 sm, 4 lg	100 g	11
parsnips, cooked	1/2 cup	100 g	10
peas, dried, cooked	1/2 cup	84 g	6
potato, baked	1 medium	100 g	13
potato, boiled	1 medium	100 g	10
potato, French fried	1 cup	136 g	30
potato chips	1 sm bag	32 g	9
pumpkin, canned	1/2 cup	120 ml	7
soybeans, dried, cooked	1/2 cup	80 g	11
spinach, cooked	1/2 cup	82 g	7
squash, winter, cooked	1/2 cup	120 ml	12
sweet potato, baked	1/2 cup	127 g	10
tomato, fresh	1 med.	150 g	9
tomato, canned	1/2 cup	120 ml	7
tomato, juice	1/2 cup	120 ml	7
tomato, puree	1/4 cup	60 ml	7
tomato paste	2 tbsp.	30 ml	7
vegetable juice cocktail	1/2 cup	120 ml	7
yam, cooked	1/2 cup	120 ml	19
Miscellaneous			
brewer's yeast	1 tbsp.	10 g	5
dulse	1/2 oz	15 g	31
mincemeat	1 serving	100 g	10
peanut butter	2 tbsp.	30 ml	5

Food rich in phosphorus

	Amount		mg P
Beverages			
beer	12 oz	340 ml	31–136
Bournvita	2 tbsp.	30 ml	70
Bovril	1 tbsp.	15 ml	118
cocoa powder	2 tbsp.	30 ml	70
Horlick's malted milk	2 tbsp.	30 ml	60
Marmite	1 tbsp.	15 ml	340
milk, cow's	1 cup	225 ml	209
milk, goat's	1 cup	225 ml	238
Ovaltine	2 tbsp.	30 ml	80
Cereals, grains & bread			
bran cereals	1 oz	28 g	107–334 (avg. 204)
whole grain cereals	1 oz	28 g	62–215 (avg. 114)
oats, raw	1/4 cup	37 g	150
self-rising flour	1/4 cup	32 g	166
soya flour	1/4 cup	24 g	134
whole wheat flour	1/4 cup	30 g	112
bran muffin	1 average	40 g	162
plain muffin	1 average	40 g	60
Boston brown bread	1 slice	44 g	70
bran bread	1 slice	34 g	78
dark rye bread	1 slice	32 g	73
malt bread	1 slice	23 g	58
whole wheat bread	1 slice	25 g	64
Meats & fish			
liver	1 oz	28 g	151
caviar	1 rnd tsp.	10 g	36
mussels	3 1/2 oz	100 g	236
oysters	3 lg, 6 med	100 g	143–153
salmon	1 oz	28 g	117
sardines	4 med.	50 g	250
scallops	2–3	100 g	208
sprats	1 oz	28 g	182
whitebait	1 oz	28 g	244
Nuts & seeds			
Brazil nuts	4 med.	15 g	104
cashews	6–8	15 g	56
filberts (hazelnuts)	10–12	15 g	51
peanuts	1/4 cup	38 g	155
pecans	1/4 cup	27 g	78
pistachios	1/4 cup	31 g	156

caraway seeds	1 tbsp.	15 ml	91
poppy seeds	1 tbsp.	15 ml	75
sesame seeds	1 tbsp.	15 ml	62
pumpkin seeds	1/4 cup	60 ml	663
sunflower seeds	1/4 cup	60 ml	243

Supplemental feeds

Compleat-B	1 bottle	250 ml	367
Enrich	1 can	235 ml	170
Ensure	1 can	235 ml	120
Flexical HN	1 can	235 ml	125
Isocal	1 can	235 ml	125
Meritene	1 can	295 ml	375
Sustacal	1 can	235 ml	317

Sweets

chocolate, bittersweet	1 oz	28 g	80
chocolate, milk	1 oz	28 g	65
chocolate, semisweet	1 oz	28 g	42

Vegetables

asparagus	5–6 spears	100 g	62
beans, white, dry, cooked	1/2 cup	85 g	126
beans, red, dry, cooked	1/2 cup	87 g	122
beans, lima, fresh, cooked	1/2 cup	84 g	106
beans, lima, dry, cooked	1/2 cup	100 g	154
Brussels sprouts, cooked	1/2 cup	76 g	55
blackeye peas, cooked	1/2 cup	84 g	123
chick peas	1/2 cup	81 g	105
corn, kernels	1/2 cup	78 g	57
lentils, cooked	1/2 cup	100 g	119
mushrooms, fresh	10 small, 4 large	100 g	116
parsnips, cooked	1/2 cup	100 g	62
peas, fresh, cooked	1/2 cup	84 g	72
peas, dried, cooked	1/2 cup	84 g	75
potato, baked	1 med.	100 g	65
potato, French fried	1 cup	136 g	151
soybeans, dried, cooked	1/2 cup	80 g	142
yam, cooked	1/2 cup	120 ml	83

Miscellaneous

baking powder	1 tsp.	3 g	253
brewer's yeast	1 tbsp.	10 g	175
mincemeat	1 serving	100 g	220
peanut butter	2 tbsp.	30 ml	126
tofu	2 oz	56 g	71
miso	1 oz	28 g	87

Some foods rich in protein

	Amount		g protein
fish	1 oz	28 g	5−7
meats	1 oz	28 g	7−9
partridge	1 oz	28 g	10
venison	1 oz	28 g	10
egg	1 lg	54 g	7
milk	8 oz	225 ml	8
cheese	1 oz	28 g	7
parmesan cheese	1 oz	28 g	10
cottage cheese	4 oz	120 ml	15.5
yoghurt, plain	4 oz	113 g	4
yoghurt, plain with milk solids	4 oz	113 g	6
Cereals			
Bran Buds	1/3 cup	28 g	3.9
40% Bran Flakes	3/4 cup	29 g	3.7
Raisin Bran	3/4 cup	43 g	4.6
Cheerios (oat cereal)	3/4 cup	21 g	3.2
Fortified Oat Flakes	3/4 cup	36 g	6.8
Granola (muesli)	1/3 cup	41 g	5.1
Grapenuts	1/3 cup	36 g	4.2
Grapenuts Flakes	3/4 cup	29 g	3.1
Nutrigrain	3/4 cup	31 g	3.4
Life	3/4 cup	33 g	6.1
Most	1/2 cup	26 g	3.7
100% natural cereal	1/3 cup	35 g	4.1
Special K	3/4 cup	17 g	3.4
rolled oats, cooked	1/2 cup	120 ml	3.0
Roman meal, cooked	1/2 cup	120 ml	3.3
Roman meal, with oats, cooked	1/2 cup	120 ml	3.6
Breads			
cornbread	1 slice	45 g	3.2−3.5
sesame Armenian cracker bread	1 oz	28 g	4.6
spoonbread with whole cornmeal	1 serving	96 g	6.4
sprouted rye	1 slice	26 g	3.1
wheat germ bread	1 slice	32 g	3.8
matzoth	1 piece	30 g	3.0
Energen rolls	1 oz	28 g	12−15
Nuts			
almonds	12−15	15 g	2.4
Brazils	4 med.	15 g	1.7
peanuts	1/4 cup	38 g	9.2

Some foods rich in protein—*cont'd*

	Amount		g protein
Seeds			
pumpkin	1/2 oz	15 g	4.1
safflower	1/2 oz	15 g	2.7
sesame	1/2 oz	15 g	2.6
sunflower	1/2 oz	15 g	3.4
Vegetables			
beans, white, dried, cooked	1/2 cup	120 ml	6.6
beans, red, dried, cooked	1/2 cup	120 ml	6.8
beans, lima, dried, cooked	1/2 cup	120 ml	7.4
beans, lima, fresh, cooked	1/2 cup	120 ml	7.0
chick peas, dried, cooked	1/2 cup	120 ml	6.5
blackeye peas, dried, cooked	1/2 cup	120 ml	4.3
lentils, dried, cooked	1/2 cup	120 ml	7.8
peas, dried, cooked	1/2 cup	120 ml	6.7
peas, fresh, cooked	1/2 cup	120 ml	4.5
potato, French-fried	1 cup	225 ml	5.8
soybeans, dried, cooked	1/2 cup	120 ml	8.8
Brussels sprouts	1/2 cup	120 ml	3.2

Some foods high in sodium

As almost all commercially prepared foods contain a lot of sodium, the following list can only be representative, not complete. Foods similar to those listed may be considered to contain a similar amount of sodium, and in general all convenience foods, snack foods, ready-to-eat foods, etc., are high in sodium.

	Amount		mmol Na
Fish			
caviar	1 rnd tsp.	10 g	9.5
cod, smoked, poached	1 oz	28 g	15
cod, dried salt, steamed	1 oz	28 g	5
cockles, boiled in sea water	1 oz	28 g	43
haddock, smoked, steamed	1 oz	28 g	15
kippered herring, baked	1 oz	28 g	12
prawns, boiled in sea water	1 oz	28 g	19.5
salmon, canned	1 oz	28 g	8
salmon, smoked	1 oz	28 g	23
shrimp, boiled in sea water	1 oz	28 g	47
shrimp, canned	1 oz	28 g	12
winkles, boiled in sea water	1 oz	28 g	14

Some foods high in sodium—*cont'd*

	Amount		mmol Na
Meats			
bacon, cooked	3 strips	19 g	13
beerwurst	1 slice	23 g	12.5
bologna	1 slice	23 g	12
Braunschweiger (German sausage)	1 slice	18 g	9
breakfast strips, cooked	3 slices	24 g	31
back bacon	2 slices	46 g	31
head cheese (brawn)	1 oz	28 g	15.5
luncheon meats	1 oz	28 g	9–23.5 (avg. 15.5)
ham	1 oz	28 g	17
corned beef, canned	1 oz	28 g	11.5
frankfurters, cooked	1 average	50 g	23.5
pepperoni	1 oz	28 g	21.5
pork sausage, cooked	1 link	68 g	44.5
salami, dry	3 slices	30 g	29.5
salt pork, raw	1 oz	28 g	17.5
Condiments			
barbecue sauce	1 tbsp.	15 ml	5.5
chili sauce	1 tbsp.	15 ml	10
chow chow sour pickle	1 tbsp.	14 g	8
bread & butter pickle	4 slices	25 g	7.5
dill pickles, cucumber	1 large	100 g	62
ketchup	1 tbsp.	15 ml	7
mustard with horseradish	1 tbsp.	15 ml	12.5
sour cucumber pickle	1 large	105 g	59
sweet cucumber pickle	1 large	100 g	25
sweet relish	1 tbsp.	15 ml	4.5
soy sauce, Kikkoman	1 tbsp.	15 ml	37.5
steak sauce, Lea & Perrins	1 tbsp.	15 ml	6.5
teriyaki sauce	1 tbsp.	15 ml	25
Snack foods			
Bacon Nips	1 oz	28 g	30.5
Bugles	1 oz	28 g	12
cheese puffs	1 oz	28 g	12.5
cheese twists	1 oz	28 g	14.5
corn chips	1 oz	28 g	9.5
dulse	1/2 oz	15 g	13.5
potato chips	1 sm pkg	32 g	14
soda crackers	2	14 g	6.5
olives, green pickled	3 med.	20 g	20.5
olives, ripe, salt-cured	3 med.	20 g	28.5

Some foods high in sodium—*cont'd*

	Amount		mmol Na
Soups			
Bovril concentrate	1 tbsp.	15 ml	41.5
Marmite concentrate	1 tbsp.	15 ml	39
Oxo	1 cube	6 g	27
soups, canned, reconstituted	1 cup	225 ml	33.5–78.5 (avg. 43.5)
soups, dried, reconstituted	1 cup	225 ml	34.5–64.5 (avg. 47)
Miscellaneous			
baking powder	1 tsp.	3 g	15.5
Big Mac	1	1	42
Egg McMuffin	1	1	39.5
quarter pounder with cheese	1	1	52.5
pizza, cheese	1, 10″ pizza	336 g	97
pork & beans	1/2 cup	125 g	25
sauerkraut	1/2 cup	75 g	24.5
TV dinners	1	1	24–65.5 (avg. 44)
spaghetti sauce with meatballs	1 serving	228 g	45.5
chop suey	1 cup	250 g	46

Appendix 2

Starting Peritoneal Dialysis with a Permanent Peritoneal Catheter (Long-term IPD)

Ramesh Khanna, Sharon Izatt,
Betty Kelman and Dimitrios Oreopoulos

Equipment required

- Dressing tray containing gauzes (10 × 10 cm), one abdominal pad, two solution containers, one plastic catheter clamp and one drape
- Sterile gloves
- Syringe (5 ml)
- Povidone-iodine solution (10%)
- Isopropyl alcohol (70%)
- Tape
- Masks

Procedure

1 Mask everybody in room.
2 Wash hands.
3 Open and prepare dressing tray using aseptic technique. Add syringe and solutions to tray. Open gloves.
4 Remove the patient's dressing. *Assess exit-site and send a swab* for culture and sensitivity if there is a discharge.

408

5 Do a three-minute surgical scrub from hands to elbows with povidone-iodine brush. Dry hands with sterile towel. Put on gloves.

6 Organize tray. Place two gauzes in povidone-iodine solution and two in isopropyl alcohol.

7 Place one of the *povidone-iodine gauzes lengthwise along the catheter*. To prevent contamination of gloves by skin or catheter, work through the gauze at all times. After soaking the catheter with the first gauze for 1½ minutes, wrap the gauze around its base.

8 Apply a second povidone-iodine gauze lengthwise along the catheter for 1½ minutes and wrap around its base on top of the first soak.

9 Arrange the sterile drape around the catheter site to provide a sterile field for the tubing connection.

10 Apply clamp to the catheter at a 45° angle approximately 1 cm from the adapter.

11 Bring in bowl of povidone-iodine and immerse the catheter's capped end in the solution for three minutes. The catheter clamp may be used to position the catheter tip in the solution.

12 Remove bowl of povidone-iodine and allow the catheter to fall onto the drape.

13 With a second sterile gauze, remove cap from catheter.

14 Attach a 5 ml syringe to the catheter, remove clamp and withdraw specimen. This should be sent for culture and sensitivity weekly on all IPD patients. Samples of 'predialysis' fluid that have accumulated after the last dialysis may also be sent for urea, creatinine and electrolyte levels; such results will be similar to serum levels.

15 Pinch catheter behind adapter using gauze. Remove and re-cap syringe. Return syringe to dressing tray.

16 While still pinching the catheter, grasp the end of the tubing with a sterile gauze and attach it securely to the catheter.

17 Continuing to work through the gauze, lift the tubing and catheter up to facilitate removal of the drape and soaked povidone-iodine gauzes.

18 Clean skin twice with alcohol-soaked gauze, starting at exit site and working outward in a circular motion.

19 Continuing to hold the catheter away from the skin, dry in the same manner.

20 Place one open gauze lengthwise on the skin under the catheter. Allow the catheter to drop on the gauze. Fold one, then the other side of the gauze over the catheter covering both the exit site and the tubing connection site.

21 Place the abdominal pad over the gauze-wrapped catheter. Tape in place. Also, tape tubing to side of bed, allowing a good length of tubing looped on bed so that patient can move freely.

Handling of samples

1 Nurse should be masked.
2 Soak the top of a vacutainer tube with povidone-iodine solution for five minutes. Dry top of tube with sterile gauze or 'shake' solution over the top of tube. Inject the sample into the tube.
3 Send 'predialysis' fluid routinely for culture and sensitivity for all IPD patients. Send a specimen of such fluid for culture and sensitivity whenever the patient complains of pain, fever and/or nausea.
4 When centre IPD patients do not have routine blood work send predialysis fluid for biochemical analysis.

Definitions

Predialysis fluid: is that which has accumulated in the peritoneal cavity following the previous dialysis. It may be sent for culture and sensitivity. Its urea, creatinine and electrolyte levels are similar to those in blood, so it can also be used for biochemical analysis.

Dialysate effluent: this is dilute fluid e.g. dialysate drainage during IPD, CAPD, or the return after catheter irrigation. It may be sent for culture and sensitivity, and Gram stain. Cell count may be done if it is fluid returned from CAPD. It cannot be used to assess a patient's biochemical status.

Discontinuing intermittent peritoneal dialysis in a patient with a chronic catheter

Equipment

- Dressing tray (same as for the connection procedure)
- Sterile gloves
- Syringe (3 ml with #21 needle)
- Heparin vial (1000 units/ml)
- Povidone-iodine solution (10%)
- Isopropyl alcohol (70%)
- Catheter sealing cap
- Airstrip dressing
- Masks

Procedure

1 Mask everybody in room.

2 Wash hands.

3 Open and prepare dressing tray using aseptic technique. Add syringe and solutions to tray. Open gloves.

4 Remove the patient's dresing. Assess exit site and, if there is a discharge, send swab for culture and sensitivity.

5 Do three-minute surgical scrub from hands to elbows with povidone-iodine brush. Dry hands with sterile towel. Put on gloves.

6 Draw up 3 ml of heparin (1000 unit/ml) from a vial held by another nurse.

7 Organize tray. Place two gauzes in povidone-iodine solution and two in isopropyl alcohol.

8 Place one of the povidone-iodine gauzes lengthwise along the catheter. To prevent contamination of gloves by skin or catheter, work through the gauze at all times. After soaking the catheter with the first gauze for 1½ minutes, wrap the gauze around the base of the catheter.

9 Apply a second povidone-iodine gauze lengthwise along the catheter for 1½ minutes and wrap around catheter base on top of the first soak.

10 Arrange sterile drape around the catheter site to provide a sterile field for the tubing disconnection. Working through a dry sterile gauze, lift the catheter connection up and hold away from the sterile field.

11 Apply clamp to catheter at 45° angle. It is essential that the clamp is applied correctly and the catheter is completely occluded.

12 Using a second dry sterile gauze, disconnect tubing from catheter. Discard the tubing and gauze.

13 Bring in bowl of povidone-iodine and immerse the uncapped end of the catheter for three minutes. To avoid touching the skin and catheter, use the clamp as a handle to position the catheter. As the catheter is being immersed in the povidone-iodine *be careful that no povidone-iodine is drawn in as the patient inhales and that no fluid leaks out into the povidone-iodine bowl as the patient exhales*. If either of these do happen, remove catheter from povidone-iodine immediately and pinch it with a dry gauze to continue procedure safely.

14 Remove bowl of povidone-iodine and allow the catheter to fall onto the drape (if the drape has been contaminated, hold the catheter with a dry sterile gauze).

15 Using dry sterile gauze, wipe the ridges of the titanium adapter. Also, tap the adapter on the gauze to remove any drops of povidone-iodine from the lumen.

16 Attach the 3 ml syringe (with 3000 units of heparin) to the catheter. Remove the clamp and inject heparin.

17 Using gauze, firmly bend catheter behind the adapter. Remove syringe. Twist on sealing cap securely.

18 Using gauze, lift capped catheter up. Remove drape and povidone-iodine soaked gauzes from its base.

19 Clean skin twice with alcohol-soaked gauze, starting at the exit site and working outward in a circular motion.

20 Continuing to hold the catheter away from the skin, dry in the same manner.

21 Place one open gauze lengthwise on the skin under the catheter. Allow the catheter to drop onto the gauze. Fold one, then the other side of the gauze over the catheter covering both the exit site and the capped end of the catheter.

22 Apply abdominal pad over catheter to hold gauze in place. Apply airstrip over gauze, removing the abdominal pad as the airstrip adheres to the skin.

Appendix 3

Manual Method
for Dialyser Re-use

Robert Uldall

At the end of dialysis the blood in the extracorporeal circuit is washed back into the patient with 400 ml sterile saline. An air rinse is not carried out because this makes subsequent cleaning of the dialyser more difficult. The blood lines are disconnected and discarded into waterproof plastic bags. The dialyser blood ports are capped and it is connected to the rinse system as shown in Fig. A.3.1. If no one is available to process the dialyser immediately, the blood and dialysate ports are capped and it is stored in a refrigerator maintained for this purpose at 4°C.

The water for dialyser re-use is purified by passing it first through reverse osmosis, next through a 5-micron particulate filter and finally through an ultrafilter (Millipore MU-60) to ensure removal of pyrogens. This water is flushed through the dialyser as shown in Fig. A.3.1 at 5 PSI for an initial 5-minute rinse. Now the dialysate outflow line (L2) is clamped and the pressure in the dialysate compartment is raised to 20 PSI. This positive pressure on the outside of the fibers creates a reverse osmosis effect and forces pure water through the fiber walls into the fiber lumens. This has the effect of dislodging blood clot from the inner walls of the fibers. After 5 minutes at a pressure of 20 PSI the clamp is removed from L2, allowing the rinse water to flow in series through the dialysate and blood compartments.

The cycle of pressurization and depressurization is repeated until the fibers appear clean. Blood clot in the end caps can usually be washed out by the fast flow of water assisted by tapping on the outside of the dialyser

413

Re-use fluid circuit

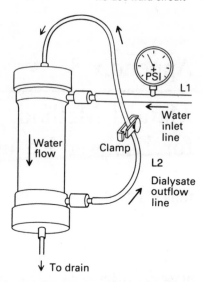

Fig. A3.1. Dialyser re-use circuit. Water is flushed through the dialyser under pressure. When a clamp is placed on the dialysate outflow line, water passes through the fiber walls into the fiber lumen, thus helping to dislodge blood clot which is then flushed out when the clamp is released and water rushes through the blood compartment.

casing. Acceptable dialysers are filled with sterilant before they are again capped and stored on a shelf till the next dialysis. We used to use 3% formaldehyde but gave it up when less noxious agents based on hypochlorite became available. At present we are using paracetic acid and hydrogen peroxide in an automated method.

Each new dialyser is indelibly labelled with the patient's name and after each use a mark is made on the dialyser casing to indicate the number of times it has been used. Details of re-use for every dialyser are recorded in a daily log.

Before dialysis is started the dialyser is flushed through the blood compartment with a litre of sterile saline. Dialysate is allowed to flow through the dialysate compartment for 20 minutes before the patient is connected. Our dialyser re-use is done by technical assistants who are employed specifically to do the job. This part of the work is supervised by the Chief Technologist.

Index